Praise for David DeKok's *Fire Underground:*
The Ongoing Tragedy of the Centralia Mine Fire

"DeKok has not only reported and written a compelling first-hand account of how an underground fire destroyed Centralia, but he even gives us an anatomy of how the disaster happened and analyzes its implications for the community, and in a sense, for all of us. A thoughtful and thoroughly engrossing read!"

—Lisa Scottoline, *author of* Dirty Blonde, *a fictional story about Centralia*

THE EPIDEMIC

THE EPIDEMIC

A Collision of Power, Privilege, and Public Health

DAVID DEKOK

LYONS PRESS
Guilford, Connecticut
An imprint of Globe Pequot Press

To buy books in quantity for corporate use
or incentives, call **(800) 962-0973**
or e-mail **premiums@GlobePequot.com.**

Lyons Press is an imprint of Globe Pequot Press.

Text design: Maggie Peterson
Project editor: Julie Marsh
Layout: Kevin Mak

Library of Congress Cataloging-in-Publication Data is available on file.

ISBN 978-0-7627-6008-4

Printed in the United States of America

10 9 8 7 6 5 4 3 2 1

To Lisa, Elizabeth, and Lydia

CONTENTS

Prelude: June 16, 1903 ix

Chapter 1: Ithaca and Its Kings 1

Chapter 2: The Boys Club 11

Chapter 3: Conflict of Interest 21

Chapter 4: Newsmen 34

Chapter 5: The Dam 45

Chapter 6: Lives of the Students 59

Chapter 7: The Valley of Death 70

Chapter 8: Typhoid, and How the Epidemic Began 82

Chapter 9: Denial 92

Chapter 10: Apocalypse 111

Chapter 11: The Fixer 121

Chapter 12: Going Home 142

Chapter 13: The Man Who Saved Ithaca 155

Chapter 14: The Man Who Saved Cornell University 173

Chapter 15: Retribution 182

Epilogue: Getting Away with Murder 196

Afterword: The Conquest of Typhoid 212

Acknowledgments 216

Endnotes 220

Bibliography 266

Index 275

About the Author 299

PRELUDE: JUNE 16, 1903

Dark water slapped against the rowboat as it drifted on Cayuga Lake, a mile out from Ithaca. It was early in the afternoon, and the sky over upstate New York was clear. Far in the distance, on top of East Hill, a soaring clock tower that today is called McGraw Tower marked the location of Cornell University for anyone on the lake. From the observation deck near the top of the 173-foot spire could be seen Stimson Hall, the new medical school building and, of late, a makeshift hospital that was the scene of student suffering and death just a few weeks before. A little closer was Sage Chapel, where angry young men and women betrayed by their elders had met to demand action against the typhoid epidemic. Finally could be seen the home of embattled *Ithaca Daily News* publisher and Cornell oratory professor Duncan Campbell Lee, who had done his best to save the school and the town, and that of Andrew Dickson White, the elderly and distinguished cofounder and first president of the university. It is doubtful anyone, even in the tower, saw the flyspeck that was the empty rowboat in the middle of the magnificent lake, unless they had binoculars or extremely keen vision. Yet the boat and the university were inextricably linked that day by events born out of reckless ambition and criminal stupidity, a combination that has brought so much sorrow to the world.

At Cornell it was Class Day of graduation week, but the students who gathered outside of former President White's home had more than diplomas on their minds. All were survivors of the typhoid epidemic that had ravaged Ithaca during the first four months of 1903. The grave diggers had been busy. At least eighty-two people died, including twenty-nine Cornell students. Another 1,350 or so Ithaca residents, including more than 381 Cornell students, contracted typhoid but survived. The exact total will likely never be known thanks to poor record-keeping. Many young people in Ithaca suffered horribly, left exhausted and awash in medical bills that could be as much as $500, nearly a year's wages for a workingman in 1903, a stiff price even for the middle class.[1]

White had been the U.S. ambassador to Germany until late in November 1902, when he tendered his resignation to President Theodore Roosevelt. The last eighteen months of his tenure were full of sorrow. His only son, Frederick, after a lifetime of medical problems growing out of his own bout with typhoid as a Columbia University student years earlier, committed suicide in July 1901. The same month, his only daughter, Clara Newberry, split from her philandering husband in an ugly, very public divorce. After leaving Berlin, White traveled to his villa in Alassio on the Italian Riviera between Nice and Genoa and was there during the Ithaca epidemic. As a result, he probably saw little of the extensive local and national press coverage. The current Cornell president, Jacob Gould Schurman, and the chairman of the university's Board of Trustees, Samuel D. Halliday, had written to him with some of the details of the epidemic, as had his daughter and grandson.[2] It was the press coverage, and the public anger it reflected, that had nearly killed Cornell. With only a touch of hyperbole, journalists had portrayed Ithaca as a charnel house. They raised pointed questions about the links between Cornell University and William T. Morris, who had purchased Ithaca Water Works in 1901. Water provided by the company had become contaminated with typhoid germs that past January. But White had been in Italy and so did not fully comprehend the shock in America that such a terrible epidemic could happen in a place like Ithaca, which had one of the country's leading universities and more physicians per capita than any other municipality in New York.

White stepped outside and assured the group of students that all was well, that Cornell would be stronger for having endured this catastrophe.[3] It was the sort of thing old people always told young people at times like this, but he was wrong. The wounds had not healed, as the disturbing and concurrent events on Cayuga Lake and the Cornell campus that day made clear. Perhaps White was thinking hopefully of his own family troubles when he spoke.

Statistically, the typhoid epidemic in Ithaca was one of the worst in American history and one of the last of note, arriving even as better sanitation was beginning to reduce typhoid's awful toll. At least that was true in Europe. But not here. Not yet. It was still a time in America when a businessman like William T. Morris could decide, for financial reasons, against building a water filtration plant for Ithaca and there was no arm of govern-ment to force his hand, no one to make him do things right. America in 1903 was on the cusp of the modern age.[4] The Wright Brothers flew their airplane at Kitty Hawk, the very first feature film, *The Great Train Robbery*, astounded audiences, and Ithaca began to seriously use long-distance telephone service, all in 1903. But corporations still had the upper hand, and American pub-lic health lagged far behind that in Britain, France, and Germany. Citizens could do little about either.

Back on the lake, one oar of the drifting rowboat dangled in the water, moving the lock and making it creak. A breeze coming from the north gen-tled the boat toward a cluster of other small craft anchored over the Hog Hole, a popular place to fish in the lake's southwest corner. As the boat drifted closer, a gentleman's derby hat could be seen on the rear seat. That spooked the fishermen, who chattered nervously across the water.

One of them, Walter L. Head, who taught blacksmithing at Cornell, rowed over and set the trailing oar back inside. His wife looked into the boat and gasped. Next to the hat lay a fancy metal matchbox and a folded pocket-knife, the accoutrement of a middle-class businessman. It was as if the owner had laid them neatly on his dresser and lain down to take a nap. But where was he? Who was he? There was water in the bottom of the boat, as if it had somehow tilted to let in the lake. But there had been no storm or heavy waves today. The name "Van Order" was stenciled on the boat. Head knew Sylvester Van Order rented boats from a livery on Cascadilla Creek, off the Cayuga Lake inlet that served as Ithaca's harbor. Assuming that one of the boatman's customers had fallen into the lake and drowned, Head tied the empty craft to his own and began the long row back to town.[5]

When the couple arrived at Van Order's, another fisherman was already there. Charles A. Zeek said he was sure the missing man was Theodor A. Zinck, proprietor of the Hotel Brunswick, the most popular student bar in Ithaca. That morning, Zeek had seen Zinck rowing down the inlet past the lighthouse at the end of the State Pier and onto Cayuga Lake. The odd thing, he said, was that the tavern keeper stopped several times to stare back at Ithaca. Ultimately he could not say what had happened to Zinck, because he had not seen him go into the water. Nor did he hear a splash or a cry for help.

Zeek had averted his eyes around 12:30 p.m. to attend to his fishing. Later, glancing back, he could see no one in the boat.

Van Order's office had a telephone, which were increasingly common in Ithaca in 1903. He raised the operator, who connected his call to the city police. It was a slow day: The police blotter showed only three arrests, one for drunkenness, one for fighting, and someone picked up on a bench warrant. Officer Alvin Sincebaugh responded. He examined the coat and vest that Zinck had left with Van Order that morning. A watch and Masonic fob were still attached to the vest, and the coat pocket held a few letters and a bank book. But there was no suicide note, nothing to explain why Zinck had decided to be his own Charon. Not that anyone in Ithaca really needed to ask. They all knew his sorrow.

Emotionally, Zinck had been dead for months, ever since his beloved daughter and only child, Louise, called Lula and aged twenty-four years, had died horribly of typhoid at the height of the epidemic. Bloody sheets were all that remained after the undertaker removed her body. Zinck had taken all of Ithaca's sorrow on himself, it seemed, and slipped into the dark water of Cayuga Lake. Officer Sincebaugh understood; two of his own children had been deathly ill during the epidemic but survived. Ninety percent of typhoid patients survived, albeit after an awful ordeal. The unlucky 10 percent, like Lula Zinck, were often young and otherwise healthy. The unfairness of it drove Zinck to despair.

He had emigrated to America in 1876, five years after his native Alsace and Lorraine were taken as prizes by Germany at the conclusion of the Franco-Prussian War. The Zinck family, despite its German name, mainly cast its lot with France. A sister stayed in the ancestral home in the village of Gambsheim, not to become French again until after World War I, but the rest of the family settled in and around Paris. Zinck himself landed in Rochester, New York, where he worked in a cousin's butcher shop for two years, saving his money. In the spring of 1878, with his brother Phillip, he moved to Ithaca and opened the Hotel Brunswick and Lager Bar at 108-110 N. Aurora St. in the downtown business district.

Every Cornell student knew Zinck's. His bar became one of the more popular places to drink, smoke cigars, and socialize during one's time in

Ithaca. Zinck, a large man with a handlebar mustache, welcomed students, professors, and townspeople alike, offering them good food and properly cooled Bartholomay's lager beer—cellar cold, not ice cold—with Gemütlichkeit thrown in at no additional charge. Although most people knew it as Zinck's, the Cornell intelligentsia insisted on calling the bar, "Theodore's, and in no other manner." So wrote Romeyn Berry, who lived through the epidemic, in his 1950 book, *Behind the Ivy*.

Among the students one might have spotted there in the months before typhoid struck was George Jean Nathan, writer for the *Cornell Daily Sun*, the student newspaper, and later a renowned theater critic, cofounder of *American Mercury* magazine with H. L. Mencken, and bon vivant in New York City. Nathan was among the few students in any given year that Zinck knew by name, but he was always "Mr. Nathan." Zinck was formal in the German manner, not prone to easy intimacy. Yet he remembered faces and would recognize old customers returning twenty years later for a class reunion. And being German, or whatever an Alsatian might choose to call himself, Zinck loved choral singing. The Cornell Glee Club would repair to his bar on Wednesday nights after practice and serenade him with one of its current favorites.[6]

The world he built for himself in Ithaca fell apart when Lula died. Nothing could bring him out of his deep depression. Two weeks after his daughter was buried in Lake View Cemetery, Zinck went to his lawyer and wrote out a will.[7] When students who fled the epidemic began drifting back to Ithaca and the Hotel Brunswick in late spring, Zinck had to relive Lula's death whenever one of them offered condolences. They were young and alive, and she was not. He told worried friends that he would stay strong for his wife, Emelie, but in the quiet of his home, the downward spiral accelerated.

On the morning of June 16, Zinck seemed in better spirits, but that is often remembered of suicides. He walked to the Hotel Brunswick at 8 a.m. and went over the books with Daniel Kelly, one of his three bartenders. Zinck seemed normal to Kelly, who took little notice when his boss left for a walk at 10:30 a.m. Through much of the spring, Zinck had taken long, intensely private morning walks up to Renwick Park along the lake. Today he walked quickly down Aurora Street to Buffalo, turning left and walking to DeWitt

Park. Here Zinck followed the diagonal sidewalk that still runs across the park, where he encountered Frank J. H. "Senator" Murphy, another of his bartenders, walking in the opposite direction. Zinck took out his pocket watch and reproved Senator for being late to work. Then he continued through the park and down Cayuga Street, reaching the Van Order boatyard at 11:10 a.m.

He explained to the proprietor that he wanted to go for a row but that his own boat, which he had not taken out in a year or two, was dirty. After climbing into the boat Van Order offered, Zinck handed back his coat and vest and asked that they be kept in the office until he returned. That was hardly unusual on a warm summer day, and Van Order thought nothing of it. When he last saw Zinck, still wearing his derby, he was rowing away from the dock, pulling toward Cayuga Lake.

All the dead young men and women in Ithaca, and especially at Cornell University, set this epidemic apart. The Ithaca catastrophe riveted America's attention during February and March of 1903. Articles about it can be found in newspapers all over the country. Other college presidents sent letters of sympathy to Jacob Gould Schurman. Typhoid touched 522 homes in Ithaca, and in 150 of those, two or more people came down with the disease.[8]

Yet it had been less an epidemic, which suggests chance, than a crime, a completely preventable catastrophe brought on by the grandiosity, greed, and stupidity of men. Morris was the principal actor, but he was aided and abetted by his wealthy Ithaca friends who sat on the boards of local banks and Cornell University. Blinded by class and personal loyalties, they arranged critical financing from the university that unintentionally set the deadly events in motion and then protected Morris against a day of reckoning. What happened in Ithaca was not simply bad luck or God's will. When a water company owner ignores the competent and well-grounded advice of his engineer for economic reasons, and suffering and death result, it is not hyperbole to label it a crime.

American sanitarians of the early twentieth century raged over the continuing death toll from typhoid. Public health doctors knew they could prevent outbreaks of the disease by keeping drinking water clean and pure. They couldn't cure typhoid—that would not come until 1949 and the discovery of the antibiotic chloromycetin. What stymied them in 1903 was the human factor, the reckless or ignorant businessman or public official who insisted on doing things his way, as if no one mattered but himself. That was still beyond their control in this era of no regulation, and it made them crazy.

In the *Atlantic Monthly* of January 1903, still in homes even as young people began dying in Ithaca, Professor Charles-Edward Amory Winslow of Yale University offered up a modest proposal. He said that for every case of typhoid, someone ought to be hanged.[9] He was far from alone in this sentiment. The great sanitarian at the Massachusetts Institute of Technology, William T. Sedgwick, referred to the hanging suggestion as "a striking saying and worth remembering, because it puts the responsibility for this disease where it belongs, namely on mankind, and not upon fate or the gods."[10]

A typhoid epidemic was like a war, senselessly reaping the lives of young people who should have lived for many decades. A typhoid epidemic cut across all social classes, because all social classes drank water. Again as in war, there was no escape except, maybe, by being old. The old were more likely to have picked up immunity to typhoid at some point during their lives and were far less likely to contract the disease.

Morris was tone-deaf to the public anger in Ithaca. He awoke the morning of June 16 thinking ahead to the Senior Dance scheduled that night in the Armory at Cornell—one of several annual social events on campus that were almost as much for the social elite of Ithaca as for students. There was no move to cancel the dance out of respect for the dead, unlike at Stanford University that spring, where the Class of 1903 had voted to cancel its Senior Dance and donate the money to the student organization that had helped contain a typhoid epidemic that broke out in Palo Alto just as the one in Ithaca was ending.

We know who was with Morris at the dance from an article in the *Ithaca Daily News* listing the occupants of the boxes that ringed the dance floor.[11] He sat in the Treman Box with his good friends Robert H. and Charles E. Treman, brothers who were members of the Cornell Board of Trustees, and their wives. Other guests included Charles H. Blood, who was a

Cornell trustee, a real estate developer, and the part-time district attorney of Tompkins County, and Thomas F. "Teefy" Crane, dean of the university faculty at Cornell. Crane became acting head of the university in 1899 while Schurman was away in the Philippines at the behest of President William McKinley, assessing the native insurrection in America's newest colony. Jervis Langdon of Elmira, a nephew by marriage of author Samuel Clemens, and Wilder D. Bancroft, a Cornell chemistry professor who sat on the Ithaca Country Club board of directors with Blood and Charlie Treman, were still other guests. They all danced, even as Zinck's body drifted in the cold depths of Cayuga Lake, just as they had in February at the Junior Prom while the first student was dying of typhoid in the Cornell Infirmary just a few hundred yards away.

We don't know what Morris told friends in private, but from his known actions we can imagine him expressing vocal anger over his negative press portrayal in the *Ithaca Daily News*, not remorse for the young people he killed. That was how he was. Narcissistic. The last victim of the epidemic was barely cold in the ground when Morris resumed an active and oblivious social life. In May, he invited friends to join him on his yacht to witness the annual Memorial Day rowing regatta on Cayuga Lake,[12] sipping cocktails as the shells glided over the dark water, their oars slashing the lake in a rhythmic frenzy.

He was already plotting revenge. Thomas M. Vinton, his general contractor on the Six Mile Creek dam project that was the proximate cause of the epidemic, signed papers a day later for a libel suit in New York City against the *Ithaca Daily News* and its managing editor, Frank E. Gannett, over a single editorial, "Nothing Less Than an Outrage," published on May 28, 1903.[13] The editorial accused Vinton's firm, Tucker & Vinton, of deliberate cost overruns and shoddy workmanship on the dam and probably did violate the much more plaintiff-friendly libel law of the day. Morris was pushing his own libel lawyer, Cornell University trustee Henry W. Sackett, who handled libel defense for the *New York Tribune*, to prepare a separate suit against the *Daily News* and its publisher, Duncan Campbell Lee. That few potential jurors in Tompkins County were likely to consider Morris an aggrieved victim of the press seemed beyond his comprehension.

Later on June 17, Cornell University took its own revenge against Lee, who was an associate professor of oratory and chairman of the department. The

Board of Trustees voted to deny Lee a promotion to full professor, a humiliating end to a distinguished academic career. The axing seemed directly tied to anger over the *Daily News* stories and editorials about the university's role in the epidemic. Among the trustees voting that day were three of Morris's fellow revelers at the Senior Dance, the Treman brothers and Charles H. Blood. His principal banker, Mynderse Van Cleef, was also there, as was his libel lawyer, Sackett. They were all trustees. Conflicts of interest didn't seem to bother them. They just didn't want Lee pointing them out.

<center>~~~~~~~</center>

After two days passed, Emelie Zinck hired "Dynamite" Dan Maloney to drop explosive charges in the lake in an effort to bring up the body of her husband. For all the things about water that were not regulated in New York, using dynamite in lakes required a permit from a state game protector because of the potential to kill fish. That permit was obtained and on the afternoon of June 18, Maloney, accompanied by the game protector, set off four charges of twelve sticks of dynamite each. He would light the water fuse, drop the charge to the bottom of the lake, then row like hell to get a safe distance away. The *Ithaca Daily Journal* described the "dull rumble and roar" of the explosion followed by an eruption of water eight feet in diameter and forty to fifty feet in height. But nothing except dead fish and "sticks, stumps, and all manner of refuse" came up from the bottom. The blasts were continued on June 19 with equally unsatisfactory results, and a rumor took hold that Zinck was not really dead. Did they think that he was hiding in the trees on the shoreline, like Huck Finn, watching the effort to recover his body?

The two Leonard brothers snagged the body with dragging hooks around 8:30 a.m. on June 22 in a section of Cayuga Lake not targeted by Dynamite Dan. The cold water at the bottom had slowed decomposition, and the body was not bloated. Zinck's face looked "perfectly natural" other than an extreme whiteness, the *Ithaca Daily Journal* reported. Believing the body would turn black if exposed to air for very long, the brothers tied a rope around Zinck's waist and attached a rock to keep him underwater. They rowed back to Ithaca, turned the corpse over to the police and undertakers, and collected a $100 reward from Mrs. Zinck. It was all in a day's work.

A Masonic funeral was held at Zinck's home the next afternoon, and he was laid to rest in Lake View Cemetery next to his daughter. Emelie would not join them until 1928, the same year Morris died. When Zinck's will was probated after his funeral, he was shown to be a prosperous businessman. There had been no reason for his suicide beyond despair over the death of Lula and the near death of his nephew, Edmond Zinck.

Given the horror of what happened in Ithaca in 1903, it is surprising that grief did not send more citizens to the bottom of that cold and dark lake. There was no justice here. The new century had not begun well. Morris was the archetype of a business executive we know all too well today, to whom profit and personal aggrandizement is everything and the public interest is a joke.

The Ithaca epidemic, too, marked the birth of a *corporation* that would long outlive its founder, challenging the public interest in America for nearly a century. In 1906, Morris organized his utilities into a holding company called Associated Gas & Electric Company. In the 1920s and 1930s, under the leadership of Howard C. Hopson, AG&E set records for corporate fraud and looting that stood for more than half a century. Many, many lives were ruined. President Franklin D. Roosevelt fought an oddly personal battle with Hopson through much of his career, and in 1940 succeeded in imprisoning Hopson, who by then was insane from syphilis. Associated Gas & Electric went bankrupt the same year and was succeeded in 1946 by General Public Utilities Corporation.

In 1949, GPU became enamored of atomic energy and set off down a road that ended thirty years later with the Three Mile Island nuclear accident and meltdown near Harrisburg, Pennsylvania. More than one hundred thousand people fled their homes, far more than in Ithaca, but unless a late wave of fatal radiation cancers breaks in central Pennsylvania, the Ithaca typhoid epidemic had by far the greater death toll. Some might argue the company was cursed, but historians and journalists rightly shy away from the supernatural and we will not go there.

We too often worship our free enterprise system in America as a fetish, taking its supposed goodness on faith. The story of this company may shake that faith. If nothing else, it drives home the need for strong regulation of those corporations with the ability to hurt the public through inept or criminal behavior. If we ignore that lesson, we risk embracing the old saw about insanity, that it involves doing the same thing over and over again and hoping for a different outcome. William T. Morris did not spring from nowhere, nor did the Ithaca catastrophe. Like so many disasters, in retrospect we can see it coming from a long distance away, finally arriving as a runaway train.

Chapter 1

Ithaca and Its Kings

LAFAYETTE L. TREMAN WAS ONE OF THOSE MEN, so common in nineteenth-century America, who built up a family business and kept on adding other businesses until he could be said, in a sense, to rule his town. The last of three brothers who came to Ithaca, New York, in the 1840s, Treman basked in the glow of respect from all who knew him, but he worried with good reason about the future of his family and his empire. Ithaca was a beautiful small town that dreamed of greatness, but which, like the Treman family itself, was beautiful and damned.

Treman and his brothers, Leonard and Elias, grew up in Mecklenburg, New York, a frontier outpost twelve miles west of Ithaca where their father operated a gristmill and where the brutal wars against the Seneca tribes were still a living memory. When their friends moved west, following the frontier into new lands, they moved east, back toward civilization. After arriving in Ithaca, the Treman brothers went into the hardware business. Treman, King & Co. evolved from a small shop into a regional hardware emporium that lasted nearly a century, closing only in 1938. Their letterhead, midway through that long reign, proclaimed themselves jobbers, or wholesalers, "of hardware, glass, paints, etc." Elias gradually became CEO of the hardware business, while L.L., as Lafayette L. Treman preferred to be known, split off into banking and Leonard into the utility business, namely Ithaca Gas Light Company and Ithaca Water Works. But they all had their hands in each other's businesses, if only as silent partners.[1]

L.L.'s story might have come from a handbook for American success, so classic was its upward trajectory. The frontier boy turned business entrepreneur became secretary of the new Ithaca & Athens Railroad in 1871, chosen for his business skills and personal appeal.[2] He became president of Tompkins County National Bank in 1873 and was a founding board member of the Ithaca Trust Company in 1891. Even the town's leading newspaper, the *Ithaca Daily Journal*, founded by his late father-in-law, state senator Ebenezer Mack, was in his camp. Mack, who had declined to be secretary of state in President Martin Van Buren's cabinet,[3] helped and inspired Treman. He repaid his father-in-law by naming his firstborn child and only son Ebenezer Mack Treman.

Over the years, L. L. Treman took over Ithaca Gas Light and Ithaca Water Works from his brothers. Elias sold his shares early on. When Leonard died of illness in 1888, his interest passed to his only child, Kate, married to John W. Bush, a lawyer in Buffalo. There was no question in that day of her running the company, so management passed to L. L. Treman and his son, who went by Eben. Kate eventually sold most of her interest to L. L. Treman, and by the turn of the twentieth century, he owned nearly all of the company.[4] Treman put Eben in charge and stuck to banking. Running the utilities was not what Eben Treman really wanted to do with his life—he should have been a musician or an impresario—but his father's word was law. He could be a bit of an autocrat to his only son.

<hr>

The city of their success, Ithaca, had 13,136 people in 1900. It lay at the head of Cayuga Lake, second largest of the eleven Finger Lakes in central New York. Dark blue, fiercely cold, and framed by steep hills, Cayuga is forty miles long, one to three miles wide, and as deep as 435 feet. Pleasure boating was common and so were drownings—the Leonard brothers, fishermen who had a cottage and boathouse along the lake, operated a grim side business of finding the drowned. They had recovered nearly a half-dozen waterlogged bodies with dragging hooks in recent years.

Geography was everything to Ithaca, both a bane and a blessing. Creeks plunged down the steep hills to the lake, creating spectacular gorges and waterfalls. Visitors marveled at the abundance of water. After a canal opened in 1828 connecting Cayuga and Seneca Lakes to the newly dug Erie Canal, and thence to the outside world, Ithaca became a major inland port. Railroads hauled anthracite coal from Pennsylvania to the upper town, where cars were shifted to an inclined plane and lowered to the docks, their cargo transferred to barges. At night, long tows of barges would depart for the north end of the lake and the canal. When they returned, they carried New York wheat—the Empire State was then the wheat capital of America—and other commodities. Ithaca's economy grew steadily, apart from the occasional national financial panic, and the Tremans and their businesses prospered accordingly.

Ithaca's first white settlers built homes on two square miles of marshy clay flats along the lake. Builders at first believed that the three hills of Ithaca were too steep for housing and insisted the city must expand to the south.[5] But by 1900, Ithaca had climbed the hills, known simply as East, South and West. It was less a problem putting the houses up than keeping fires from burning them down. Getting enough water to the fire hydrants in the upper reaches of Ithaca was a constant challenge for Ithaca Water Works, but that did not stop the growth of the city. Fires or no fires, Ithaca grew and the Tremans continued to prosper, especially after the advent of Cornell University. The brothers sent their sons to Cornell to be educated but not their daughters, even though the university was a pioneer from the start in the coeducation of young women.

The university opened in 1868 atop East Hill, looming over Ithaca and Cayuga Lake like a fortified Tuscan hill town. Andrew Dickson White was the first president. Cornell University was built on what had been the three-hundred-acre farm of its founder and benefactor, Ezra Cornell, who endowed the university in 1865 with his land and a sizable portion of his Western Union fortune. He had discovered a better way to run the telegraph wires, and at the peak of his wealth owned one-sixth of Western Union's immensely valuable stock.

One of the first philanthropists to come out of the phenomenal American industrial boom in the nineteenth century, Cornell believed that because his fortune came as much from opportunity—the Civil War and its carnage— as hard work, he had an obligation to use it to help the public. The magnificent public library Cornell built for Ithaca in 1863 (it was demolished in 1960 and replaced by a useful, if decidedly modern structure) was an inspiration to Andrew Carnegie, who as a young man was a telegraph operator for Western Union. After he prospered in the steel industry, Carnegie went Ezra Cornell several times better and built scores of public libraries in towns large and small across the land. He joined the Cornell University Board of Trustees in 1890. But as Cornell well knew, libraries were not the only thing communities needed to grow and prosper. Trained, talented people were just as critical, and not only from the upper classes.

Cornell and White, the cofounders of the university, became acquainted in 1864 as members of the New York State Senate. Cornell was fifty-seven years old, self-educated, and at heart a farmer and mechanic. White was thirty-one years old, a college professor educated at Geneva College (today called Hobart and William Smith College) in Geneva, New York, the Sorbonne, and Yale, who had been deemed too slight to carry a rifle in the Civil War. But they stood as one in their desire to create a large, modern university open to students of all social classes, offering a wide range of courses of study, financial aid, and freedom from control by a religious denomination. They built an educational utopia atop East Hill in Ithaca and threw open the doors to the nation and the world.

White wanted to protect his university from pedants and philistines. He wrote in his autobiography, "I took pains to guard the institution from those who, in the higher education, substitute dates for history, gerund-grinding for literature, and formulas for science; as to the latter, I sought to guard it from the men to whom 'Gain is God, and Gunnybags his Prophet.'"[6]

White aimed to spare his new university from the Greco-Roman classicism that dominated American higher education before the Civil War and had largely become a system for turning out new clerics and schoolmasters. After four years of brutal and bloody war, that approach to higher education seemed quaintly inadequate to Americans eager to get on with building a modern industrial nation. White did not abandon Greek and Latin but made them optional and added courses in science, engineering, agriculture, and modern European languages. He and Ezra Cornell suffered merciless attacks from traditionalists who were horrified at the idea of mixing science and the classics and from clergy convinced the university was "Godless" because it had no church affiliation and taught the works of liberal thinkers condemned by conservative churchmen.

But other people showered Ithaca and the university with praise. What better place to acquire knowledge, they enthused, than this earthly paradise? A letter written to the *New York Times* in 1872 rhapsodized that in Ithaca, "the man or woman with soul to appreciate the work of nature can commune with nature's God—can drink and be full." The writer—seemingly a man, but not identified beyond his initials—climbed up Fall Creek Gorge during his visit. After passing the 150-foot Ithaca Falls, "higher than the American Fall at Niagara," the writer scrambled up a one-hundred-foot cliff and came upon the sixty-foot Forest Falls, "a perfect gem of a waterfall, set, as it is, in a framework of rocks and evergreens." After climbing past Rocky Falls, Foaming Falls, Thune Falls, Beebe Falls, and finally Triphammer Falls, the writer emerged from the gorge into the Cornell campus, rejoicing, "That young literary giant, the pride of the state, and justly so. Four years in bringing a faculty of about 40 and 700 students, and with endowment, buildings, library and cabinets that other institutions have been generations in trying to acquire, and where the lover of science can drink to repletion."[7]

The two founders persevered in the face of their critics. White sailed to Europe to hire leading professors and to purchase scientific equipment that Cornell University needed to realize his vision.[8] Ezra Cornell never wavered from his financial commitment to the university that bore his name, even after criticism of his motives—detractors said he wanted merely to line his own pockets—became slanderous.

He lost much of his remaining Western Union fortune when economic panic swept the land in 1873. Cornell invested a huge sum—$2 million, or the equivalent of about $36 million today—in the construction of four short-line railroads intended to give Ithaca better connections to the outside world. The most important was the Ithaca & Athens, which connected to the Lehigh Valley Railroad at Athens, Pennsylvania, and thence to the rest of the East Coast. In this venture he was a partner with, among others, L. L. Treman, who seems to have emerged relatively unscathed. The railroads were finished but carried Ezra Cornell to the brink of bankruptcy. He was forced to sell the rest of his Western Union stock to ensure the final driving of the spikes and died in December 1874, shattered by his losses. His eldest son, Franklin C. Cornell, managed to salvage $560,000 by selling his father's interest in two of the connections to the Lehigh Valley Railroad.

White lived on until 1918. Perhaps his greatest failure as Cornell president was allowing local alumni too much control over the business affairs of the university. They dominated the Executive Committee of the Board of Trustees, the committee that made day-to-day business decisions for Cornell. The arrangement may have made sense when the university was young, but had become ever less tenable, as the university became a realm apart from Ithaca, a wealthy institution recognized far and wide for its academic prowess. Students came from all over America and the world, and eminent guest lecturers graced the halls. Yet Cornell University was controlled by a small, often parochial group of Ithaca businessmen who were personal friends, or worse, had interlocking business interests they saw no harm in advancing through their membership on the board. White and his successors had no power to veto a decision of the Board of Trustees or Executive Committee. The president could vote or remonstrate against it, but in the end the majority ruled.[9]

For all their achievements, the men who ran Cornell University seemed prone to gross errors of judgment. Consider the case of the University Library. Erected in 1891 and regarded as one of the two or three best in the United States, the library had 160,000 books and room for 500,000. The building was topped by a 173-foot spire that was among the last things Theodor Zinck saw from Cayuga Lake on June 16, 1903.[10] At the top were chimes donated by Jennie McGraw Fiske. Yet the library was also a symbol of the fallibility of this great institution.

McGraw's tragic life could well have inspired Henry James and his 1902 novel, *The Wings of the Dove*, which concerns a doomed heiress and the people who try to grab her money. In 1877, Jennie McGraw inherited a lumber fortune from her father, John McGraw, a Cornell University benefactor and business partner of Henry W. Sage, then chairman of the university's Board of Trustees. She immediately became a target for fortune hunters, despite or perhaps because of having an advanced case of tuberculosis. In fact, her health was in steep decline. Fearing the McGraw fortune would not come to Cornell, President White shamelessly pushed his good friend, Daniel Willard Fiske, the university librarian, to woo and wed Jennie. He provided money to Fiske in 1880 so he could travel to Italy in pursuit of his quarry. It is an astonishing story. White even paid for the engagement ring. She died a little over a year after the wedding, and as White hoped, left a large bequest to the university to build a magnificent new library for her beloved husband.

But legal technicalities in the university charter delayed settlement of the estate. Fiske grew tired of waiting for his own bequest and professed to be angry over White's conniving scheme, despite his central role. He sued to break the will. Nine years later, the U.S. Supreme Court ruled in his favor. By then he was living in Florence, Italy, and working as a rare book dealer. Sage was angered by the litigation and donated money to allow the library to be built.[11] Jennie McGraw Fiske was entombed in a sarcophagus in Sage Chapel on the campus, and Willard Fiske was entombed next to her after he died in 1904. That angered the Sage family, which resigned their seats on the Board of Trustees. Fiske left Cornell $400,000 in his will, and that trumped the Sages' hurt feelings.

The president of Cornell at the beginning of the twentieth century was Jacob Gould Schurman, a prominent intellectual of his day who looked out from his office in Morrill Hall to the nation, not down the hill to Ithaca. Trained as a philosopher, he wrote many books and was highly intelligent, almost scarily so. He was as much a king of Ithaca in 1900 as L. L. Treman. They simply ruled different realms.

Schurman was the great-grandson of William Schurman, a slave-owning American Loyalist who was jailed for a time by the revolutionary government. In 1784, he fled the country with his family, first for Nova Scotia and then for Prince Edward Island, traveling in his own ship.[12] Schurman acquired large land holdings on the island. He was in the shipping, cooperage, and lumber businesses and served in the provincial legislature and as a magistrate.[13] But his wealth, spread among too many descendants, was mostly gone by the time Jacob was born in 1854.[14] Young Schurman grew up in Freetown, Prince Edward Island, a tiny hamlet surrounded by potato fields that is seemingly as remote and rural in the twenty-first century as it was in the nineteenth. His parents were solid, hard-working farmers but by no means wealthy. Nevertheless, they encouraged his education. He left home at age thirteen, his quest for learning taking him as far as London, Heidelberg, and Berlin. Much of the costs were covered by scholarships and fellowships. He was a bright, ambitious boy.

Schurman was forty-six years old in 1900 and in his eighth year as Cornell president. A handsome man with princely features, he was a superstar intellectual of his day and much in demand for public lectures around the country. Of late, he devoted his speeches to his opposition to the U.S. takeover of the Philippines after the 1898 war with Spain and the bloody guerrilla war with Filipinos that followed, a subject on which he had firsthand knowledge after heading a presidential investigating commission in the islands. In this he matched the views of the wealthiest man on the Cornell Board of Trustees, steel magnate and philanthropist Andrew Carnegie.

Schurman rarely shied from controversy. Earlier in his career, he struggled to resolve the conflict between science and the traditional Protestant faith of his rural Canadian childhood.[15] He took up the cause of evolution, controversial then and now, arguing that one did not have to choose between God and Darwin. Schurman said belief in God grew out of rational thought, not the turbulent and shaky roller-coaster of faith. That was far from his only controversial statement. He once even pronounced America commercially strong but intellectually weak because it had produced "no really great creative minds" such as Darwin or Shakespeare.[16] Schurman longed for the national stage. It was a pleasant diversion from the little problems of Ithaca.

He was austere in manner and difficult to approach, despite what we might now call a movie-star handsome face. Romeyn Berry wrote that Schurman's "outward demeanor did not invite student intimacy." Morris Bishop, another Cornell historian, recalled Schurman's advice to students to "always study in a straight-backed, hard-bottomed chair." Yet to students he was a popular lecturer during his four years as a philosophy professor before becoming president, and he was able to form warm mentor relationships with some of them.

In winter, a traditional time for fun at Cornell, Schurman donned his Sutherland tweed jacket, strapped on his ice skates, and headed out onto frozen Beebe Lake, which Ezra Cornell had created in 1828 by damming Fall Creek. Then, wrote Berry, Schurman was "a different man. He was an expert skater and knew it. On the ice he was all smiles and ever the center of a circle of admiring undergraduates." They did not care about his intellectual attainments, only that he skated better than any other university president they could imagine. Schurman cut a fine figure in his tweed jacket, "like a duke off for an afternoon's tramp over the moors," Berry wrote. Thomas F. "Teefy" Crane, the dean, skated reasonably well, but wore the same clothes he did in the office. Andrew D. White did not skate at all but would stand at the edge of the lake in his fur-lined overcoat and felt topper and smile at the happy scene before him.[17]

Yet despite the different realms ruled by L. L. Treman and Jacob Gould Schurman, there was really no separating Cornell and Ithaca. The city's bankers and businessmen dominated the Board of Trustees. Most students lived off-campus in rooming houses on East Hill. They may have taken their lessons atop East Hill and thought themselves a breed apart, but they came back down to eat and drink with the rest of Ithaca.

For Treman, his pleasant, orderly world was not without problems. Ithaca Common Council was up in arms, as it always seemed to be, about low water pressure in the hill sections of the community. There had been a disastrous fraternity house fire in January 1900, made worse by a lack of water. The clamor for a better water system, preferably owned by the town, grew louder. But he had shrugged that off before and might well do so again. What could you do when the biggest source of water in the region, Cayuga Lake, was too polluted to drink? All he could give them was water from two creeks, Six Mile and Buttermilk, and that wasn't always very much. What came out of their taps could be muddy and disgusting, and more than 1,500 Ithaca residents still had private wells. Cornell freshmen often suffered stomach disorders, though rarely typhoid, until they adjusted to the water.

Treman had family problems, too. The succession issue crept up on him as insidiously as the thick wisteria vine winding around the columns of his stately, thirty-room Greek Revival mansion near downtown Ithaca. He seemed always to fear the worst. Who would take over the Ithaca gas and water companies if his son passed from the scene? Eben, forty-nine years old, had no surviving children. His first wife, Eugenie, and their newborn son died a day apart in 1886. His second wife, Belle, was childless after nine years of marriage. L. L. Treman's two daughters, Jeannie and Louisa, were not expected to have either the ability or inclination to take over the family business. What if sudden, accidental death took Eben just as it took his uncle Elias?

Elias died in a carriage accident in 1898 on his way to his summer cottage on the western shore of Cayuga Lake. His driver whipped a snake to keep it from scaring the horse, but the horse was scared by the whip and bucked, tipping the carriage and breaking Elias's neck. He lingered for almost four months, but complications from paralysis finally killed him. At least he had two sons, Robert H. and Charles E. Treman, ready to take over the hardware business. And Rob already had a son in line to take over from him. Even Elias's daughter, Elizabeth, was taken care of—she was married to Mynderse Van Cleef, general counsel for Cornell University and a prominent local banker.

That friend of his son, William T. Morris of Penn Yan, inquired more than once about purchasing the gas company, but L. L. Treman brushed him off. He wanted his family business to continue down the generations and had no interest in selling to Morris. And why should he? When L. L. Treman walked from his mansion to his office, he was still a king of Ithaca. Men in suits would offer respectful greetings, and women in long dresses and broad hats would tell their children, there goes Mr. Treman. But even kings grow old and die, and now on April 27, 1900, that had happened and nothing would be the same for his family, his community, and scores of people he would never know.

Chapter 2

The Boys Club

STEPPING THROUGH THE OPENING IN THE GIANT WISTERIA VINE that wrapped around the columns, William T. Morris found himself at the front door of the L. L. Treman mansion at 210 N. Geneva St. in Ithaca. The porch was crowded with mourners here for the funeral of the patriarch, who had lived here for half a century. Morris came for that reason, too, but he looked for Eben Treman, the only son of the man in the coffin. Eben grew up in this house, and Morris had visited many times. They had become friends through the Chi Phi fraternity at Cornell University in the late 1860s but developed a deeper friendship after Eben returned to Ithaca from the Midwest in 1884 after many years away.

Entering the parlor, where the coffin lay on a bier, Morris spotted Eben with his mother, Eliza A. Treman, and his sisters, Jeannie Waterman and Louisa Treman. Nearby were Eben's cousins, Robert H. Treman and his younger brother, Charles E. Treman. Rob was about to succeed L. L. Treman as president of Tompkins County National Bank in Ithaca and would be a director of the New York Federal Reserve Bank from 1916 to 1929. Charlie was president of the board of the Ithaca Conservatory of Music, today Ithaca College. Mynderse Van Cleef, who was married to their sister, Elizabeth, was also there. Morris knew the trio nearly as well as he knew Eben. Indeed, many of the important people in his life were here in the parlor. It was a nice little boys club Morris had joined. They helped him, protected him, and followed him into hell. But none of them was closer to him than Ebenezer Mack Treman.

The Tremans in 1900 were a wealthy and accomplished family, and the patriarch's grand funeral reflected as much. They "epitomized the enterprising upward mobility of the American population," wrote Carol U. Sisler, an Ithaca historian, in *Enterprising Families, Ithaca, New York.* "They were well educated, they were well mannered, they were cultured with interest in music, the arts, and the theater, and by Ithaca standards, they were wealthy."[1] Indeed, Rob and Charlie Treman and Mynderse Van Cleef were about to begin construction of adjoining mansions on East Hill, overlooking the city and lake, to celebrate their ascendancy to Ithaca's ruling elite. Rob Treman and Van Cleef sat on the Board of Trustees of Cornell University, and Charlie would join them in June 1902. Van Cleef also did important legal work for the university. He was treasurer and a director of Ithaca Trust Company and had even probated Ezra Cornell's will, no easy task.

Morris was an unmarried, darkly handsome, forty-six-year-old lawyer and gas company owner from Penn Yan, a small town about fifty miles northwest of Ithaca on Keuka Lake, another of the Finger Lakes. Known to his friends as Will, or even, when quite old, as Billy, Morris moved through life with a sense of entitlement found in certain people who have inherited their good fortune. His father was a U.S. congressman, and young Will received a grand start in life from his father's wealth. He seemed to have little ability to appreciate the impact of his actions on people outside the boys club. It was all business to him. Narcissistic and intelligent, his fatal flaw was a reckless willingness to cut corners to get what he wanted. What he wanted now was to live closer to Eben.

By the spring of 1900, Morris had acquired nine small-town gas companies, including four in just the previous six months. He was looking to buy more. The economy was booming. Now that L. L. Treman was dead, Morris intended to make Ithaca Gas Light Company the crown jewel in his empire. He had long dreamed of moving his headquarters from Penn Yan to Ithaca, a far more convenient, cosmopolitan, and interesting place for a man like himself, who was wealthy but had no wife or children to occupy his time. He had been rebuffed in previous attempts to buy the company and knew better than to bring up the subject today. But his mind was calculating. He walked over to the Treman family and offered his condolences.

Morris was born in 1853 and spent his youth in the village of Rushville at the northern end of Yates County, where the buckwheat fields came up to the edge of town. The Senecas who first settled this land were long gone. His father, Daniel Morris, served as the Yates County district attorney from 1847 to 1850, then was elected as a Republican to the New York State Assembly. In 1860, he moved his law practice to Penn Yan, perhaps so his son could enroll in Penn Yan Academy, a private school.[2] Daniel Morris served two terms in Congress during and immediately after the Civil War. In December 1865, he added his "D. Morris" signature to the Thirteenth Amendment to the U.S. Constitution outlawing slavery.[3] He was a Lincoln man through and through.

Young Will showed early promise, doing well at Penn Yan Academy and passing an entrance examination to Cornell University in the spring of 1869, when he was only sixteen years old. That fall he joined the second class of freshmen to enter the new school.[4] Morris was drawn to athletics, playing third base for the Cornell baseball team as a junior and senior and rowing second position in the number two crew for eight-oared barge. He had a flair for the arts, too, serving as treasurer of the Adelphi Literary Association and playing B-flat cornet in the Geneva Street Cornet Band. He didn't join the Chi Phi fraternity until his senior year, but once he did, his fraternity brothers became the most important people in his life. He would turn to them again and again over the years.[5]

After graduation in 1873, Morris read law, which in the parlance of the time meant he studied case law in the office of a practicing attorney. When he had studied enough, he took the bar exam to prove he had mastered the profession. That was how most lawyers trained prior to the early twentieth century, when law schools became ascendant. Morris studied first with his father and then with the Foster & Thomson law firm at 69 Wall St. in New York. A prominent firm specializing in corporate and railroad law, Foster & Thomson first appeared in the New York city directory in 1852 and was still listed as late as 1934. Little about Morris's early law career has survived. He was admitted to the bar in Brooklyn on February 17, 1876, but stayed with Foster & Thomson one more year as managing clerk.[6] Morris returned to Penn Yan in the fall of 1877 and briefly joined his father's law firm. In 1879, he moved out and became junior partner in the new firm of Wood, Butler, and Morris.

This star-crossed law firm had a short life, just four years. The reason seems silly, an upturning of common sense, but here is what happened: On February 28, 1883, J. P. Farmer, a client, turned over a $500 note drawn on Baldwin's Bank of Penn Yan to Ralph T. Wood, one of Morris's partners, in payment for legal services. It was supposed to be payable only to Farmer's company, but he signed it over to the law firm and Wood endorsed it in the name of the law firm. He then took it to the bank, cashed it, and placed the proceeds in the law firm's account. Morris, who was in charge of office accounts, immediately spent the money on new linoleum floor covering and other office expenses. The Penn Yan bank's correspondent bank in Brooklyn rejected the note because Morris's law firm had cashed it and Baldwin's Bank was left holding the bag.

Each partner refused to return the money, about $11,000 in present value. Butler and Morris said Wood had no legal authority to endorse and cash the $500 note and claimed that shielded them from responsibility. But the law said that if the partners knew and acquiesced in spending the money, which the record showed they had, they were just as guilty as Wood, who resigned from the firm on March 3, 1883. Butler stayed on until June 1884, when he left to grow wine grapes. Morris continued as a solo practitioner and for the next seven years refused pleas from the bank to pay back the money. Baldwin's finally went to court in 1889, winning an embarrassing judgment from a jury in Yates County that stood up on appeal in 1892.[7] It was a high price to pay for new linoleum, but Morris seemed too stubborn to care.

Whether the controversy damaged his reputation as a lawyer in Penn Yan or he simply decided he wanted to do something different is unknown. His finances appeared to improve with the probating of his father's will in 1889, and Morris turned his attention to the gas industry. Not natural gas as we know it today, but the dirty, factory-made gas extracted from coal or oil and used for decades by Americans to light their homes and fuel their stoves. Electric lighting was making big inroads in some areas, but the market for gas in New York State was still significant and profitable.

Morris made his first acquisition, his hometown Penn Yan Gas Light Company, in 1892. Further deals were put on hold by the economic panic of 1893, which culminated in a brutal stock market collapse. William

McKinley's victory over William Jennings Bryan in the presidential election of 1896 seemed to spark a rally, so Morris resumed the hunt, buying gas companies in other small New York towns. But the economy slumped again in 1897 and did not fully recover until 1899 and the end of the Spanish-American War.[8] Morris shut down the remainder of his law practice in 1898 to devote all of his time to buying gas companies. He bought and bought, believing the day of the small-town businessman who owned one or two utilities was over. It was a trend of the times.[9] Men who bought the companies built by others and ran them as an empire would rule the business world in the new century. Of that Morris and many others were certain.

He could have accomplished none of this, of course, without access to capital. Although he borrowed from many banks in the Finger Lakes region and on Wall Street, one of his regular and more important funding spigots was Ithaca Trust Company, where his Cornell classmate Mynderse Van Cleef was treasurer and counsel. Eben, Rob, and Charlie Treman sat on the board. Much of his correspondence with Van Cleef has survived, mostly handwritten in Morris's distinctive Gothic, inky style. Van Cleef doesn't seem to have turned him down very often, although the record shows that he and the bank were not complete pushovers. But the motto of Ithaca Trust Company seems mainly to have been: *What are friends for?*

Morris certainly had legitimate business reasons for moving his base of operations to Ithaca. Banks in those days liked to have their big borrowers close by. The rail connections between Ithaca and the rest of the Northeast and Midwest (Morris acquired the Van Wert Gas Light Company in western Ohio in 1899) were better than those in Penn Yan thanks to Ezra Cornell. But there was a personal reason as well. Ithaca was where Eben lived. Morris never failed to visit when he was in town. In Treman's own words, they were "very close."[10] The two had been friends since their days at Cornell in the late 1860s, although Treman was three years older than Morris. Both were members of the Chi Phi fraternity and were now officers of the Chi Phi House Association, a kind of alumni auxiliary that kept them in contact with Cornell students who joined the fraternity. Eben, Rob Treman, Morris, and several other local alumni had organized the house association in 1890.

A photograph of the Chi Phi house, built in the English Tudor style, would be featured in *Cosmopolitan* magazine in March 1903, at a time when at least two students in the house lay prostrate with typhoid.

The relationship between Morris and Eben Treman, which is the back story of the Ithaca disaster, might have been as simple as a strong, adult male friendship. Or perhaps it was more complex and intimate. We are forced to fall back on stereotypes to consider this question, but to ignore it seems detrimental to our understanding of how the epidemic occurred. Of the two, Morris seemed the more likely to have been gay. He was handsome, wealthy, and intelligent, sometimes went out with women in group situations, but never married. Indeed, on his alumni card at Cornell University, he wrote in a bold, defiant hand, "Unmarried," when asked for his marital status. Morris's interests leaned toward the traditionally feminine. He obsessed, for instance, about interior decoration, like the linoleum in his office in Penn Yan. Regarding the new offices for one of his acquisitions, the Seneca Falls & Waterloo Gas Light Company, he wrote to the landlord, who happened to be Mynderse Van Cleef: "Of course, I would like to have a little something to say in regard to the color paper that goes on the room." The matter of the wallpaper preoccupied Morris for nearly two months, and he finally agreed to bear half the cost of replastering the walls so the wallpaper he wanted for the office—which he himself would only visit, not use on a daily basis—would lay smoothly and look its best.[11]

And what of Eben Treman? Despite his two marriages, was he also a closeted gay man or perhaps bisexual? As a young man, he seems to have had a more-than-usually troubled relationship with his father. Although L. L. Treman wanted Eben to become a businessman like himself, Eben was far more interested in music and the arts. In 1865, when Eben was fifteen, his father transferred him from an Episcopal boarding school in Vermont to the Eagleswood Military Academy in Perth Amboy, New Jersey.

Eagleswood was founded in 1861 by two Quaker abolitionists, Marcus and Rebecca Spring. The idea of a Quaker military academy isn't quite as odd as it sounds—Quaker meetings and their members during the Civil War became deeply divided over whether fighting the South to end slavery was a greater good than following the strict precept of their faith to shun participation in war.[12] Rebecca Spring was a fervent supporter of the radical abolitionist John Brown. She ministered to him in prison before his execution for organizing and leading the abortive Harpers Ferry raid of 1859, which was intended to seize arms for a slave uprising. She even arranged to move the remains of two of Brown's executed coconspirators to a cemetery near Eagleswood, where cadets training as officers for the Union Army could presumably venerate them.[13]

Eben Treman cannot have found the school a congenial place. Eagleswood was modeled on West Point and enforced "strict military discipline" on all students, according to a course catalogue.[14] Packing a teenage boy who loves music and the arts off to military school is rarely a sign of parental happiness. While no letters home from Treman about the school have surfaced, the record of another unhappy boy sent to the same school by an overbearing father leaves no doubt about the nature of Eagleswood or the motives of some fathers. Charles Tiffany, the renowned jeweler, considered his son, the future stained-glass artist Louis Comfort Tiffany, "careless, forgetful, and dreamy." He was especially galled by Louis's poor handwriting and spelling, and wanted Eagleswood to whip him into shape so he could eventually take over the family jewelry business.

Louis Tiffany arrived at the school at age fourteen in the fall of 1862, three years prior to Treman. "Eagleswood was an infinite emotional distance from home," wrote Michael J. Burlingham, one of the family biographers. "He [Tiffany] awoke to reveille, slept after taps, and spent the hours between 6:00 a.m. and 8:30 p.m. never far from misery. He suffered all the usual humiliations of the plebe; outranked, outflanked, and out of step, his every move was dictated by bugle blasts and flourishes of the snare drum." Tiffany remained at Eagleswood for three years, graduating in 1865, and still told friends in middle age how much he hated the place.[15]

Treman spent two years at Eagleswood. When the school closed for good at the end of the 1866–67 academic year,[16] he returned to Vermont Episcopal for one more year and then was accepted into the first freshman class at Cornell University. He stayed for only the 1868–69 academic year. The reasons he dropped out are unknown. Eben went to work for his father but stayed active in the Chi Phi fraternity, where he met and befriended both Morris and Frank Thornburg, who was five years his junior. Thornburg spent two years at Cornell, leaving in 1876. He and Treman headed west to his hometown of Clinton, Iowa, on the Mississippi River, where they organized "Thornburg & Treman, lawyers and insurance."[17]

Both men took wives in 1884, and the partnership ended. Eben, who was thirty-four, married Eugenie MacMahan of nearby Lyons, Iowa, daughter of a former riverboat captain turned banker. After a honeymoon of several weeks, the couple settled back in Ithaca. She died in childbirth two years later and was buried with her newborn son in the Treman family plot in Ithaca City Cemetery. Five years later, at age forty-one, Treman married Belle Norwood, adopted daughter of Miles L. Clinton, foreman of the Cornell University machine shop. They had no children, and after Treman died in 1915, Belle Treman departed Ithaca for New York City.

It is unclear when Morris and Treman resumed their friendship. It could have been in 1884, when Treman returned to Ithaca with his first wife, or it could have been as late as 1889. In that year, J. Herbert Ballantine, nephew of the president of the Peter Ballantine & Sons Brewing Company of New Jersey, revived the Chi Phi fraternity's Xi chapter at Cornell University, which had been inactive for ten years. Both men became active as alumni in the revived fraternity and the Chi Phi House Association, a sort of alumni auxiliary.

As his father aged, Eben took over management of the gas and water companies. Whatever energies Treman devoted to business, his heart was in music and theater. He had a fine tenor voice and was choirmaster of St. John's Episcopal Church in Ithaca; president and patron of the Lyceum Theatre, an opera house in Ithaca that drew top talent and traveling theater productions; and president and founder of the famed Ithaca Band. He persuaded Patrick Conway—one of the band leaders immortalized by actor Robert Preston in his spoken introduction to "76 Trombones" in the film *The Music Man*—to come to Ithaca in 1895 to be the leader of his band. Treman's library of music and books about music was said to be immense.

It would not have been unusual at that time for Treman to lead a dual life. The closet was typical for nineteenth-century gay men, says Graham Robb, author of *Strangers: Homosexual Love in the 19th Century*. Marriages of convenience were common. "Nineteenth century homosexuals lived under a cloud, but it seldom rained. Most of them suffered, not from the cruel machinery of justice, but from the creeping sense of shame, the fear of losing friends, family and reputation, the painful incompatibility of religious belief

and sexual desire, the social and mental isolation, and the strain of conceal-
ment. Loveless marriages caused more lasting grief than laws, and still do,"
he wrote.[18]

Whatever the nature of the relationship between Morris and Treman,
there is no doubt that the bond between them was extraordinary and close
and that one of the primary factors driving Morris to acquire the Ithaca Gas
Light Company was so he could move his world to Ithaca.

There were other members of the boys club. Charles H. Blood was the
part-time district attorney of Tompkins County. Son of a well-to-do Ithaca
haberdasher, banker, and New York National Guard general, he became a
director of Ithaca Trust Company after his father's death in 1898. Blood's
best friend was Charles E. Treman—they had been fraternity brothers at Cornell and served together on the board of the Ithaca Conservatory of Music—
and he was nearly as close to Robert. A longtime bachelor, Blood lived with
his mother and owned a club for bachelors called Umphville in a cottage
along Cayuga Lake. Men had to be unmarried to belong, and young Cornell
men were encouraged to visit. Many of the Umphville photographs in an
album in the archives of the History Center of Tompkins County could have
come straight from an edgy fashion shoot today. In 1905 at age thirty-nine,
Blood married a young South Carolina woman who had been working as the
assistant to the warden of Sage College, as the residence for women students
at Cornell was known. He moved her into his mother's house. A year into
the marriage, Louise Blood ran home to South Carolina to her family and
wouldn't come back. Charles was discouraged from visiting. She eventually
did return, however, and the couple continued to live with Blood's mother
until she died in 1912.[19]

Finally there was Jared Treman Newman, a cousin of Rob and Charlie
who was a lawyer and future mayor of Ithaca. He and Blood were real estate
developers. They had their eyes on a tract of land adjoining Cornell University with nice views of Cayuga Lake. The development became known as Cornell Heights, and while it had nice views of water, it didn't have much water
for homebuyers to drink. They hoped to remedy that if they were successful
in acquiring the land.

L. L. Treman's casket was flanked by sprays of flowers sent by community groups he supported, including the Ithaca Band and the Chi Phi fraternity, and by employees of Ithaca Gas Light and Ithaca Water Works. The white-robed choir of St. John's Episcopal Church, which Eben directed on Sundays, sang "Abide With Me." L. L. Treman was one of the parish's more prominent members, serving as a vestryman for forty years. After the Episcopal priest read the service for the dead, the casket was carried out by the pallbearers, among them Treman's old friend George E. Priest, copublisher of the *Ithaca Daily Journal.* They passed through the wisteria to a horse-drawn hearse. Eliza Treman and Eben boarded a carriage.

The procession climbed slowly up the steep mile to Ithaca City Cemetery, led by fifty uniformed members of the St. Augustine Commandery, a Masonic organization to which L. L Treman belonged. Hundreds of people followed on foot. At the graveside, Treman's granddaughter, grandnieces, and grandnephew scattered flowers on evergreen boughs that hid the dirt from the grave. The first quartet of the St. John's choir sang, "Leave We Now Thy Servant Sleeping." Then the mourners, among them Morris, drifted away.[20] He wondered how best to approach the Treman family about selling Ithaca Gas Light Company.

Chapter 3

Conflict of Interest

> *The situation of 1901 was one which turned men's heads. The country seemed to have reached a pinnacle of prosperity from which nothing could dislodge it. The profits of our incorporated enterprises seemed to have no assignable limit. American capital pressed upon every avenue of investment. The most reckless and foolish speculation was apt to achieve success.*
>
> —Alexander Dana Noyes,
> Forty Years of American Finance, 1909[1]

William T. Morris bided his time for nearly a year, but in the summer of 1901, more than a year after L. L. Treman's death, he began serious negotiations with Eben Treman and his extended family about acquiring Ithaca Gas Light Company.

The time was ripe. America had won its brief and boisterous war with Spain in 1898. President William McKinley, Republican and pro-business, sat in the White House. New York financier J. P. Morgan created U.S. Steel early in 1901, causing the Wall Street bulls to run wild and making Andrew Carnegie, who sold his steel company to Morgan, one of the wealthiest men in the world. And thanks to rising gold production around the world, notably in the Alaskan and Canadian Yukon region, the money supply had risen dramatically. Plenty of money was available to finance speculative deals. Even though the most frenzied period of postwar financial speculation was over by the summer of 1901, the underlying causes and general market excitement were still there.

Morris had just concluded his part in a six-investor deal to create the Inter-Ocean Telephone and Telegraph Company, capitalized at $2 million, or more than $51 million in today's money. The company planned to provide long-distance telephone service among more than three dozen cities, mainly in New York but also in Ohio and New Jersey.[2] With that out of the way, Morris was ready to realize his Ithaca dream. He already owned manufactured-gas companies in Penn Yan, Hornellsville, Canisteo, Cortland, Seneca Falls, Waverly, and Newark in New York, as well as in Van Wert in Ohio and Sayre in Pennsylvania. Half had been acquired during the postwar boom. Investors were acquiring the small companies of the nineteenth century and merging and improving them for the new century.[3] Bigger was better. Investors were particularly enamored of energy producers. American manufacturing seemed unstoppable, just as the Internet and the companies that profited from it seemed to promise endless earnings a century later.

For Eben Treman, the decision to begin negotiations came down to family. What may have changed his mind was the final illness and death on July 14, 1901, of his aunt, Elizabeth Lovejoy Treman. She was the mother of Rob and Charlie Treman and the mother-in-law of Mynderse Van Cleef. Her death seems to have fanned fears in Treman about his own mortality. As he testified in 1906, Ithaca Gas Light Company and Ithaca Water Works were "good paying" companies, so there was no pressing need to unload them. But as the only man in his immediate family, there would be no one to look after the investments for his mother and sisters if he were to die suddenly.[4] Needless to say, it was an era of different expectations for women.

Treman invited Morris to his private office for negotiations. The office was at the rear of the Ithaca Gas Light Company headquarters in a four-story brick building on the corner of Green and Cayuga Streets. Once it had been the site of the foundry for the neighboring Treman, King & Company hardware emporium.[5] Eben was not simply negotiating on behalf of his mother, sisters, and himself, but also for the extended Treman family, many of whose members stood to gain or lose financially depending on how the deal turned out. His mother, Eliza A. Treman, and sisters, Jeannie M. Waterman and A. Louisa Treman, owned nearly as much of the gas company stock as he did and a slight majority of the water company stock. His cousin, Kate Bush, also owned some of the gas stock, the remainder of the legacy from her father, Leonard Treman. The children of Elias Treman, namely Rob and Charlie and their sister, Elizabeth Van Cleef, may also have owned stock in Ithaca Water Works. As did Kate Bush, they definitely owned water company bonds. Treman had little room to maneuver. Any deal he cut had to keep his family happy. Morris, his good friend, would get no special favors. If anything, Eben extracted top dollar. Perhaps all that military drill at Eagleswood had left him with some backbone.

Treman wanted twice the face value of the capital stock, or $150,000, for Ithaca Gas Light company, about $3.8 million in current value. There was a condition, however. If Morris wanted to buy the gas company, he would also have to buy Ithaca Water Works. Eben wanted face value, or $100,000, for the water company capital stock, plus assumption by Morris of $250,000 in outstanding bonded indebtedness dating from 1891.[6] That $350,000 is about $8.9 million today, so the present value of the price demanded for the two companies came to more than $12.7 million.

Treman had tried to sell the water system to the city of Ithaca a few weeks before his father died in 1900. This was his response to a fire on January 29, 1900, that destroyed the Delta Chi fraternity house at 315 Huestis St., today called College Avenue, killing one Cornell student and injuring nine others. The house had no fire escape. Some boys jumped from third-floor windows onto a stone sidewalk thirty feet below to escape, suffering terrible injuries. While the speed of the fire and the inability of anyone to find the key to the alarm box for several minutes were important factors, so was the lack of hydrants within hose range of the fire. Ithaca Common Council, in comments to the *Ithaca Daily Journal*, demanded more hydrants and higher water pressure in the hill neighborhoods.

Bad fires were old news in Ithaca. The Kappa Alpha fraternity house had burned on December 30, 1898, and before 1900 was over, fire would destroy the main building of the Cornell Veterinary College. Treman knew it was a problem, but he didn't want to undertake a major project to fix it. He told the council he was willing either to sell Ithaca Water Works outright for $100,000 in cash plus assumption of the $250,000 bond issue or enter into a long-term contract to supply water to the city at less than he was charging now. If the city didn't want to buy the system, his alternate idea was a half-way measure, another big tank to hold water in reserve for firefighting.[7]

Some on Common Council were receptive to Treman's proposal to unload the company, especially after nearly three hundred East Hill residents petitioned council for better fire service.[8] Inevitably, old grievances arose. Ithaca residents paid 40 percent more for their water than did most Americans served by water companies, according to a report published by the council finance committee.[9] The finance committee thought either option was good. "It is supremely important that every community should be able to guarantee to its citizens, at all times, an abundant, safe, wholesome and agreeable supply of water, and at a moderate cost," the committee's report stated.[10] But the full council could not come to a decision, so the matter was tabled and Treman did little or nothing to improve the system.

As Morris left the Ithaca Gas Light offices in the summer of 1901, Eben's demand that he buy the water company must have given him pause. For one thing, he had never run a water company or been responsible for providing safe drinking water. For another, did he really want to be responsible for quickly making the improvements the city demanded? Even some members of the extended Treman family, notably John W. Bush, husband of Kate, thought the price Eben asked was unrealistic.[11] But Morris wanted Ithaca Gas Light so badly that he kept on talking.

Morris, it should be noted, could be a sucker for bad ideas. At the beginning of 1900, he became enamored of Niagara Falls, New York, and a promising new technology, electricity. The city by the falls was a boomtown in a boom era. The Niagara River generated an estimated six million to nine million horsepower as it plunged down a one-mile race course, dropping 336 feet as it cascaded over the falls and continued down to Lake Ontario. Properly harnessed, it was enough to power all the factories in the nation provided a way could be found to move the energy to where it was needed.[12] As it turned out, long-distance transmission of electricity was far in the future, not even fully realized today. In the meantime, investors set about turning all that water power into cheap electricity for regional use, and manufacturers flocked to the region around Niagara Falls. But speculators looking to make a quick buck ran up against a wall: Rights to all that water power were locked up by the existing producers and their licensees.

Hoping to cash in anyway, Morris, Frank A. Dudley, and four other investors acquired Niagara Falls Gas Company and the Power City Illuminating Company and combined them into the Niagara Falls Gas & Electric Light Company.[13] The "electric" in the company's name referred to a dubious plan to use the flow in the city's main sewer line to generate electricity before the sewage dropped, untreated, into the Niagara River below the falls. That was to be the new company's source of electricity to serve local customers. The proposal was almost a parody of the huge hydroelectric operations at the falls, which employed man-made tunnels to divert water out of the river and turn electric turbines before emptying it back into the Niagara downstream from the falls.[14] The company eventually faded into obscurity.

Back in Ithaca, Morris needed to find someone to back the deal now that Treman had agreed to sell. Mynderse Van Cleef was a logical candidate. Van Cleef, who graduated from Cornell in 1874, a year after Morris, had financed a number of his previous deals, including Niagara Falls. Born in Seneca Falls, New York, he moved with his parents to Ithaca in 1869, a year before he started at Cornell. After graduation, he studied law at Columbia University at the same time Morris was reading law at Foster & Thomson on Wall Street. It does not stretch the imagination to suppose they went drinking together a few times in the taverns of lower Manhattan. They were both admitted to the bar in 1876.

Van Cleef was on an up-escalator to the Ithaca establishment. He became a member of the Cornell Board of Trustees in 1881 and married Elizabeth Lovejoy Treman (her mother had the same name) in 1882. In 1891, soon after Ithaca Trust Company was founded by Franklin C. Cornell, Ezra's eldest son, he joined it as treasurer and a member of the board of directors. The bank was closely connected to the Cornell family and the university. Francis Miles Finch, Ithaca Trust's vice president, had offered eloquent courtroom defenses of Ezra Cornell when he was under attack near the end of his life for the complex Wisconsin land deals that had provided operating funds for the young university under the Morrill "Land Grant College" Act. Now Finch was dean of the Cornell Law School. So it was that Van Cleef, married to a Treman at home and to the Cornell family and its university at the office, lived at the heart of the Ithaca establishment.

In a letter to Van Cleef on August 3, 1901, Morris wrote that unnamed financiers, presumably on Wall Street, were willing to provide the money he needed to acquire the gas and water companies but that he "would prefer to deal with home people if they would like to take it up."[15] That may have been true, or it may have been the first indication that Morris was either having trouble persuading disinterested investors that this was a good deal or was hedging his bets. Ithaca Trust Company was anything but disinterested. Besides Van Cleef, members of the board included Eben, Rob, and Charlie Treman. They all would benefit if the companies were sold to Morris at a high price.

Not that conflicts of interest were something new for the Treman family. A report by a federal bank examiner in April 1900 on the other Ithaca bank in which the Tremans had a major stake, Tompkins County National Bank, noted that the third largest outstanding loan on the bank's books, $11,000 (more than $281,000 in current money), was to Ithaca Water Works and that bank president L. L. Treman (who died just before the report was issued) and bank board member Ebenezer M. Treman also ran the water company. Morris might well have believed the Treman family would do whatever it took to make the sale happen. For a time, there was no need to find out. Late that summer, Fisk & Robinson, a leading Wall Street bond house of the period, took a shine to the deal and began due diligence, looking at the numbers to see if they made sense.

~~~~~~~~

In America and especially in New York State, the main event of the summer of 1901 was a world's fair. The Pan-American Exposition in Buffalo ushered Americans into the modernity of the twentieth century. Visitors could marvel at the Tiffany & Company fountain, ride an Otis Elevator to the top of the Electric Tower, see their own bones via an actual X-ray machine set up in the U.S. Patent Office exhibit, and take a midway ride called "Trip to the Moon" in a rocket ship that from its appearance could have been designed by H. G. Wells or Jules Verne.

The fair opened on May 1 and drew more than eight million visitors by the time it closed six months later.[16] From Ithaca and every part of America and Canada, visitors came to this Emerald City of Oz, actually known as the "Rainbow City" for the rainbows that formed over nearby Niagara Falls. Trains from Ithaca were convenient and cheap. Ticket sale statistics seemed to show that more Ithaca residents went to the fair than actually lived in the city. In fact, the fair was so popular that some people went two or three times.[17]

They were eager to see the modern world of wonders in the exhibition halls and especially the dazzling nighttime display of "incandescent brilliance."[18] Electricity from Niagara Falls was king at the Pan-American, and every sort of electrical machinery save the electric chair—which had debuted at Auburn Prison in New York in 1890—was on display. Cornell University student Isabel Dolbier Emerson pasted the official fair booklet, with the Electric Tower on the cover, into her scrapbook.[19]

John W. Bush wrote to Mynderse Van Cleef on June 28, expressing happy wonder that fifty-one thousand people had passed through the turnstiles the day before. Kate Bush was a member of the women's board of the exposition, and she and her husband were as caught up in the excitement of the fair as everyone else.[20] Inspired by what he saw, Bush decided to have their Buffalo home wired for electricity.

The glory of the fair ended on September 6, 1901, when President William McKinley was shot and mortally wounded by a lone gunman, Leon Czolgosz, who claimed to have been inspired by the writings of the anarchist Emma Goldman. McKinley, who was receiving the public in the Temple of Music, was hit by two bullets as the building's pipe organist reached the climax of a work by Bach. It was a fitting beginning to the violent twentieth century. Yet the modern technology of the fair did not save McKinley. Despite the working X-ray machine in the Patent Office exhibit, doctors were afraid to use it to find the bullets in his body. Dr. Matthew Mann, a gynecologist who lived nearby, insisted on operating on the president in makeshift facilities on the exposition grounds rather than remove him to Buffalo General Hospital, which had just opened a new operating amphitheater for its renowned surgeon, Dr. Roswell Park. McKinley died of gangrene eight days later. Modernity held out the promise of much that was good but could not yet overcome the backwardness of American medicine at the beginning of the twentieth century.[21] McKinley might as well have been back with his Army unit during the Civil War.

President Jacob Gould Schurman of Cornell, in his speech on September 27 to two thousand students in the Armory, a large gymnasium-like building on campus, decried the growth of anarchy in America, which he defined as defiance of established law. But he said social and political inequality was one of the chief reasons anarchy was growing. Men of great wealth needed to "wisely disseminate their fortunes for humanitarian purposes," Schurman said. "It is my honest belief that Mr. [Andrew] Carnegie is doing more to repress anarchy than any state or all states combined would be able to do by legislative enactment."[22]

Carnegie, one of the world's wealthiest men, was his new best friend. The steel magnate had been on the Cornell Board of Trustees since 1890, but in 1896 he had rejected a request from Cornell University for a major gift. Much of his wealth was illiquid, Carnegie explained, and in any case Pittsburgh, where he made his fortune, was his top priority.[23] But after he sold his steel company to the new U.S. Steel conglomerate in the spring of 1901, he had more money than he knew what to do with. Carnegie began making large philanthropic grants for libraries and university education.[24]

Perhaps because of this, or perhaps because fighting between American troops and Filipino insurrectionists was raging, Schurman had taken up Carnegie's anti-imperialist cause with a vengeance. It became the topic he talked about the most in his many public lectures outside Ithaca. The war was not going well. An American unit at Balangiga on the island of Samar was ambushed and nearly annihilated at the end of September 1901. U.S. Army General Jake Smith ordered a campaign of terror on the island, demanding it be turned into "a howling wilderness" and deeming civilian males over the age of ten fair game for the Gatling guns. Besides the killings of civilians, villages and rice fields were burned. Many in the United States were outraged and ashamed. Schurman, a leader of the anti-imperialist cause, publicly favored a policy of building up the Philippines economically and socially and quickly granting independence. American generals all but called him a traitor.[25]

~~~~~~~~~

In September, probably around the time of the McKinley assassination, Fisk & Robinson developed cold feet and began finding fault with the Ithaca gas and water deal. Bond houses, especially as prominent as this one, did not handle paper of problematic companies. If they were unfamiliar with a company, they sent experts to do a white-glove inspection. That was when things went south. The papers were supposed to be signed on October 1, but a day before that, Bush received a telegram from Eben Treman telling him the closing had been postponed until November 1.[26] No explanation was given, and Bush expressed bewilderment at the course of events.

Fisk & Robinson had been unable to get a certified public accountant to issue an opinion that the companies were a sound investment. That, in turn, may be related to a discovery that the Tremans had increased the amount of capital stock in Ithaca Water Works to nearly three times the amount allowed by its charter. The amount of bonded indebtedness was more than ten times the limit. No reputable bond house would put its imprimatur on a corporation that engaged in that kind of funny business.

Instead of accepting this as the kiss of death, Morris wrote to Van Cleef on October 2 that "Menken," Wall Street lawyer S. Stanwood Menken, was insisting that Fisk & Robinson intended to go forward with the bond sale "on the opinion of two experts instead of an expert and public accountant, and they will arrange to have the expert come on at once." Menken insisted to Morris that the deal "was in better shape than ever" and that he had every reason to believe it would go forward.[27]

Menken, like Morris, was a member of the Chi Phi fraternity at Cornell.[28] He had graduated from the university in 1890, one year behind Charlie Treman, and had a long and varied career. He was a partner in the Wall Street law firm of Philbin, Beekman, Menken & Griscom, which counted J. P. Morgan among its clients. Menken appears to have been a close friend of Harvey E. Fisk, one of the name principals in the bond house. A Jew who converted to Christianity—his first name was Solomon, but he now went by his middle name—Menken moved in the upper reaches of New York society. He is remembered today as a leading internationalist who publicly urged the United States to enter World War I on the side of Britain and France and as founder of the National Security League. When Fisk & Robinson went belly up in 1910, his law firm became counsel to the receiver appointed by the court.

Morris seems to have remained confident that Fisk & Robinson would salvage the deal and began making plans. He decided that Ithaca Light & Water Company would be the name of the new holding company that would own the two utilities. He even vetted some candidates for the board of directors with Van Cleef. One should be Eben Treman, he said, and state senator Edwin C. Stewart, a dedicated but somewhat naive public servant who represented Ithaca in Albany, would be another. "I would also like to have the opinion of yourself, Rob and Charlie as to what other two [directors] might be desirable," Morris wrote.[29]

Despite what Menken told Morris or what Morris wanted to believe, Fisk & Robinson had given up on the Ithaca Light & Water Company bonds. Bush, in a letter to Van Cleef on October 12, made reference to a broken contract and how he did not "have much faith in the deal going through." In desperation, Morris again approached Van Cleef and asked Ithaca Trust Company to provide the financing. This forced his old friend to confront all the problems in the proposed deal. First and foremost was the valuation Morris wanted for the two companies, which would determine the amount of money he could borrow. Sounding all too modern, Morris argued to Van Cleef that the gas and water mains of Ithaca Gas Light and Ithaca Water Works ought not to be valued simply at the cost of the pipe, but also at the cost to put them under streets today. "If this were done in the present instances, it would easily add $100,000 to the value of the two systems," Morris insisted.

That $100,000 figure wasn't picked out of thin air. It was what Morris needed to close the deal, but Van Cleef and Ithaca Trust Company weren't prepared to loan it to him. Eben Treman was not willing to cut his price. Where would he get the remaining investment capital that he needed? Enter a surprise investor—Cornell University.

When the smoke cleared on November 12, 1901, Morris owned Ithaca Gas Light Company and Ithaca Water Works, and the university had invested $100,000, or more than $2.9 million in present dollars, in Ithaca Light & Water bonds. That amounted to 18 percent of the total deal, although looked at another way, it was 100 percent of the price Treman had asked for Ithaca Water Works.[30] Treman received his asking price for the two companies, which included retirement of the charter-busting $250,000 in bonds issued by Ithaca Water Works in 1891. Ithaca Light & Water Company issued $550,000 in new obligations, with an extra $50,000 tacked on to pay for improvements. They were backed by an equal amount of first mortgage bonds of the water company and gas company.[31] The university's investment in the bonds was the final piece of the financing deal.

What part of Cornell's educational mission was served by investing in the water company? The university had its own water system for campus buildings, drawing water from Fall Creek instead of Six Mile Creek and Buttermilk Creek as Ithaca Water Works did. True, the university invested its endowment funds in many corporations around the country, including other water companies. But this was a deal that had been rejected as unclean by a leading Wall Street bond house. Nor had Mynderse Van Cleef and Ithaca Trust Company been willing to finance the full amount the Tremans were demanding. There were many companies with less risk in which the university could have invested its money.

If there was no valid investment reason to buy the bonds of Ithaca Light & Water Company, we must assume that the Cornell University Board of Trustees, and more to the point, its Executive Committee, did so for other, less savory reasons—namely to help out the Treman family and their good friend, William T. Morris. The chairman of both the Board of Trustees and the Executive Committee in 1902 was Samuel D. Halliday, a local attorney who had been a classmate of Morris's during the 1869–70 academic year at Cornell. Who pushed the investment? The record doesn't provide an answer but gives enough clues to allow conclusions to be drawn.

The investment in the water company took place in late October or early November of 1901, after Morris incorporated Ithaca Light & Water Company on October 24. When we look at the attendance rosters for the Executive Committee during that period, they include the names of several men with an interest in seeing the sale of the gas and water companies to Morris go forward. Among those attending the Executive Committee meeting of October 29 were Mynderse Van Cleef, who chaired the meeting; Franklin C. Cornell, president of Ithaca Trust; Robert H. Treman; and Jared Treman Newman, whose significance will be discussed momentarily.

If there was any local bank with close ties to the university, it was Ithaca Trust Company. Besides the people already mentioned, the bank board included Francis Miles Finch, revered dean of the Cornell Law School; Emmons L. Williams, secretary-treasurer of the Cornell Board of Trustees; and Ebenezer M. Treman. Van Cleef and the two Tremans were Morris's closest friends. All the elements were present for a classic conflict of interest. Is this what happened? Often the most likely explanation is the correct one.

There is an alternate, or perhaps complementary, road map to follow to the university investment, and it involves valuable real estate. On October 23, a day before Morris incorporated Ithaca Light & Water Company, Jared Treman Newman and Charles H. Blood, both core members of the Executive Committee, bought into and took over the Cornell Heights Land Company that had been incorporated in 1897 by Herman Bergholtz, who had built Ithaca's streetcar line, and Edward G. Wyckhoff. Cornell Heights was then a mostly undeveloped tract of land adjacent to the campus, immediately north of the Fall Creek gorge with stunning views of Cayuga Lake. Newman and Blood envisioned a planned, parklike subdivision of thirty acres with curving streets that would appeal to Cornell professors and other upscale professionals.[32]

Cornell Heights was not presently served by Ithaca Water Works and would face the same water pressure problems as East Hill if the current mains were simply extended without any other measures being done to increase the water supply and water pressure. The fact that Blood and Newman were close friends of Morris's and signed their land deal a day before he incorporated Ithaca Light & Water suggests that they may have had a promise from Morris to provide them with all the water their homebuyers would need. An article about the new subdivision in the *Ithaca Daily News* on November 20 made much of the planners' work to ensure good streetcar connections for Cornell Heights residents. It makes no sense that they would have ignored the water issue. It would not have been prudent to move ahead with so large a development unless the water issue had been resolved.[33]

Did Blood and Newman prevail on the rest of the Executive Committee to invest $100,000 to make certain Morris was able to buy Ithaca Water Works? This scenario, at least, offered some legitimate attraction to the university, as its professors would be able to buy nice new houses within walking distance of campus.

In the end, for whatever reason, Cornell University did invest $100,000 in the bonds of Ithaca Light & Water Company. In the late autumn of 1901, Morris's deal went through and the Treman family was very happy. "I am so glad on the Elias Treman family account as it will put them in good shape," wrote John Bush to Van Cleef on November 13, referring to the family of Rob and Charlie Treman and Van Cleef's wife, Elizabeth. "It will also be very acceptable for Kate. Kate has $7,000 of the [1891] water bonds and as I understand they have sold around 110. She may be inclined to sell them."[34] Bush wrote to Van Cleef again on December 2 saying that his wife had received payment for her Ithaca Water Works capital stock, "and I feel so glad for her and for the L. L. Treman family. I have never understood how anyone could pay par for the stock."[35]

Morris had paid too much for the water company and would need to find a way to recoup his investment. Cornell University was now inextricably tied to Morris and Ithaca Water Works, for without its investment the deal would have collapsed. Today such a deal to acquire a public utility would be subjected to careful scrutiny by a state public utility commission, but those did not yet exist and so the public could only hope that bankers and businessmen would rise above their pocketbook interests to make sure the public interest was protected as well. It was a fleeting hope.

Chapter 4

Newsmen

Word of the Morris-Treman deal leaked to the local press. Ithaca in 1901 had two modern, competing daily newspapers. If the *Ithaca Daily Journal* didn't report something, chances were the *Ithaca Daily News* would. Both papers had good, sometimes uncommonly good editors and reporters. The difference was their publishers. No matter how talented a newspaper staff, a newspaper publisher plays a critical role in determining how well the news is reported. Publishers have their own interests, prejudices, and friends. Sometimes that influences the articles they allow or don't allow into their newspapers, for better or for worse. It certainly did in Ithaca.

The upstart *Ithaca Daily News*, founded only in 1895, had been owned for the past two years by Cornell University oratory professor Duncan Campbell Lee, who was also editor-in-chief. An unrepentant Anglophile, Lee had gone on sabbatical to England for the 1901–1902 academic year. Frank E. Gannett, the *Daily News* managing editor and a future giant of American newspaper publishing, was in charge when reporters learned of the deal. He broke the story on October 31, 1901. Today's journalist would judge the story to be a good, workmanlike effort to flesh out a rumor the newspaper believed to be true. The *Daily News* reported that at least one of the purchasers was believed to be from Penn Yan but did not identify Morris. It even had Eben Treman swatting away a pesky reporter with an over-the-shoulder remark that he would issue a statement when he had anything definite to announce. Some things never change.[1]

Journalists stalk the no-man's-land between insiders and outsiders. They hope to explain to their readers what the insiders are doing and try to keep the door cracked open, hoping to see or hear a little of what is going on. If that is impossible, or if the door is slammed shut, they instinctively seek out relevant facts wherever they can find them. They publish what they know, even partial stories, fully expecting that the complete story will be coming soon. This may infuriate the more controlling members of the insider camp but is standard practice and arguably what most newspaper readers expect.

Two days after that first article, the *Daily News* reported, "Local Water and Gas Plants Sold," saying that "despite the denials" by Eben Treman, the sale of the plants took place on October 31. Citing "a special dispatch to the *News* from Penn Yan," the newspaper identified Morris as the buyer and Thomas W. Summers as his general superintendent. The article provides such a detailed account of Morris's plans and background that we suspect Morris or Summers was the unidentified source. President Treman "refused to be interviewed regarding the sale" when a *Daily News* reporter came to see him, the newspaper noted. Several days later, Treman issued a statement denying the companies had been sold, at which point the *Daily News* revealed that Morris indeed *was* its source for the previous story.

The *Ithaca Daily Journal* was the establishment newspaper with long and close ties to the Treman family. Founded in 1816 by Ebenezer Mack, the father-in-law of L. L. Treman, it had changed hands a number of times during the nineteenth century but was still friendly to the Tremans. George E. Priest, one of the *Journal*'s two publishers (Charles M. Benjamin was the other), had even been a pallbearer for L. L. Treman. The *Journal* remained silent on the sale of the gas and water companies until November 12, when it was forced to acknowledge the obvious. The *Journal* heaped scorn on its competition, which it did not deign to name, alleging that "much that has been said [by the *Daily News*] was news to members of the company," meaning it wasn't news until the Tremans said it was news. "No authentic information had been given out by the company until this morning when the deal was consummated, and then only to a reporter of the *Journal*, who was called in to interview E. M. Treman, of this city, and W. T. Morris, of Penn Yan," the *Journal* huffed. It then proceeded to reprise much of what the *Daily News* had already reported, adding a few details of its own.[2]

Crusading newspaper editors are the stuff of legend, but they really did exist. Duke Lee, editor and publisher of the *Ithaca Daily News*, was one of them. If this story were a Western movie, Lee would be the brave small-town editor or sheriff taking on the corrupt businessmen and politicians who were hurting the public. He was intelligent, athletic, dashing, and willing to put himself on the line for his beliefs. He would probably find twenty-first century journalism and its rules puzzling, because he drew few distinctions between journalism and politics. Like many publishers of his day, Lee was openly active in party politics, in his case the Democratic Party. Yet he was no party hack. Lee was dedicated to the truth, and in the end that destroyed him.

Ithaca had a considerable number of journalists for so small a town. Besides the newspapers already mentioned, there was the weekly *Ithaca Democrat*, founded in 1874 and near the end of its life, and the *Cornell Daily Sun*, the student newspaper, founded in 1882 and given over mostly to reports of campus sports and social events. That would change. Cornell students with an itch for real journalism worked as stringers for the big New York City dailies, including the *Times*, *Tribune*, *Sun*, and *Evening World*. Anything of interest that happened in Ithaca quickly made its way via these student stringers or the Associated Press bureau in the *Daily Journal* building to the outside world.

Lee, though, was in a class by himself. Born in 1869 in rural Bovina Center, New York, his father was Rev. Dr. James B. Lee, a minister in the Presbyterian Church, at that time as dour and conservative a denomination as there ever was. Two of his brothers, Rev. J. Beveridge Lee and Rev. John Park Lee, became Presbyterian clergy. At age fifteen, Duke Lee found work as a telegraph operator for the Bankers and Merchants Telegraph Company in New York City.

He wanted an education and gained admission to Delaware Academy, a college-preparatory school near his hometown, graduating as valedictorian in 1887. Next stop was Hamilton College in Clinton, New York, where he excelled as an orator and in Latin and Greek, winning several prizes at a college renowned for its oratory program. On the playing fields, he captained the football team and was named the college's best all-around athlete. Lee graduated from Hamilton as salutatorian of his class in 1891.

Like many college graduates, he wanted to stay near his friends, so he turned down a college teaching job in the West that fall to become vice principal of the Cascadilla School, a college-preparatory academy in Ithaca. Popular with students, Lee drew the attention of faculty at Cornell. When Professor Brainard G. Smith, chairman of the Department of Elocution and Oratory, resigned to accept a similar position back at Hamilton College, he recommended the twenty-four-year-old Lee to replace him as department chairman. President Jacob Gould Schurman and the Executive Committee of the Board of Trustees approved, and Lee was hired for the fall term in 1893.[3]

Lee and Smith had oddly parallel careers and one can only wonder if there was a rivalry between them. Both were Hamilton graduates. Smith was a reporter and editor for fifteen years at the New York Sun, where he worked closely with Charles A. Dana, the Sun's legendary editor. He left in 1887 when Andrew D. White hired him to build up a department of public speaking at Cornell and, abortively, a journalism school. Although his former colleagues at the Sun thought it a good idea, most newspapers across the United States hooted at the "College of Journalism," not believing their craft could be taught in the classroom. Twenty-five students enrolled, but the Cornell Board of Trustees, upset with the laughter, placed such severe restrictions on Smith's journalism program that he ended it. Returning to Hamilton in 1893, he taught oratory for five years. But journalism ran in his veins, and he left Hamilton in 1898 to become editor of the Utica Herald-Dispatch, followed by a six-year stint beginning in 1899 as editor of the Ithaca Daily Journal. That was the same year Lee acquired the Ithaca Daily News.[4]

Duke Lee revived Cornell University's intramural debate clubs and turned the intercollegiate debate team from a persistent loser into a regular winner. It captured four out of five annual contests beginning in 1896. In the classroom, he taught his students the principles of analysis, the nature of evidence, and the writing of briefs and oral delivery, "until today it is safe to say that no college or university in the country surpasses Cornell in thorough and systematic training in the art of debate," Lee wrote in a letter to President Schurman of Cornell. His system of arranging and preparing arguments for a debate was dubbed the "Cornell system of debating" by a writer for another university.[5] The syllabus for his extemporaneous speaking course during the 1897–98 academic year promised to "awaken deeper interest in American institutions through study and research; to give training and practice in logical and forceful arrangement of thought; to develop accuracy, fluency and grace in speaking the English tongue; and to enlarge the vocabulary." One longs for a course like that today.[6]

〜〜〜〜〜〜

But Lee had grown restless in academic life and longed to pursue his ideals out in the world. After Congress declared war on Spain on April 22, 1898, he volunteered for two years of Army service. In all likelihood, he charged into the war with the noble aim of helping to free Cubans from Spanish colonial oppression. President Schurman granted him a leave of absence, and he enlisted as a sergeant in Company M, 203rd Regiment, New York Volunteers, later moving to Company C. The idea of a college professor enlisting in the Army to fight in the war caught the fancy of the *New York Times,* which ran a small story about him.[7]

It was a much different war from what he expected. Lee traveled with the 203rd New York Regiment from Syracuse to Camp Black on Long Island in late July. They drilled and trained, and Lee was promoted to second lieutenant. Fighting in Cuba was over by late summer, but the Puerto Rico campaign was under way and the occupation of the Philippines was just beginning. The 203rd departed on September 11 by train for Camp Meade near Middletown, Pennsylvania, and again by train for Camp Weatherill near Greenville, South Carolina, on November 11. There the regiment stayed until mustered out on March 25, 1899.[8]

Yet despite seeing no action, the regiment waged a losing war against an unseen enemy, typhoid, that killed at least eleven soldiers and possibly as many as eighteen if common misdiagnoses of other diseases such as pneumonia or malaria were, in fact, manifestations of *bacterium typhosa.*[9]

Most of the deaths occurred during the two months in Pennsylvania. Sanitation in all the Army camps was appalling, and Army medical investigators found that volunteer soldiers unaccustomed to Army life were the worst offenders. The latrines, or *sinks,* quickly filled up. To avoid the horrible stench, men defecated anywhere they could find a little privacy. It was a deadly situation, even if the consequences were not understood at the time.

Major Victor C. Vaughan, who served with Major Walter Reed and Major Edward O. Shakespeare on the Surgeon General's Typhoid Commission, wrote: "We were able to show that in 1898 typhoid fever was so widely distributed in this country that in the assembling of a volunteer regiment, about 1,300 men, there would be from one to four men already bearing the infection. These brought the infection into the camp."[10] And this was four years before the concept of typhoid carriers—seemingly healthy people who unknowingly spread the disease through defecation—was even understood, and then only in Germany. Physicians knew only that typhoid lurked everywhere, waiting for the recklessness of man to unleash its fury.

Duke Lee's Company C was especially hard hit, losing four soldiers to typhoid in October while the regiment was in Camp Meade. Since 10 percent of typhoid patients typically died, we can assume that as many as thirty-six other soldiers in Lee's company contracted the disease but survived. Lee was discharged from the Army on October 21, 1898, the same day as one of the Company C deaths and a day after another.[11] Was this because he was ill with typhoid? While that would be a fair assumption, it appears that the conclusion of the Cuba campaign and the freeing of the Cuban people had dampened Lee's appetite for war. He was opposed to the bloody new war in the Philippines against native insurrectionists and refused a posting there.[12] He was also trying to get out early to ease the burden on Cornell University caused by his absence.[13]

Lee returned to Ithaca with a healthy respect for the damage typhoid could do and laughed off the ribbing he took from students in the yearbook about going off to war and never coming under fire.[14] There were many ways to die in war, and bullets were only one. Although he quickly resumed the professorial life, it was not enough for him. He wanted to be a voice in Ithaca, his adopted hometown, and vowed to find a way to do that.

~~~~~~~~~

On November 22, 1898, Andrew Carnegie traveled by train to call on President McKinley at the White House. Carnegie had opposed the war with Spain. He remonstrated with the president not to annex any of Spain's former colonies, especially the Philippines. Carnegie was opposed to America becoming a colonial power in the manner of Britain, France, or Germany.

Writing in the August issue of the *North American Review*, Carnegie said becoming a colonial power would force America to build a navy equal to that of Britain or France and divert dollars from real needs, such as a Central American canal or what, fifty years later, would be called the St. Lawrence Seaway. Nor should America trample on the moral rights of the Philippine people for independence. McKinley did not agree, and a furious Carnegie, who had supported McKinley over William Jennings Bryan for election in 1896, now spoke out publicly against him. Because Carnegie was one of the world's richest men, the press paid attention.[15]

Seeking to dampen opposition to the Philippine annexation, McKinley decided to appoint a fact-finding commission to go to the islands, which were so far away that getting to Manila required a three-week sea voyage from California. Secretary of State John Hay summoned President Schurman of Cornell to a meeting with McKinley in January 1899. Carnegie had become a member of the Cornell Board of Trustees in 1890, two years before Schurman became president, so they knew each other well and were on the same page when it came to the Philippines. Schurman had used his speech to students at the start of the 1898–99 school year to condemn the war. Nevertheless, McKinley asked him to lead a Philippine study commission that would examine every aspect of life in the islands. When Schurman protested that the Philippines should be returned to Spain in exchange for U.S. Navy bases in the islands, McKinley hastened to assure him that he himself had not really wanted to keep the islands but had found no alternative.[16]

Leaving the White House, Schurman sent a telegram to a young Cornell graduate he knew well, Frank E. Gannett, asking him to come along to the Philippines as his personal secretary. Gannett would found a media empire that today includes the national newspaper *USA Today*. But in 1899, he was just a poor, striving young reporter.

Son of a failed innkeeper, Gannett moved with his family from town to town in upstate New York before winning a scholarship to Cornell and enrolling in the fall of 1894. From the start, he wanted to be a journalist. He met and impressed the notoriously distant Schurman, who opened up to him and became a mentor, if also an imperious father figure. Rarely lacking an opinion on matters academic, Schurman sat Gannett down and told him to take more Greek and Latin, more literature, more history, and plenty of science if he wanted to be a journalist. And he should also study political science, economics, law, statistics, and public speaking.[17] Gannett apparently followed that advice. To master the craft of journalism, he wrote for the *Cornell Daily Sun* and then became a reporter for the *Ithaca Daily Journal*. Summers, he worked for the Syracuse *Herald*. After graduating in 1898, Gannett continued reporting for the *Journal*, worked as a stringer for other newspapers, and contemplated a master's degree. But in early January 1899, he set all that aside after receiving the telegram from Schurman asking him to work for the Philippine Commission as his private secretary.

Schurman and Gannett traveled through the Philippines and even made a side trip to the island of Borneo, today divided between Malaysia and Indonesia, to compare British and Dutch colonial rule. Ever the demanding mentor, Schurman instructed Gannett on what to do in just about every waking hour of every day. Schurman returned to America in time for the start of the fall term at Cornell, leaving Gannett in Manila in charge of the commission's office there.

Early in 1900, he cabled Gannett and directed him to return home. Gannett sailed back by way of the Suez Canal and Paris, where he received another cable from Schurman informing him that President McKinley had appointed a Second Philippine Commission. This one was headed by Judge William Howard Taft, who had been appointed governor-general of the Philippines. Taft wanted Gannett to return to Manila in the same job as he had before. Gannett, unsure of what to do, continued on to Ithaca, where Schurman, as always ready with advice, told him that remaining a civil servant was not in his best interests. He should find a job at a newspaper if he hoped to be a journalist. Gannett complied but added the episode to a growing store of resentments against his mentor.[18]

The story Gannett told his biographer was that, after he left the telegraph office in Ithaca, where he had cabled Taft to decline the offer, he started up the hill toward campus. He planned to spend the night in a friend's room.[19] Almost immediately, he ran into Professor Lee on the street. Duke Lee was looking for a managing editor for his newly acquired newspaper. Gannett, whom he knew from his work for the *Ithaca Daily Journal* to be an "enterprising, reliable reporter of news," was Lee's first choice for the job. They talked on the sidewalk, and Lee persuaded him to take the job. "I shall write the editorials," Lee supposedly said. "I have employed a reporter. But I need a city editor to boss the reporter. What about it?" They were not that far apart in age. Lee was thirty and Gannett just twenty-three, but Lee seemed much older, as mature and successful men often do.

He was pleased with Gannett, whose title on the masthead was actually managing editor, almost from the start. The *Daily News* expanded from a four-page newspaper into an eight-page edition that was "newsy," in journalistic parlance. Circulation nearly doubled in the first year of his tenure, from 900 to 1,884, and reached 2,929 by the beginning of 1902, exceeding that of the rival *Ithaca Daily Journal*. "Mr. Gannett has been the largest factor," Lee wrote in a job reference for him in 1903. "He has been the active head of the City Department and has written nearly all the editorials. He has proved himself to be the best newspaper man the city has had. His English is particularly strong and racy [lively]. He can weigh news and determine its value more quickly and with better judgment than any young man I know. He moves among men; is a member of F. and A.M. [the Masons] and B.P.O.E. [the Elks] and is socially popular. He is also absolutely temperate, regular, and reliable."[20]

Duke Lee had one foot in the world of upstart journalism and the other in the Ithaca establishment. And he was handsome. The New York *Tribune* described him as five feet, ten inches tall, weighing about 165 pounds, with dark-brown wavy hair and blue eyes. He married Elizabeth Williams, whose aunt was married to Jared Treman Newman, a member of the boys club surrounding Morris. His father-in-law was George R. Williams, the wealthy president of First National Bank of Ithaca and a member since 1883 of the Cornell University Board of Trustees. The wedding took place on July 8, 1899, in the ornate and Gothic Sage Chapel on the Cornell campus. The couple lived in a house in the heart of campus at 23 East Ave., near the chapel, and he found ways to balance his teaching, newspaper work, and family. Lee did much of his editorial work between five and eight o'clock in the morning before heading back uphill to teach his classes.[21]

He was a Democrat and made no bones about it, just as the publishers of the *Ithaca Daily Journal* were unabashed Republicans. Charles M. Benjamin was the Tompkins County treasurer and George E. Priest chairman of the state Board of Tax Commissioners. Neither job was available to someone who was not popular with the party in power. Nor was it likely Lee could have been president of the William Jennings Bryan Club in Tompkins County if he only stood back and commented editorially. We cringe today at the idea of newspaper publishers directly involved in politics, and rightfully so, but at least in Lee's day they were open in their support of one party or the other. You rarely had to guess whom they supported by analyzing the sort of news they reported or suppressed. And when they did participate in politics, no one batted an eye. If you didn't like their politics, there was often as not a newspaper to buy that supported the party you liked. Unless of course there wasn't.

Lee caused a sensation on September 11, 1900, when he introduced a resolution at the New York State Democratic Convention in Saratoga Springs denouncing the Ice Trust.[22] It was a perfect example of his idealism and public spirit. The Ice Trust had raised prices beyond what poor New Yorkers could pay, and the threat of children dying from spoiled food was real. Charles W. Morse, president of the American Ice Company, achieved monopoly control of the market in New York City beginning in April 1899. These were not the bags of ice cubes we purchase today at gas stations and convenience stores, but rather large blocks of ice cut in the winter from the Hudson River around Manhattan or as far away as Maine. The ice was stored in icehouses and delivered daily by icemen to New York apartments for placement in iceboxes to cool perishable food. Ice was a critical public health commodity. Deny it, or price it beyond the reach of the poor, and doctors could almost chart the food poisoning and infant mortality that would occur as milk warmed and spoiled.[23]

Morse and his Ice Trust were able to maintain their monopoly through a corrupt partnership with Richard Croker's Tammany Hall Democratic organization, which controlled New York City government. City employees helped eliminate Morse's few remaining competitors by revoking their docking privileges on the Hudson or wrecking their ice. Morse finally took advantage of his monopoly in April 1900, when he remorselessly doubled the price of ice, cut deliveries from daily to three times a week, and eliminated the nickel and dime chunks that were more affordable to the poor.

Public outrage erupted, but with no government regulation of the ice industry, little could be done. Then, in June, 1900, a list emerged of stockholders
in the American Ice Company, and the public was shocked to learn that the
mayor of New York was a stockholder, as were several city judges, one of Boss
Croker's top deputies, and the two city dock commissioners who held the
power of life and death over competing ice companies.[24]

Lee waved a piece of paper in his hand and told the state convention
that he had a resolution he would like to have read and referred to committee, not saying what it contained. A messenger brought it to the clerk, who
started to read it and then stopped. He looked nervously at the party chairman, who shook his head. The resolution was never read and never adopted
either, but Lee gave copies to the press and it made front page news. He had
written:

> Resolved: that we especially condemn and denounce that illegal
> corporate combination known as the Ice Trust, which particularly
> oppresses the poor and arbitrarily raises the prices for one of the
> necessities of life, and we demand that the Republican attorney gen-
> eral of this state proceed with diligence for the legal destruction of
> said trust.[25]

Lee's bravery was not so much in criticizing the Ice Trust, which many
had done, but in bearding the beast in its lair, daring to publicly humiliate
Croker and his Tammany organization at their very own state convention.
His bravery contributed to Tammany mayor Robert Van Wyck's defeat for
reelection as mayor of New York in November 1901. Van Wyck lost to former
Columbia University president Seth Low, who ran on the Republican/Citi-
zen Action ticket. Boss Croker resigned as Tammany chairman in the wake
of the defeat.[26]

But mainly Lee crusaded on local Ithaca issues, especially water. He
wanted good clean water to drink and a plentiful supply for fighting fires in
the hill neighborhoods. When Lee went on sabbatical to England, Gannett
carried on the crusade in the publisher's absence.

Chapter 5

The Dam

EMILE M. CHAMOT HAD BEEN CONCERNED ABOUT ITHACA'S water almost since his first days as a student in the chemistry laboratories of Cornell University. He was thirty-three years old, short, quiet, and friendly. In a photo from the period, Chamot sported a thick mustache, a tweed jacket and a pince-nez, looking a bit callow yet still professorial. He did not look like an activist, but a fire to save the city from a health catastrophe burned within him.

Chamot graduated from Cornell in 1891 and stayed to finish his PhD in 1897. Then he went to Europe for a year to polish his education, as many American scholars did in the late nineteenth century. After studies in France and the Netherlands, he returned as an assistant professor on the Cornell chemistry faculty and became a recognized expert in use of the microscope, which he employed for chemical analysis and for studying the "little beasties" in Ithaca's drinking water. That was how the great Dutch microscopist Anton van Leeuwenhoek referred to bacteria after observing them for the first time in the seventeenth century. Like Duncan Campbell Lee, Chamot yearned to make an impact outside academia. In 1899, he proved that most wallpaper sold in America contained dangerous levels of arsenic. In 1902, his examination of organs from an exhumed corpse helped the Syracuse police convict a seventeen-year-old girl of murdering her late husband's brother with strychnine after he spurned her advances.

But his passion was safe drinking water. Chamot followed the testing protocols of the American Public Health Association, drawn up by a committee of leading American and Canadian bacteriologists, including Dr. Veranus A. Moore of Cornell University, between 1894 and 1897 in an effort to bring order to a chaotic science. The protocols covered all aspects of water testing, from turbidity to the biological, and were as specific as requiring that glass stoppers rather than corks be used on sterilized water-sample collection bottles.[1] Chamot mapped the location of private wells in Ithaca, tested well and creek water samples in his laboratory in Morse Hall, and worried that the city was heading toward disaster.[2]

Students in each new freshman class at Cornell became ill with intestinal disturbances from drinking the water during their first months in Ithaca, seemingly no matter which of four sources it came from.[3] If they drank water from a tap or fountain at the university, it came from Fall Creek, which ran through campus. Downtown, or in their boardinghouses, it was either Ithaca Water Works water, coming from Six Mile Creek or Buttermilk Creek, or from a private well. Illnesses were often blamed on "a change of water." This was an old folk belief, heard even today, that water drunk in a different place can make you ill merely by having different mineral content from the water you are used to. In fact, Chamot said, it was polluted water that made freshmen rush to the lavatory with diarrhea or nausea.

The Ithaca Water Works deal both worried and intrigued him. Would William T. Morris do what needed to be done? After years of private well testing, continuing work begun by the Cornell chemistry department in 1880, Chamot was convinced that the wells were an abomination and that the Treman-owned water company provided "far superior" water. Sometimes it was a little better, sometimes a lot. But so far, the city had made no move to condemn the wells and require all residents to be customers of Ithaca Water Works. For one thing, the system did not reach all Ithaca homes, and even hooking up everyone in reach of the present mains might overwhelm the system. Profound improvements were needed, and Chamot had reason to hope they were coming. A company source told the *Ithaca Daily News* on November 16, 1901, that Morris was planning "many elaborate improvements" to provide purer water and more water pressure, especially on East Hill.

Chamot decided it was now or never, so he made plans to address the November 26 meeting of the Ithaca Board of Health. Water was on everyone's mind. The Board of Health, which had been given new powers when the state legislature reformed the state sanitary code that summer, was concerned about a few recent cases of typhoid and whether contaminated residential wells might be to blame. In October, the board ordered an end to the use of outhouses in a major portion of the city by May 1, 1902, which meant those homes that had them would need to connect to the public sewer lines running under their streets. It also asked the Board of Sewer Commissioners to extend sewer lines to more of the city. Yet the city had no sewage treatment plant and ultimately discharged untreated wastes into Cayuga Lake, supposedly "a safe distance" from Ithaca. There was talk of building a second discharge pipe once the rest of the city was connected to the system.[4]

Unlike some in academia, Chamot had little difficulty talking at a level average people could understand. An account in the *Ithaca Daily News* reported that he held the rapt attention of the Board of Heath and a score of citizens for nearly two and a half hours while keeping his lecture mostly free of technical and scientific jargon. That was a stamp of approval from the reporter who wrote the story. Reporters, even well-educated ones, rarely had science degrees then or now. At the end of the night, the board chairman commended Chamot "for the very entertaining evening," even though what he had to say was doubtless unpleasant to hear.

Chamot told the board that all wells in Ithaca less than one hundred feet deep ought to be condemned because nearly all of them were contaminated with sewage from homes not connected to the public system. Those in the East Hill neighborhoods, where many students lived, tended to be the worst. Effluent from toilets and latrines, instead of sinking deep into the ground, tended to flow downhill beneath the surface until it entered and polluted somebody's well, the *Daily News* reported. A home owner would sometimes insist his well was in fine condition, arguing that his family had drunk the water without incident for forty years. That might well be, Chamot said, but only because they gradually became immune to the bacteria. Newly arrived Cornell freshmen did not have that immunity.

When he spoke of bacteria and disease, Chamot was referring to *E. coli* bacteria originating in the intestines of humans and animals. Some strains are harmless, but others can cause nasty intestinal upsets of the type experienced by travelers in Third World countries. Victims without access to antibiotics are typically prostrate for two or three days with intense stomach pain, weakness, and diarrhea. That is not to minimize this sort of ailment in any way, but only rarely does it kill otherwise healthy young adults, as typhoid could and did in 1901. Despite the Board of Health's recent concern, Ithaca had relatively few typhoid cases, just a handful each year, and some of those may well have been misdiagnosed given the varying skills of local physicians.[5] Chamot worried about typhoid being brought to Ithaca from elsewhere. What would happen, he wondered aloud, if an epidemic broke out in a distant farming community along Six Mile Creek, the main source of the drinking water provided by Ithaca Water Works?

Chamot's knowledge of waterborne diseases seemed fairly up to date for an American scientist in 1901. He based what he told the Board of Health on his own observations under the microscope and did not subscribe to the moralistic and fallacious belief that diseases like typhoid sprang to life from the miasma, meaning dirt and filth. We will discuss this fallacy more fully in a future chapter. Yet he was not completely free of erroneous beliefs. Chamot readily acknowledged, for example, that the two creeks were subject to occasional farm pollution. But he did not believe this was a significant threat by the time the water reached Ithaca. That may have been a manifestation of a mistaken belief, common into the twentieth century, that if pollution flows far enough in a river, it will be diluted into insignificance.[6] Or he may have so badly wanted a safe alternative to the foul Ithaca wells that he was willing to overlook problems with the quality of Six Mile Creek and Buttermilk Creek water.

He told the Board of Health that the best thing that could be done to eliminate the risk of something deadly like typhoid coming into the streams from the distant country would be to install "mammoth filters," either an English-style sand filter or the American-style mechanical filter. Filters had been proven to save lives, greatly reducing typhoid and cholera outbreaks in European cities and in Albany, New York. Otherwise, the *Daily News* reported, the city water "is reasonably pure and is good to drink."[7] But Chamot's warning that the water ought to be filtered fell on deaf ears. Fires and having enough water to fight fires were what worried people the most.

The Treman family had considered several plans for building a new dam and reservoir for Ithaca but rejected all of them as too costly.[8] Shortly after Morris took over Ithaca Water Works, a member of the Cornell University Board of Trustees—never identified—asked Professor Gardner S. Williams of the engineering faculty to meet with Morris "with a view to an engagement." Williams had designed and built dams all over the Midwest. He had come to Cornell in 1898 from Detroit, where he was chief engineer for the city water board.[9] There were many engineers who could do this sort of work, but Williams was experimenting with designs and materials he hoped would reduce the cost of a dam without compromising safety.

Williams was in charge of Cornell's hydraulics laboratory.[10] Built next to Triphammer Falls, the laboratory, one of the largest in the world of its day, was for "the study of water's behavior." Cornell University liked to hire teachers for its engineering schools who already had a professional reputation and were familiar with the ways of business. As we shall see, Williams was a bit of a cowboy. He would build dams for anyone who paid his fee and does not seem to have been overly particular about whom he worked for. Indeed, he ended his career in 1930 designing a massive and misconceived dam for Josef Stalin at Magnitogorsk in the Soviet Union as part of the First Five-Year Plan.[11] Williams and Morris signed a contract on November 27, 1901, the day after the Health Board meeting at which Chamot spoke.[12]

"I made an investigation of the water supply of the city of Ithaca," Williams later testified. "It was realized at the time that the works were not in a suitable condition to meet the requirements and I was asked to give the company the benefit of my advice to best produce a supply that would be satisfactory to the citizens of Ithaca."[13]

Many in Ithaca believed that Morris would build a new reservoir atop East Hill. The *Ithaca Daily News* on November 16 speculated it would be built near the Lehigh Valley Railroad's East Ithaca Station, which was then located on Maple Avenue near Cascadilla Creek. But Morris quickly gave up on that idea, if it ever even reached that stage, and thereafter went silent about his plans for nearly two months, causing immense public frustration.

Williams worked two months on the design. He considered nearly every major water source in the region. Taking water from Cayuga Lake was ruled out because it was polluted with Ithaca's sewage at its southern end and would cost too much to pump uphill in any case. Fall Creek, Cascadilla Creek, Enfield Creek, Buttermilk Creek, and artesian wells tapping pressurized pockets of groundwater also failed to pass muster. Williams finally settled on Six Mile Creek. Ithaca Water Works already drew the major part of its water supply from the stream but had done almost nothing to tap its potential.[14] Williams was attracted to a location two miles above Ithaca where Six Mile Creek flowed through a deep gorge only 90 feet wide. Here, he told Morris, was the perfect location for a ninety-foot-high dam that would back up a sixty-acre lake in the valley beyond the gorge. Ithaca would have all the water it needed, more than twenty million gallons per day. Without the dam, there would be no more water than there was now.

The professor was not as sanguine as Chamot about the safety and quality of the water from Six Mile Creek. After storms, tap water was muddy. And as he later testified, the amount of bacteria in the water was "considerably higher than I would think desirable." He had looked at the map of Six Mile Creek's forty-seven-square-mile drainage area and feared for the safety of his family. Williams had no illusions about the sanitary habits of "country people," some of whom had outhouses that emptied directly into the stream. He ordered all the water used in his household to be boiled and advised friends to do the same. So it came as no surprise when he made a strong recommendation to Morris to build a filtration plant for Six Mile Creek before he put up the new dam. He surely told him about the high bacteria count in Six Mile Creek water samples.

But why build the filtration plant before the dam? That had to do with the typically foul sanitary habits of construction workers in the field, so common a problem in 1901 that some engineering and public health books of the day contained warnings to anyone building a reservoir. Amory Prescott Folwell, for example, wrote in his 1900 book, *Water Supply Engineering*, that "care should be taken that the soil is not polluted by the workmen upon the reservoir; to prevent which, [outhouses] should be provided below the dam site and the workmen compelled to use them." William T. Sedgwick wrote in *Principles of Sanitary Science and the Public Health* in 1903 that "serious pollutions . . . may occur in surface [water] supplies from the temporary residence on the watershed of thousands of laborers, some of whom may be walking cases of infectious disease."[15]

So Williams proposed building a sand filter for Ithaca's drinking water.[16] Sand filtration plants had become relentless typhoid fighters in Europe since the first one was built for the London water system in 1829. In Hamburg, Germany, the death rate from typhoid plunged from 34 per 100,000 in 1892, the last year before filtration, to 6 per 100,000 in 1894.[17] Yet filtration was a hard sell in America, where the population used five to six times as much water per capita as Europeans did, and where it was long assumed that new supplies of unpolluted water could always be found, or if not, so what?[18] This indifference to pollution when an easy solution from Europe existed was a source of frustration to American sanitary engineers. "Still, curiously enough, there are some who discuss sand filtration as practiced abroad very much as they do the subject of air navigation and the *mobile perpetuum* [perpetual motion machines]—things very interesting in themselves, but quite impossible of practical results," wrote John W. Hill in his 1898 book, *The Purification of Public Water Supplies*.[19] Old Europe's advanced practices were no more welcome then than they are in the national health-care debate today.

Part of the problem in 1901 was that American courts almost never held water companies liable for deaths caused by water they delivered to customers, so there was no financial incentive to improve. Anyone who did bring a lawsuit faced daunting hurdles, having to prove first, that the water company intended to defraud or deceive the public about the quality of its water; second, that it was guilty of criminal negligence; third, that there was no doubt that the water was the cause of death; and finally, that the victim had not negligently contributed to his or her own demise by drinking the water in the face of public knowledge that it was polluted.[20]

Nevertheless, increasing numbers of American cities, motivated by public health more than profit, embraced water filtration in the late 1890s. Albany's plant, the largest European-style sand filtration plant in America, began processing Hudson River water in the fall of 1899. Typhoid had been rampant in New York's capital city, but deaths dropped dramatically after the filters began removing 99 percent of bacteria in the river water. In Elmira, New York, just thirty-three miles from Ithaca and where Morris had friends, the results were equally dramatic. Some 287 typhoid cases attributed to city water were reported in 1896, the year before filtration began, and just thirty-eight in 1898, the first full year afterward.[21]

Other Americans took notice and wondered why they could not have the same precautions. On January 4, 1901, a U.S. Senate committee held a hearing at the Waldorf-Astoria Hotel in New York City to consider whether the nation's capital should filter drinking water from the Potomac River. All the best experts attended. The main issue quickly became not *whether* to filter, but which filtration system to use. The choices were the "English" slow sand filter, which mimicked the natural filtration of the Earth and had been used successfully in Europe for seventy years, or the "American" mechanical filter, which was somewhat speedier and used coagulant chemicals to remove more dirt particles from water than sand filtration did. Each filter had its proponents and detractors—sand filter proponents, for example, claimed that mechanical filters made water look nice but didn't remove as much bacteria—and arguments could be intense.

In the end there was no way to force a water company or local government to filter water, because no law or regulation required anyone to do so. Too often, filtration was seen as an unnecessary expense. As Allen Hazen, designer of the Albany filtration plant, wrote in 1895:

> The one unfortunate feature is the question of cost. Not that the cost is excessive or beyond the means of American communities; in point of fact, exactly the reverse is the case; but we have been so long accustomed to obtain drinking water without expense other than pumping that any cost tending to improve quality seems excessive.[22]

Morris did not make an immediate decision on the filtration plant. He approved the ninety-foot dam on Six Mile Creek when Williams showed him the final plans early in January 1902, and he must have marveled at how slight it appeared on the drawings, just eight feet wide at the base and jammed between the walls of the gorge. Williams had designed America's first dome dam, so named for its curvature, and was able to make it smaller and more cost-effective because of that design and because he would use reinforced concrete. He was supremely confident that his dam was safe, and Morris gave the go-ahead to begin construction.[23]

The two-month silence on what he intended to do with Ithaca Water Works, though, had the city in an uproar, mainly because people really cared about what the answer might be. Finally, on January 14, 1902, the Ithaca

Business Men's Association approved a resolution calling for the city to "own and operate a first class system of waterworks." The following evening, Ithaca Common Council debated the question, giving every indication that it was amenable to the idea. Probably in response to the growing agitation, Morris released Williams's plans for Ithaca Water Works on January 26—minus the recommendation for the filtration plant—and soon found himself in a full-scale battle to prevent the city of Ithaca from taking over the system by eminent domain.

An interesting part of Williams's report is his outright mendacity about Six Mile Creek and its suitability for use as drinking water. First he diverts attention to Fall Creek, which ran through the Cornell campus and provided the unfiltered drinking water used at the university. He called it "unfit for drinking purposes" and stated that filtration would cost as much as pumping water uphill from Cayuga Lake. Then he gave his stamp of approval to Six Mile Creek, the same water he boiled at home because it was full of bacteria. "As to the quality of the water, Professor Williams raises no question, but says that it will be improved by storage for considerable periods" the *Ithaca Daily Journal* reported.[24] Council was not impressed. A week later, citizens jammed its chambers. Petitions in favor of a public takeover were presented by three local unions, the Masons, the Tinners, and the Journeymen Tailors, along with one signed by some 120 Ithaca women. Council voted to hold a municipal referendum on February 27 on the question, "Shall the city acquire its own water works system both for fire purposes and the use of its inhabitants?"[25]

Morris was not about to have his investment taken away, and over the next three weeks, mounted an aggressive campaign to win a "no" vote in the referendum. Because of either naïveté or foolishness by the Common Council—news stories do not reveal its thinking on this question—the election was limited to property owners, who could vote as many times as the number of properties they owned in the city. And they didn't even have to go and vote themselves—they could send agents to vote for them. It was tailor-made for Ithaca's landlord class, who stood to benefit from Morris's plan to improve fire service. We are so used to the concept today of "one man, one vote" that this voting system seems almost cartoonishly wrong, but in fact not until the 1960s did the U.S. Supreme Court enshrine the concept.

Even as the people of Ithaca agitated for public water, the Treman establishment began to fight back. On February 4, Judge Francis Miles Finch appeared at the Ithaca Common Council finance committee meeting along with Morris, Mynderse Van Cleef, and Williams to denounce the idea of Ithaca running its own water system. Finch, of course, was vice president of Ithaca Trust Company, which had financed Morris's acquisition of Ithaca Water Works, but no one called him out on the conflict of interest.

"Every such step is a drift toward socialism," said the elderly Finch, sounding at times like a twenty-first-century Tea Party member in his comments to the *Ithaca Daily Journal*. "The people are governed too much already, losing their personal freedom, and multiplying tyrants." He predicted a municipal takeover would bring oppressive increases in debt and taxation. "If an effort is made to ruin the company and despoil its bond holders, who are mainly our own tax paying citizens and the University . . . by the destructive competition of a new city works, we must expect the company to fight for its life to the ultimate tribunal of the United States Supreme Court," Finch said. "Why should it not? Any of us would do the same."[26]

If the public needed more reason to vote for public water, it came on February 11 when Professor Chamot released the first results of water testing he had done under contract for the Board of Health. He gathered samples at City Hall and the East Hill School, carefully sealing them in sterilized glass bottles and taking them back to his laboratory. There, he drew out a small amount of each sample, placed each in separate petri dishes, and added agar, a gelatinous material derived from algae that acted as a sort of fertilizer for the bacteria. Then he placed the petri dishes in a warm, damp incubator for forty-eight hours to grow the bacteria in the water. When the "baking" was done, he examined the samples under his microscope and counted the bacteria colonies that had formed. The City Hall sample had 800 colonies per cubic centimeter, Chamot said, and was "of very poor quality." Indeed, that was eight times the level of bacteria allowed in London water after filtration. The bacteria, he said, came from "putrefying organic matter of objectionable quality," meaning human or animal feces.[27] There were wicked things in the water.

Perhaps in response to Chamot's report, but also in response to much public comment on the poor quality of Ithaca water, Judge Finch on February

11 told the *Ithaca Daily Journal* that if Common Council would only stop its efforts to take over the water system, Ithaca Water Works was prepared to build a water filtration plant. Morris certainly authorized him to make that statement. Had Professor Williams finally convinced Morris of the need to incur this extra expense?

In the days leading up to the referendum, Morris employed "opposition talkers" to buttonhole voters on the street and persuade them to vote against public water. An inflammatory pamphlet, "Yes or No?," opposing the takeover was widely distributed. Among its arguments was one asserting that Ithaca Water Works had "invested its capital freely, and did not let its work out to Dago [Italian] contractors, or do its work on a cheap-John plan." Those words would come back to haunt Ithaca Water Works and Morris.

On election day, Morris's people boasted that they had a list with the names of eight hundred people who said they would vote no in the referendum. The water company hired carriages to bring its voters to the poll. Problems developed at the polling place. Some would-be voters discovered that they not only had to be property owners and taxpayers to cast ballots, but that the properties had to be listed in their own names on the assessment rolls. So even if they paid the taxes on an inherited property, they could not vote if the house was still listed in their father's name. The man in charge of the official voter list, assessor J. P. Merrill, was an outspoken opponent of public water. And of course, there was the multiple voting. Some agents for landlords cast ten to thirty-seven votes, and it came to be believed by proponents of public water that this odd electoral system had turned the tide in Morris's favor. The final tally was 718 opposed to public water, 583 in favor.

Morris quickly set up shop in Ithaca. Thomas W. Summers, his manager and superintendent, had been living in Ithaca since December, but now Morris's attorney, George S. Sheppard, rented an office above 123 E. State St. from a Common Council member and a house at 111 W. Green St. from Mary King, who planned to travel abroad with her daughter. Sheppard was a longtime friend of Morris's from Penn Yan who had attended Columbia University Law School for two of the three years Van Cleef was there. Morris took a room in the house with Sheppard and his family. Williams continued work on his design for the ninety-foot dam. Ithaca residents did not yet know how high the dam was going to be.

They had reason to believe, though, that their longtime complaints about the poor quality of the water would finally be addressed. Less than a week after the referendum, the *Ithaca Daily News* published an article—clearly based on an interview with Professor Williams—that discussed Ithaca Water Works's plans for improving its system. "It is also announced that a sand filtration plant will be constructed for the purpose of purifying the water. The plans for the filter have not been completed, but it is said the much needed improvement will cost nearly $100,000," the newspaper reported. Judge Finch's comment that Ithaca Water Works would build a filtration plant if Common Council stopped its harassment seemed to be coming true. Finally Ithaca would have water purified with the same technology that had been keeping London's water clean for more than seventy years.

But it was all a lie, perhaps not that day but quickly enough. Morris soon rejected filtration, and in doing so doomed many in Ithaca to death by typhoid. Anyone inclined to excuse his behavior as innocent ignorance should consider another incident from the winter of 1901–02 that goes to his cavalier attitude toward customers and the kind of businessman he was. Morris could not be trusted to do the right thing if it cost him more money than doing the wrong thing.

Pressed by Ithaca Common Council to do something now about the fire problem, Morris agreed to install additional badly needed hydrants. But instead of purchasing new ones, he paid $5,000 to the city of Canandaigua, New York, for seventy-three used hydrants as well as some old water mains that had to be dug out of the ground. Morris charged Ithaca Water Works $15 each for the hydrants, even though the man doing the repairs was charging him only $4. Similarly, he sold the used water mains to the company for $20 a ton, the price of new. Some of the mains that Ithaca Water Works couldn't use were resold, but for only $11 a ton.[28]

In court testimony in 1905, Williams started to explain Morris's decision not to build the filtration plant but was brought up short by objections. We know not from which side, but it is not hard to imagine. Nor is it difficult to guess why Morris did not want to build a filtration plant. Like the businessmen of Allen Hazen's acquaintance, he clearly saw it as a needless expense, an investment that would bring no return on equity. This was the classic rationale of polluters in any age and is why government laws and regulations to control pollution are necessary.

And even if he had wanted to build the filtration plant for Ithaca, Morris was out of money. He had paid the Treman family too much for the water company, and now had to build a ninety-foot dam that would cost him an estimated $150,000, or about $3.8 million in present value. Something had to give, and the first expense to be discarded was the $100,000 filtration plant.[29]

None of this was known at the time. Williams did not go public with his concerns—his first loyalty was to Morris, his client—but he may have complained privately to some of his students. One of them, Herbert E. Fraleigh, wrote a concluding paragraph to his June 1902 thesis on municipal water supplies that seemed out of step with the rest of the text, almost an editorial comment. "In past years the design and control of the public water supplies has, in very many instances, been left to politicians and business men with no technical training or skill," Fraleigh wrote. "But, with the enormous and complicated systems of the present, the services of a skilled engineer are indispensable." Williams could only wish.[30]

～～～～～～

On May 2, 1902, Morris and Sheppard escorted Laura Hosie Treman, wife of Rob Treman, and Mary Bott Treman, wife of Charlie, to a ceremony honoring the eminent Scottish physicist Sir William Thomson, a.k.a., Lord Kelvin, in the Armory on the Cornell campus. Sheppard found the ceremony "an interesting occasion." President Schurman welcomed the white-bearded scientist to the platform, where several members of the Board of Trustees, including Rob Treman and Mynderse Van Cleef, were seated. Charlie Treman, not to be elected to the board for another month, was elsewhere, probably chaperoning the Ithaca Conservatory of Music orchestra, which performed at the ceremony. He was president of the board of that school.

Lord Kelvin was renowned for his work in electricity and thermodynamics and had been a scientific adviser to the corporation that laid the first transatlantic telegraph cable in 1866. Schurman and members of the Cornell faculty laid on the praise, basking in the glory the eminent scientist had bestowed upon the university and its science programs by agreeing to visit.

The dream of Ezra Cornell and Andrew D. White had been for a university where science was cherished and nurtured as much as the classics, and there was no doubt that dream had been fulfilled. Indeed, without the first-rate scientists on the Cornell faculty, the people of Ithaca would have fared even worse than they did in the coming epidemic.

As he left the building, Lord Kelvin was treated to the rousing Cornell Yell from students lucky enough to get inside to hear him, probably a far more excited response than he would receive that August, when he was among the small group of notables receiving honors on the occasion of the coronation of King Edward VII. They had sacrificed a pleasant spring afternoon for the opportunity to see and hear a hero of world science. Their cry, *Cornell! I yell! yell yell! Cornell!* shook the rafters of the Armory.[31] The students were bright, enthusiastic, and full of life. One of them, junior Elsie Hirsch, even cut out Lord Kelvin's picture from a local newspaper and pasted it into her Cornell scrapbook. They were typical college students of their era—and the unlikeliest of victims.[32]

Chapter 6

Lives of the Students

NEARLY EVERYONE ARRIVED AT CORNELL UNIVERSITY by train in 1902. Students who traveled via New York City could choose between the Lehigh Valley or the Delaware, Lackawanna & Western. Both railroads chugged west through the Pocono Mountains and anthracite coal country of Pennsylvania before turning north to Owego, New York, in the case of the DL&W, or the border town of Sayre, Pennsylvania, a major hub for the Lehigh Valley. At either location, Ithaca-bound students changed to one of the spur lines on which Ezra Cornell had spent the remainder of his Western Union fortune in the early 1870s. The line from Owego passed through the poetic towns of Catatonk, Candor, Willseyville, and Caroline before arriving in Ithaca, inspiring a later Cornell student, the writer E. B. White, to admit, "There is no use minimizing the magic of this particular journey."[1]

Of the 3,300 students who made the journey to Cornell in that last year before the typhoid epidemic, many were sons or daughters of middle- or even working-class parents, the first in their families to attend college. Among these were Floyd L. Carlisle, son of a sewing machine factory mechanic and politician from Watertown, New York.[2] He was junior class president and a member of the debate team. Oliver G. Shumard, the bright, overachieving son of a farmer in Bethany, Missouri, came to Cornell for graduate study in philosophy. He had won a $300 scholarship to Cornell upon graduation with honors from the University of Missouri, where he was senior class president.[3]

The Clark family—Zella Marie and Annie Sophia and their brothers, John Artemas and Judson—were devout Baptists who, like President Jacob Gould Schurman, hailed from Prince Edward Island. Their father was a farmer near Bay View on the island's beautiful north shore, and they lived near and doubtless knew the young schoolteacher Lucy Maud Montgomery of Cavendish, who wrote *Anne of Green Gables* in 1908. The two sisters and John Artemas were allowed to share an apartment in a university-owned building at 603 E. Seneca St.; Judson, who was married and an assistant professor of forestry at Cornell, lived across the street with his wife. Zella was here for premed studies and intended to become a physician and medical missionary.[4]

George A. Wessman had grown up in poverty in New York City after his father died at a young age. He was at Cornell studying mechanical engineering on a four-year Pulitzer Scholarship, awarded by newspaper publisher Joseph Pulitzer to a dozen or so New York City boys each year who did well on a competitive exam. Skeptics, notably U.S. Senator Chauncey Depew (R-NY), the former president of the New York Central Railroad, called Pulitzer a fool, proclaiming that poor boys couldn't be turned into scholars and would end up as paupers on the street. Pulitzer proved him wrong. Wessman was now a senior at Cornell and on track for a good job in a large engineering firm. His mother and siblings had finally been able to move out of the city to suburban Passaic, New Jersey.[5]

Ezra Cornell had this kind of student in mind when he founded the university in 1868. The university awarded a full merit scholarship to a deserving student in each of New York's legislative districts. James Francis McEvoy, son of a widowed mother with five other children, won from Wyoming County in 1901. He was now an active debater at Cornell, well known to Duncan Campbell Lee, the oratory professor and publisher of the *Ithaca Daily News*. George Hill of Gouverneur, New York, also had parents of modest means and had likewise won the Cornell scholarship. Like McEvoy, he was active in debate. Addison P. Lord, raised in an orphanage—the Masonic Home in Utica—was another winner. For students like these, four years in Ithaca was the apex of their dreams.

Not that the sons and daughters of the better-off families of the Gilded Age ignored Cornell. Arthur Garfield Dove, named (in reverse order) for the Republican presidential ticket of 1880, was the son of a prominent builder and brick maker in Geneva, New York. He arrived at Cornell after two years at Hobart College, also in Geneva, mainly because his father wanted him to study law. Instead, Dove took art courses. He drew illustrations for the *Cornellian*, the university yearbook, that bore scant resemblance to the style he developed a few years beyond the university. He traveled to Paris late in the decade, was influenced by the Fauvists, and was transformed. Around 1909, he became a protégé of photographer and art gallery owner Alfred Stieglitz and has good claim to be the first American modernist painter, the first to embrace abstract, nonrepresentational art.[6]

Graham B. Wood arrived at Cornell in the fall of 1902 to study civil engineering, accompanied by his good friend, Charles Worthington Nichols Jr. Both boys grew up in Camden, New Jersey, at a time when that city was still a fine place to live. Wood was the only son of a Philadelphia advertising executive who had done well for himself. The father, Jarvis A. Wood, rose from modest origins. He arrived in Philadelphia from New York at age twenty-two in 1876 to attend the Centennial Exposition and decided to stay. In 1888, Wood was hired by N. W. Ayer & Son, a pioneering advertising agency in downtown Philadelphia, and moved up to be head of the copy department and assistant to F. W. Ayer, the founder's son. Executives and coworkers liked him, calling him "genial, friendly, and gifted with a ready flow of words." They paid tribute to his "tact and fatherly manner." He made partner in 1898—by then Ayer was the largest ad agency in America—and could afford to send Graham to Cornell when he came of age in 1902. It was a point of pride for him. Wood did not consider himself a rich man and scrimped on other expenses to pay the tuition, room, and board bills. He was pleased that his son was keeping his part of the bargain by holding down his living costs and studying hard.[7]

Edna Huestis, whose father owned a shirt and collar factory in Troy, New York, was a party girl with a weakness for chocolate sundaes—invented in Ithaca at the Platt & Colt Pharmacy in 1892. But she was also a talented artist, drew illustrations for the *Cornellian*, and would become a leading American miniature painter.[8]

Andrew White Newberry seemed twice privileged. His father was Spencer B. Newberry, a former Cornell chemistry professor who became a prominent cement manufacturer in Sandusky, Ohio. That was no small matter. Spencer

Newberry helped to break the European stranglehold on the engineering-quality cement market, producing Portland cement as good as that imported from Germany. Young Andrew was also the grandson of Andrew Dickson White, cofounder of Cornell University and its first president. He was now the U.S. ambassador to Germany. His mother, Clara, was White's only daughter, and his uncle, Frederick, had been the ambassador's only son.

Yet it was a profoundly troubled family. Andrew Newberry spent several weeks during the summer of 1901, his last before entering Cornell, with his grandfather in Berlin while his parents went through an ugly, very public divorce. His father had been carrying on an affair with Nellie Francis, his pretty stenographer. In the midst of this, Frederick White shot himself to death in the depths of depression said to have been brought on by chronic health problems he had suffered since nearly dying of typhoid while a student at Columbia Law School in 1883. Transatlantic travel being what it was in 1901, Ambassador White did not attend the funeral and was not able to return to settle his son's affairs until the fall.[9]

Then there were the Vonneguts of Indianapolis, Walter, '04, Anton, '05, and Arthur, '06. Vonnegut Hardware Company was as much an institution in Indianapolis as Treman, King & Company was in Ithaca. Apart from Anton, who was elected junior class president in the fall of 1903, we know very little about them. But their grandnephew, Kurt Vonnegut Jr., who came from the architecture side of the family, followed them to Cornell in 1940 before joining the Army in 1943. In 1945, as a young prisoner-of-war in Germany, he set out from the ruins of fire-bombed Dresden on a road that led to literary immortality.[10]

Perhaps the most notorious of the upper-class students of that era were Richard Croker Jr. and his brother Herbert, sons of the fabulously wealthy Tammany Hall political boss Richard Croker Sr. The Croker brothers were legendary; one oft-repeated story was that they brought a stable of horses, and Richard Jr., his Westminster champion bulldogs, to Ithaca to keep themselves amused during their college days. One of the dogs, Rodney Stone, was valued at $5,000 and the other at $4,000, more than ten times the average annual salary of a workingman at the time. The brothers quit Cornell in the fall of 1901, supposedly weary of being hounded by the press and pestered by country folk who wanted to see the dogs. In truth, their father suffered a mortal blow in 1901 when the incumbent Tammany mayor of New York, Robert A. Van Wyck, lost to the reform candidate Seth Low, former president of Columbia University. Professor Duncan Campbell Lee's denunciation of the Ice Trust at the 1900 Democratic State Convention in Saratoga Springs helped bring down the Tammany machine.

The Croker boys were on a course to somewhere else. In February 1903, at a time when his former Cornell classmates were dying of typhoid, Richard suffered the humiliation of seeing Rodney Stone lose first place in the bulldog category at Westminster to Chibiabos, a bulldog owned by Harry Billings. Four years later, Herbert was found dead on a train, victim of an opium and alcohol overdose. Richard spent much of the rest of his life battling his remaining siblings over their father's estate after he died in exile in Ireland, the land of his birth, in 1922.[11]

〜〜〜〜〜

No matter if you were a student or townie in Ithaca, Cornell University was like a shining city on the hill, looking out over the world. It was literally true. With few exceptions, no matter where you lived in Ithaca, you looked upward to Cornell and climbed up Buffalo or other steep streets, or one of the various footpaths, to get to classes if you could not afford the streetcar. Young men and women arriving for their freshman year in September were met at the station by students in white felt hats bearing a red "S," meaning they worked for the Student Agencies. The new arrivals were bundled into carriages and driven around to the approximately twenty-five student rooming houses on East Hill. Cornell had but two dormitories in 1902, housing about 235 women students of Sage College, which despite its name was a dormitory for women students at Cornell, not a separate, degree-granting institution like the position Radcliffe once occupied in the orbit of Harvard. Not all the women students could be accommodated in Sage. The remaining 165 or so women and all of the men lived and ate off campus in rooming houses or one of twenty-four fraternities that had their own houses. Hendrik Van Loon of Rotterdam, the Netherlands, arrived in Ithaca on the night train in the summer of 1902. He recalled being driven by carriage up to the Cornell campus, where he marveled at the starry sky and students burning the midnight oil in the brightly lit library under the clock tower.[12]

Most students lived on East Hill, although a few found rooms in the first two blocks of the "Flats," as the non-hilly part of Ithaca bordering Cayuga Lake, including the downtown, was known. The housing situation would have warmed the heart of a free marketeer. Morris Bishop, in his history of Cornell University, recalled how landladies boasted of the particular comforts of their boardinghouses, such as bathrooms on every floor or steam radiators, when he made the carriage tour that day he first arrived in Ithaca. The university made no attempt to regulate or certify boardinghouses or the food or water they served. It was all up to the student, who had little but first impressions on which to base a decision.

Without the imposed equality of the dormitory and dining hall, the gap between rich and poor students at Cornell was evident. A survey taken during the 1896–97 school year, and cited by Bishop, found that 16.8 percent of male students paid a dollar or less per week for their rooms, the author commenting that these "were surely very wretched, cold and bare." At the other end of the scale were the sumptuous fraternities for upper-class students, which resembled clubs for wealthy men in New York and other large cities. Chi Psi's quarters in the mansion built for Jennie McGraw Fiske were the best, at least until the Alpha Delta Phi lodge opened in 1903. Poor students got by on a dollar or less per week for food, while the upper crust ate well at $4.50 per week, according to the 1896–97 survey. Those same poor students might be their waiters. President Jacob Gould Schurman longed for more democratic treatment of all students and pushed for building dormitories—only about a third of male students joined fraternities—but the Board of Trustees would not agree.[13]

Cornell University, despite its location atop East Hill, could not help but have deeply entwined relationships with the city of Ithaca. The university was a major part of the Ithaca economy, employing local residents as both professors and staff and purchasing goods and services. Students acquired room and board from local landlords and bought much of their clothing in downtown Ithaca. Berry wrote that "it took a score of merchant tailors to provide the distinctive garments of Cornell at the turn of the century." Bishop wrote that students tended to be well-dressed in class, with males in tailored jackets, stand-up collars, and cravats, and women in the wide hats of the day and gloves.[14]

Decisions made at Cornell could seriously impact downtown businesses. In the fall of 1901, the Department of Military Science and Tactics changed the uniform color of the Cornell cadet corps—military drill was then a part of the curriculum for men—but only informed one of the half-dozen merchants who had sold uniforms to students for the past twenty years. The rest were stuck with old-style uniforms they could not sell and appealed to President Schurman to have the color change delayed for two years. Major William P. Van Ness, in his reply to Schurman, accused the merchants of providing poor-quality, ill-fitting uniforms that damaged corps morale, and argued that mail-order firms in Philadelphia and elsewhere had offered to provide quality, good-fitting uniforms if local merchants could not.[15]

Conflicts between the town and the university did arise. Boys from Ithaca playing baseball on the campus green on Saturday mornings greatly annoyed some of the professors. On May 3, 1902, a Saturday, Burt G. Wilder, professor of neurology, vertebrate zoology, and physiology, dashed off an angry letter to Emmons L. Williams, secretary-treasurer of the Board of Trustees Executive Committee, demanding that the university take action to stop the ballgames. He complained that games were played every Saturday and that one was going on even as he wrote. "I consider that my class, myself, and all others who are trying to perform their appropriate work in what is supposed to be an institution of learning are subjected to an outrage, and I earnestly recall your attention to it."[16]

But on the whole, the two worlds coexisted peacefully. Students ate and drank in downtown bars and restaurants, especially Theodor Zinck's Hotel Brunswick. Moviegoing was not part of student recreation, but that was about to change. The new "Edison moving pictures" were demonstrated at Library Hall on campus in December 1901 "for a large and well-pleased audience." For group recreation, especially at the fraternity level, students might rent a tally-ho—a large, horse-drawn coach—at Cornell Livery on Tioga Street and take twenty friends on an outing to Rogue's Harbor or Dryden. In winter, students rode toboggans or skated on Beebe Lake on campus or on the Cayuga Lake inlet. If the lake itself froze over, wrote Emily Barringer, ice boats would appear along with sharp-shoed horses pulling sleighs. Winter could be a magical time.[17]

Women students had been present at Cornell since 1874, six years after the first freshman class entered. Sage College was endowed by Henry W. Sage, Barringer's great uncle, who believed Cornell should offer equal opportunity to women students. The cornerstone for the ornate, Second Empire–style building was laid on May 15, 1873. In the 1892–93 academic year, Cornell had 225 women students. Now, in 1902, the number had reached 400, still only one-eighth of the student body but more than enough to be noticed, not always favorably. The New York *Herald* reported in 1894 that Cornell women students were ostracized by fraternity men, who were put off by their high intelligence and earnest approach to their studies. Barringer both acknowledged and dismissed the problem, writing, "While the men students affected to frown, somewhat, upon the coeds, nevertheless we women managed to have a more than average worthwhile existence." She thrilled to the memory of the men's glee club serenading the women of Sage College one moonlit winter night, and of her arms filled with American Beauty roses at the Junior Prom in February, the social event of the winter.[18]

Sage College women loved basketball and tennis, especially the former. Three interclass games were played that year in the Armory. Male students were banned from the bleachers for propriety's sake, but male faculty members were allowed. Women were permitted to invite men to their dances in the Sage gymnasium, provided that the warden, Margaret Harvey, or her assistant were present. The Sage College Dramatic Club put on an outdoor performance of Alfred Tennyson's *The Foresters*, based on the Robin Hood and Maid Marian story and with music by Arthur Sullivan. It was first produced in New York in 1892 and remained popular in regional theater. Harvey wrote in her section of the 1902 annual report that the performance "delighted a large audience by its naturalness, its beauty, and its artistic fidelity."

Even in 1902, women students worried about crime. That year, professor of Greek George P. Bristol wrote to Schurman "to protest most seriously the dark condition of the campus walks . . . I am not speaking on my own behalf but for the women, some of whom have told me that they feel very timid about going around the campus evenings on account of the darkness." The electric arc street lamps that lined the campus roads were often turned off, Bristol said.[19]

Cornell's male students, at least in the freshman and sophomore classes, were caught up in serious rivalry and high jinks in the winter of 1902. Members of the sophomore class kidnapped William P. Allen, a future federal prosecutor who was to be the toastmaster at the freshman banquet. They held him for several days before he was freed by seven freshmen who forced their way into the house where he was being held, overpowered his guards, and spirited him to freedom at the Chi Phi fraternity house. President Schurman issued a stern warning to stop the nonsense. "What you look upon as a huge joke is in reality doing great harm to the university every hour that it proceeds. The disorders must cease at once."[20] It was probably a speech every college president delivered at some point.

Schurman had to step in again on March 1 when the freshman class finally held its banquet at the Lyceum Theatre in downtown Ithaca. Sophomores kidnapped freshmen and painted their faces half black and half red, with the number "'04" written on their foreheads. Some were dressed in women's clothing. Sophomores threw rocks at the caterer attempting to bring the food through the back door of the theater until they were driven away with a water hose. After three sophomores were arrested, Schurman called a "council of war" and ordered the attacks to cease, and they did. The banquet was held in peace, and some 260 freshmen attended.[21]

Famous people came to Ithaca. Students and town residents alike filled the Lyceum Theatre on the evening of March 6, 1902, to hear a long speech by William Jennings Bryan, who had been the Democratic Party's presidential candidate in 1896 and 1900, losing both elections to William McKinley. He denounced tax evasion by rich Americans and corporations that forced the poor and working classes to pay more, sounded a warning about "the danger caused by the combination of great financial interests unrestrained by law," and infused all of it with his own devout brand of Biblical morality. The next morning, Bryan had lunch with a group that included Manton M. Wyvell, a student who had worked on his campaign in 1900 and who would work for him again as private secretary when Bryan became President Woodrow Wilson's first secretary of state in 1913; Frank E. Gannett, managing editor of the *Ithaca Daily News*, who was running the paper that spring in the absence of Duncan Campbell Lee; and Charles E. Treman and others. The next day, Gannett wrote an editorial attacking the *Ithaca Daily Journal* in angry terms over its coverage of Bryan's visit. The *Daily Journal* was Ithaca's Republican newspaper.[22]

Winter and spring sports for male students were as popular at Cornell as anywhere else. Basketball was new, having just been recognized as an intercollegiate sport by the Athletic Council. Baseball had been played almost since the university's founding in 1868. The track team had triumphed at the Inter-Collegiate Games held in conjunction with the Pan-American Exposition in 1901. But more popular than any of these (excepting football, a fall sport) was the sport of crew. The rowers had a most formidable coach, Charles E. Courtney.

Courtney was the type of coach who today we would call old-school. Despotic, a disciplinarian, he tolerated no dissent from any of the rowers, but delivered a winning program. In June 1897, he kicked five students off the team before the all-important Poughkeepsie Regatta for violating his ban on eating strawberry shortcake. He replaced them with benchwarmers and still emerged victorious. In 1901, one of his crews achieved a record time in the four-mile Hudson River course at Poughkeepsie: 18 minutes, 53.2 seconds, which stood until 1928. Now, on June 21, 1902, Cornell would defend its title against crews from Wisconsin, Columbia, Syracuse, the University of Pennsylvania, and Georgetown.[23]

The Poughkeepsie Regatta was hugely popular, drawing a large number of spectators from the closer schools and surrounding region. Some stood at the river's edge while an estimated three thousand others packed an excursion train—adorned with the flags of the six schools—that moved along the east side of the Hudson. Others still were in a small flotilla of steam yachts anchored offshore to watch the rowers as they rhythmically powered their shells toward the finish line. Cornell spectators on the shoreline let loose with the Cornell Yell just as students on campus had done for Lord Kelvin. They stayed despite the weather. Rain clouds hung over the Hudson Valley for much of the day, and for a time that morning, rain pelted the race course. Umbrellas popped up, and both the "young women in their light summer gowns" and young male collegians put on their rain gear, the *New York Times* reported. When Cornell's boat crossed the finish line to win each of the three events, "day fireworks" erupted from the Poughkeepsie Bridge and cannons fired from yachts.[24]

Back in Ithaca, the scene was no less frenzied. By 3 p.m., a large crowd gathered around the bulletin board outside the telegraph office where race results wired throughout the day from Poughkeepsie were posted. Even as races were in progress, word sped over the wire to Ithaca reporting who was in the lead. Young men with megaphones shouted the news to the assembled fans, who responded with loud cheers. The *New York Times* reported:

> Every heart beat warmly for "Old Man" Courtney. He and his crews were cheered until all throats were hoarse. Cornell flags and red and white bunting decorations of all kinds were in evidence on all residences, and parading and noise-making were kept up until nearly midnight.[25]

This was the student life at Cornell University in the last happy year before the great epidemic. To many, whether students or not, life in Ithaca was something just this side of paradise. As Frank E. Gannett wrote in an editorial, "An Ideal City," in the *Daily News* one day that spring, Ithaca was nearly free of both serious crime and "the pestiferous tramp," meaning a stranger bearing a contagious disease. But Gannett could not contain his enthusiasm for his adopted city, and wrote on:

> If a person is looking for an ideal place to reside where he can enjoy all the beauties of nature, breathe the atmosphere of intellectual refinement, have nearly all the pleasures that can be bought in the largest cities and at the same time be freed from the disagreeable sights of the poor and suffering such is everywhere in evidence in large centers of population—if a person cares for all of this he should come to Ithaca.[26]

Perhaps Gannett should have headlined his editorial, "Tempting Fate."

Chapter 7

The Valley of Death

LOOKING BACK AT THE TRAGEDY MORE THAN A CENTURY LATER, we want to shout to the people of Ithaca and the students of Cornell, you are in grave danger! But all we can do in the twenty-first century is watch the tragedy play out.

On August 25, 1902, with construction of the dam and reservoir on Six Mile Creek about to commence, William T. Morris and Mayor William R. Gunderman of Ithaca signed a contract requiring Ithaca Water Works to provide more fire hydrants, meet very specific targets for increased water pressure for firefighting, and cut the high water rates that Ithaca residents were paying. The city was quite satisfied with the deal.

But there was more. Ithaca Water Works in the contract "covenants and agrees that the water supplied shall be clear, pure and wholesome [and] shall be at all times free from disease producing organisms." Given that Morris had rejected Gardner Williams's proposal to build a water filtration plant for the city, and given that Williams believed the Six Mile Creek water to be filthy and full of bacteria, the mendacity of Morris in signing that contract was breathtaking. He simply didn't care. The purity clause, no doubt insisted upon by the city of Ithaca, could be neutralized with the lie that Six Mile Creek was clean now and would be in the future. Did he never think it would come back to haunt him?[1]

Six weeks after Morris signed the contract, Williams told the *Ithaca Daily News* that Six Mile Creek "is unquestionably pure." Morris even approached his friends on the Cornell Board of Trustees in June about switching the campus water supply from Fall Creek to Ithaca Water Works once the reservoir on Six Mile Creek and a new pumping station were completed. He was hoping the board was ready to make the switch. The more one thinks about the willingness of Morris and Williams to tell these blatant lies, the more criminal what happened becomes.[2]

In early September, Williams collected bids from six construction companies that wanted to build the dam. The low bidder was Tucker & Vinton of New York City at $34,224, or $969,000 in current dollars. It edged out a well-known and established Ithaca firm, Driscoll Brothers & Company, which bid $35,360.[3] Thomas M. Vinton was the latest member of Chi Phi to be pulled into Morris's world, although he joined at the Massachusetts Institute of Technology rather than Cornell. He probably knew Morris through Chi Phi events at the national level.

Low bids, even from fraternity brothers, can have consequences. Tucker & Vinton quickly ran into problems hiring local workmen to build the dam for the low wages the bid and contract dictated. The company offered only $1.50 for a ten-hour day ($390 a year assuming full-time employment), with wages docked for downtime during rainstorms. That might have worked during economic hard times, but it failed miserably during a boom when construction work was available all over the region. The City of Ithaca, for example, paid $1.50 for an *eight-hour* day, or 25 percent more per hour.[4]

So Tucker & Vinton made the fateful decision to hire immigrant labor to build the dam. Perhaps that was the plan all along, despite the statement made by a supporter of Morris's during the referendum campaign that the water company did not hire "Dago contractors, or do its work on a cheap-John plan."[5] The order went out for sixty "sons of Caesar," as the *Ithaca Daily News* put it. There has always been some question about the real ethnicity of the dam workers, with the news coverage referring to them as either "Italians" or "Hungarians." "Italians" were generally Italians, but sometimes Greeks, and "Hungarian" was a catchall term for immigrants from Eastern Europe and the Austro-Hungarian Empire, which then included all of what became the separate countries of Austria, Hungary, Czechoslovakia, and Yugoslavia after World War I. The immigrants working on the Six Mile Creek dam were most frequently referred to as "Italians," so it seems more likely they were part of the vast influx of poor Italians who came to the United States in the late nineteenth century.

From 1880 to 1924 "there was a virtual hemorrhaging of people from Italy to America," Jerre Mangione and Ben Morreale wrote in *La Storia: Five Centuries of the Italian American Experience.* Indeed, between 1900 and 1910, more than two million Italians, many from backward and impoverished southern Italy, entered America. They were too late for much of the free land given to immigrants of other nationalities in the nineteenth century, so they tended to stay in or near the cities where they came ashore. Cheap, unskilled labor was in great demand in urban factories and on big infrastructure projects. More than three-quarters of Italian immigrants ended up in the Northeast industrial states like New York. They built the Brooklyn Bridge and burrowed the Lexington Avenue subway tunnel in New York City. Many traveled back and forth between America and their villages in Italy, especially during the winter here, when construction work was suspended. Immigration officers in America called them "birds of passage."[6]

Ithaca was no stranger to xenophobia. Much of New York State in April 1900 had been subjected to hysterical newspaper headlines during a strike by seven hundred Italian laborers at the New Croton Dam construction site four miles north of Sing Sing (now Ossining), New York. The strikers were universally identified as "Italians," although almost none of their names made it into the articles. They went on strike after the contractor refused to pay the local prevailing wage for public projects required by a new state law. Governor Theodore Roosevelt, soon to become President William McKinley's running mate in the 1900 election, made matters worse by sending National Guard troops to break up the strike. One soldier was killed by gunfire. The Italian strikers were widely portrayed in the press as sinister and foreign, and it was little surprise that the Ithaca public was suspicious of them when they came to work on the Six Mile Creek dam.[7]

~~~~~~~

But Ithaca's citizens were far more scared of the dam itself. Until a story appeared in the *Ithaca Daily Journal* on September 11, 1902, they had no idea it would be ninety feet high and, thanks to Williams's radical design, a bare wisp of a thing. The dam would be just eight feet thick at the base, a few inches less in the middle, and two feet thick at the top, and it would hold back a mile-long reservoir with enough water to wipe out Ithaca if it all came raging down the valley. Williams planned to use brilliant engineering and reinforced concrete—then a relatively new material that was a Tucker & Vinton specialty—to safely reduce the bulk of the dam, but the public was having none of it. Their imaginations went wild. All they could think of was the terrible Johnstown Flood of 1889. Thirteen years was not long enough to forget.

The Johnstown disaster in Cambria County, Pennsylvania, killed 2,209 people, including ninety-nine entire families, after an earthen dam burst and a thirty-foot wall of water swept down the narrow Conemaugh Valley to Johnstown. The poorly maintained dam held back a private fishing lake owned by the South Fork Fishing and Hunting Club, whose members were wealthy Pittsburgh industrialists, including Andrew Carnegie and Henry Clay Frick. A screen placed in the dam's outflow pipe to prevent escape of game fish had allowed dangerous accumulations of sediment behind the dam, and the spillway, or waste weir, was too small, the result of lowering the dam's height by several feet to allow the road across its top to accommodate the larger and more luxurious carriages of its members. Six to eight inches of rain fell on May 30 and 31, 1889, and the dam could not hold back the rise in the lake. Late in the morning of May 31, water began to spill over the top, which should never have happened. Just before 3 p.m. that afternoon, a huge piece—four hundred feet long and forty feet deep—broke away, and the catastrophe began. The Johnstown Flood was arguably the biggest news event in America between the Lincoln assassination and the sinking of the *Titanic,* and it left many Americans skeptical about dams and the people who built them.

So it is not hard to understand why people were scared of the proposed dam on Six Mile Creek. Ithaca, somewhat larger than Johnstown, was barely two miles below the dam site, far less than the fourteen miles separating Johnstown from its doom. Johnstown's dam was shorter, at seventy feet, but much thicker: 265 feet at the base, eighteen feet on top. If such a large dam could give way, what possible assurance could Professor Williams offer that his design was safe? Had they known the truth, that Williams came up with his radical design because Morris and Ithaca Water Works couldn't afford a more conventional dam, which he confessed to an obscure professional journal in 1904, they might have rioted.[8]

Williams believed that the narrow gorge where he intended to build the dam was nearly ideal for his design, but he could do nothing to assuage public fears. "Many citizens are opposed to the construction of the dam under any circumstances," the *Ithaca Daily News* reported on September 29. "They regard it as a perpetual menace to the lives and the property in the lower sections of the city." An unidentified Cornell professor told the newspaper that Williams's design worked on paper but that he would hesitate to trust it. One member of Ithaca Common Council began agitating to have the design examined by an independent third party. Morris told the *Ithaca Daily Journal* that he had no problem with that proposal provided "a competent engineer" conducted it.[9]

In the middle of October, with work on the dam already begun, downtown Ithaca businessmen petitioned Common Council to appoint that engineer. They worried that the city was insecure "on account of the great height, length, and comparative thinness of the dam . . . and realizing the vast volume of water that will accumulate and the horrible deluge and the loss of life that must occur in this city by the breaking of that dam." A letter to the *Daily News* questioned whether any sane person would "trust to the feeble device of man to avert a calamity which is too horrible to consider."[10] Some people likened Ithaca to St. Pierre, Martinique, which had been wiped out the previous spring by the eruption of Mount Pelée. More than twenty-eight thousand people died. They wondered why the additional water the reservoir would provide was even needed, given the many streams in the region and the vast amount of water in Cayuga Lake.[11]

The arguments in Ithaca foretold, at least in style, the debate over the construction of nuclear power plants in the 1970s, especially the Three Mile Island nuclear plant in Pennsylvania. General Public Utilities Corporation, the ultimate owner of that nuclear plant, was the direct corporate descendant of Ithaca Water Works and the rest of William T. Morris's utility empire. In both eras, in both debates, citizens could not find a way out of the thicket of their fears, and scientists could not admit there was any risk worthy of serious discussion.

In the case of the dam, matters came to a head on the evening of November 6, 1902. Professor Williams appeared at a meeting of Ithaca Common Council and answered questions about the dam for more than two hours.

"Throughout he strenuously insisted that the dam will be perfectly safe, and that it will never give way," the *Ithaca Daily Journal* reported. Williams scoffed at the idea that another Johnstown disaster would result even if the ninety-foot dam broke. He said that at most, the wave of water would be no more than a foot high by the time it reached downtown Ithaca, and damage would be minimal. Few believed him, just as seventy years later GPU's nuclear engineers changed few minds among their critics when they insisted that a nuclear core meltdown was impossible at Three Mile Island.

The events of 1979 proved the nuclear brotherhood wrong, but Williams was quite correct. His design for the dam, while radical and scary to the citizens of Ithaca, was brilliant. The threat to Ithaca came not from the dam itself but from the workers imported to build it, and the typhoid they carried.

<hr />

Although surveying for the dam began within days of the referendum, actual construction did not begin until late September. During the summer of 1902, Ithaca Water Works built a 275-foot tramway for lowering pipes and other supplies to the bottom of the gorge from the Delaware, Lackawanna & Western switchback. Hills were unavoidable obstacles in Ithaca, whether in taking the railroad down to where the city was or in getting supplies to the gorge where the dam would be built. Once the general contract for the work had been awarded to Tucker & Vinton and approximately sixty Italian workers along with a number of striking Pennsylvania anthracite coal miners had been hired, work began to clear trees and brush from what would become the bottom of the mile-long reservoir that would form behind the dam. Once the ground cover was removed, rainwater raced down the hillsides to Six Mile Creek, carrying along dirt and anything small that got in the way.[12]

By early October, workers were digging into the soft shale at the dam site, getting down to the bedrock on which the dam would rest. Vinton, who was supervising the overall work, hoped to have seventy feet of the ninety-foot dam in place before winter weather suspended construction. He had the Italians working day and night.[13] Some workers quit around October 17 to return to their old jobs in the Pennsylvania anthracite mines. A long coal strike had been settled, and the miners were going back to work on October 23.[14] Tucker & Vinton hired more Italians to replace them.

About a dozen of the Italians lived in a bunkhouse near the dam, and both the bunkhouse and the outhouse that served it were close to Six Mile Creek. The outhouse, which was also used by the workers who commuted in each day, quickly became filled and foul, based on eyewitness accounts. The workers—as construction workers, soldiers, and anyone who toiled in the outdoors were wont to do in 1902—simply defecated wherever the spirit moved them, often near the stream. It is entirely likely that they washed their hands in the creek afterward. Six Mile Creek, of course, was the source of most of the drinking water that Ithaca Water Works provided to customers. The intake pipe was about a half-mile below the worker camp.

One Sunday in early November, Holmes Hollister, fifty-eight, a planing-mill owner who was a member of the Ithaca Board of Public Works, walked out to the construction site. He was hardly the only Sunday visitor. "Hundreds and hundreds" of men, women, and children, taking advantage of Indian summer weather, turned out on November 2 and 9 to watch the never-ending work on the dam or the turning of the eight large pumps that kept water out of the work pit.[15] Some of them managed to drive their carriages close to where the work was being done. But Hollister strolled away from the main work area and was appalled by what he found. About two hundred to three hundred feet below the shanty where the workers lived, "I observed human excretions on the bank and adjacent to the creek in different places from 15-20 feet of the creek bank extending for some distance up and down the creek," he wrote in a letter to Veranus A. Moore, professor of bacteriology in the Cornell Veterinary School. But the letter was sent much later, during the epidemic. Hollister was concerned enough, though, that the following morning, he went to the office of Dr. Edward Hitchcock Jr., the health officer of the city of Ithaca, to let him know what he had observed.

Hitchcock was the son of Edward Hitchcock Sr., director of the Department of Hygiene and Physical Culture at Amherst College in Massachusetts and considered a nineteenth-century pioneer in physical education in colleges. The Hitchcock system made physical and health education mandatory for all Amherst students.[16] The younger Hitchcock, who never achieved anything close to his father's fame, graduated from Amherst in 1878 and from Dartmouth College School of Medicine in 1881. He practiced for a time in the village of Amherst but then was appointed an instructor in physical culture under his father at the college. He taught the same class at Massachusetts Agricultural College [today the University of Massachusetts] before joining the Cornell faculty in 1884. His duties included teaching physical culture and hygiene, running the gymnasium, and acting as the Cornell medical officer. Hitchcock had not had an active medical practice since his early days in Massachusetts.

When Hollister confronted him with the news, Hitchcock displayed the shortsightedness seen too often on the road to catastrophes. Because the fouled area was outside the Ithaca city limits, Hitchcock proclaimed, he had no jurisdiction. Nor is there any evidence that he raised the issue with Ithaca Water Works.[17]

Hollister was not the only local resident to witness the ground littered with human excrement along Six Mile Creek near the dam site. Emile M. Chamot, the clean water crusader who was conducting water quality tests under contract to the Ithaca Board of Health, saw the mess around the same time. So did Professor Elias J. Durand, who taught botany at Cornell, and two of his graduate students, Herbert H. Whetzel and James M. Van Hook, who observed the filth on several plant-specimen-collecting hikes through the Six Mile Creek valley. Even Gardner S. Williams, who had designed the dam, admitted in court testimony in 1905 that Six Mile Creek had been "used" by the workers hired to build the dam.[18]

Tucker & Vinton had agreed in its contract with Ithaca Water Works to provide sanitary facilities for the workers and "so enforce their use, as will preclude the possibility of fecal or other contamination of the water of the creek." The contract specifically prohibited "committing of nuisances" at or near the work site.[19] So why was this not enforced?

The construction firm hired a young Cornell engineering graduate, Shirley Clarke Hulse, to supervise the workers at the dam. Hulse, one of Williams's former students, graduated from Cornell with a civil engineering degree in 1902, and Williams got him the job. Hulse later claimed that he was always under the direct supervision of his professor at the dam site. From the piles of human excrement observed along Six Mile Creek and overflowing from the single outhouse, it is logical to assume that either Tucker & Vinton had little interest in enforcing sanitation or young Hulse was unable to work his will over the foreign workers. He probably couldn't speak their language, but he also appears to have been an arrogant upper-class jerk, qualities that would come to the fore during the typhoid epidemic. One has little sympathy for Hulse by the time all is said and done. The consequences of the failure to enforce the contract's sanitation provisions were too awful to excuse his youth and inexperience, even if the ultimate line of responsibility goes all the way up to Morris.

~~~~~~~~

Cornell University and its president, Jacob Gould Schurman, were at the top of their game in the fall of 1902. Total enrollment at the main campus in Ithaca and the medical school in New York City topped three thousand for the first time. Stimson Hall, which was to house the Ithaca branch of the College of Medicine, had been finished in time for the start of the fall semester. On October 8, speaking to the state convention of the Women's Christian Temperance Union, Schurman announced the location of the new Rockefeller Hall of Physics. And he urged the Board of Trustees to approve the construction of a hall for the arts and humanities to be named after Goldwin Smith, who taught English history at Cornell from 1869 to 1894. Schurman called Smith "the most illustrious exponent of liberal culture who ever sat in the Cornell University."[20]

All the buildings, new and old, were to be tied into a grand, new master plan for the campus approved by the Board of Trustees on October 25, about a year after it approved the university's fateful investment in the bonds of Ithaca Water Works and Ithaca Gas Light Company. The board employed the architectural firm of Carrère and Hastings of New York City, considered one of the best Beaux-Arts architecture firms in the United States. The architects would realign the campus to take advantage of the beautiful views of Cayuga Lake and "the lovely valley toward Newfield." The master plan was aimed at making the Cornell campus "undoubtedly the grandest in the world."[21]

Cornell University in the fall of 1902 had a good, but not great football team that ended its season with an 8-3 record. While the game looked somewhat different—players wore leather helmets and quilted pads that evoked ancient Japanese battle gear—it was no less exciting than it is today. The season's most anticipated game came on October 18, when Cornell lost at home 10-6 to Carlisle Indian School in Carlisle, Pennsylvania. Open from 1879 to 1918, Carlisle was a federal government boarding school for young men and women from Indian tribes in the West. The purpose of the school was to forcibly assimilate Indian children into white culture. The great athlete Jim Thorpe would first make his name as a football player at Carlisle a few years later. The opposing teams were coached by brothers, the immortal Glenn S. "Pop" Warner for Carlisle and Bill Warner for Cornell.[22] They were sons of a Union Army captain who had been a wheat farmer in New York but later moved to Oklahoma. Glenn graduated from Cornell in 1894 and coached the football team at the school until 1898. Bill was both a player and a coach—the rule, adopted the previous season, was that the team captain would be the head coach, assisted by three recent graduates.[23]

Freshman Graham B. Wood went to his first Cornell football game at Percy Field on September 27 when the Big Red opened their season against Colgate University, winning 5-0. He wrote in his diary that it was the first chance he had to let off any yells as a Cornell man. And the songs! "After the game, every mother's son of a Cornellian rises, doffs his hat, and sings, or does the best singing he can. The tune which evokes such reverential feeling is no other than 'Alma Mater.' There is no joking while that is going on. Even the pipes and cigarettes are for a time forgotten. You certainly feel glad that you are in college."[24]

By the end of the season, even with losses to Princeton and Carlisle Indian School behind them, Cornell students were as excited as ever about the Big Red team. Andrew Newberry wrote to his mother on November 26, gushing about the excitement of the previous night when the football team departed on a southbound train to its final game, against the University of Pennsylvania. He called the festivities "the grandest ever" and continued:

> Our class drew the float by a rope a block long on which every man had a hand. The seniors and juniors marched in front and the 'frosh' brought up the rear. Red lights and Roman candles blazed and popped all the way from the Ithaca Hotel to the Lehigh Valley Station. The yelling was immense. . . . After the team went to bed on their car, we came up town and lapped up a few beers, the first time this fall for me."[25]

Or so he told his mother. Yet this night of happiness and celebration was also tragic. A young restaurant cook in downtown Ithaca, who could only be a spectator of these college frolics, was caught up in the excitement and climbed to the rooftop of a building across from the Ithaca Hotel, according to Newberry's letter to his mother. Following the procession, the young man ran across the roof in the darkness and then jumped onto the roof of the adjoining building. But instead of landing on the roof, he crashed through a skylight and fell to his death. The parade did not stop, and probably few knew of the tragedy until the next day. Cornell narrowly lost to Pennsylvania, 12-11, at Franklin Field in Philadelphia.

Workmen that fall finished building the adjoining mansions of Robert H. Treman, Charles E. Treman, and Mynderse Van Cleef. These grand homes were located along University Avenue (today Stewart Avenue) with magnificent views of Cayuga Lake and the valley toward Newfield. William H. Miller, the architect, intended to make the three mansions "symmetrical" and to decorate their grounds with formal gardens. Each would have "a beautiful rolling lawn sloping to the west, and so arranged as to catch the lights and shadows of the afternoon sun."[26] Miller was a member of Chi Phi, a fraternity brother of Morris and Rob Treman.

As much as the Treman brothers and Van Cleef had profited from their connections to Cornell and its students, they did not want the students intruding into their personal lives. On November 18, 1902, the Executive Committee of the Board of Trustees approved a "reservation." In return for a payment of $8,500, or about $219,000 in twenty-first-century dollars, the board agreed to never build any athletic field near the mansions. And for fifty years, no fraternity house or dormitory could be built nearby. The Treman brothers and Van Cleef were members of the Executive Committee and were at the meeting when the "reservation" was approved, as were their good friends Charles H. Blood and Jared Treman Newman. There is no indication any of them recused themselves from the vote. That was just not how things were done on the Cornell Executive Committee, whether they were helping their friend William T. Morris by investing in Ithaca Water Works or keeping annoyances out of their own lives.[27]

Work on the Six Mile Creek dam ended for the season in late-November when the weather turned cold and wintry. The Italian workers left the gorge around the middle of the month, although they labored on other projects for Ithaca Water Works. All but a dozen were gone entirely by December 12, and the rest a week later. The U.S. Weather Bureau station on the Cornell campus recorded ten inches of snow on December 4 and 5, the opening salvo to one of the snowiest Decembers in Ithaca memory. Andrew Newberry wrote to his grandfather that he took advantage of the storm by going skiing.[28] The snow covered the human excrement along the banks of Six Mile Creek in a thick blanket of white, hiding, freezing and preserving the wickedness it contained.

Chapter 8

Typhoid, and How the Epidemic Began

THERE WERE FEW GODLIKE FIGURES IN THE WORLD OF MEDICINE in 1902, but Dr. Robert Koch was one. He was known far beyond his native Germany and was arguably the most famous healer in the world. Short, bearded, and bespectacled, he did not resemble a deity, but his pioneering achievements as a bacteriological and epidemiological researcher put him squarely atop the medical Mount Olympus.

Koch achieved his fame by taking on the big diseases, the ones that killed significant numbers of people. In 1882, he discovered the microbe that caused tuberculosis, the leading cause of death in nineteenth-century Europe and North America, killing one of every seven people. The German government created the Institute for the Investigation of Infectious Diseases for him in Berlin ten years later. It remained under Koch's direction until his death in 1910, after which it was renamed after him.[1] "Personally, Koch is a most approachable man, kindly in his relations with his associates and assistants, and a most industrious and enthusiastic worker," wrote Dr. Hermann M. Biggs, the New York City health commissioner in 1901. "He has the power, to a remarkable degree, of inspiring his pupils with his own scientific spirit and enthusiasm."[2]

Koch studied anthrax, tuberculosis, cholera, and malaria and learned how they lived and died. He used that knowledge not to cure those dread diseases, which would await the coming of antibiotics after World War II, but rather to contain their spread, to stop them from infecting new human hosts. In so doing Koch stopped epidemics, saved countless lives, and gave the public hope. Biggs and the Health Department used his rigorous methods to contain a cholera outbreak in New York in 1892 after infected ships arrived from Hamburg, Germany, where an epidemic was raging, and spawned new cases in the densely populated tenement districts of the Lower East Side.[3] Now it was the turn of typhoid fever, the world's third-leading killer disease, to be subjected to rigorous research and analysis by Koch and his associates. Finally, he was ready to report his findings and scheduled a speech to military doctors at the Kaiser Wilhelm Institute in Berlin. To say his speech was much anticipated in the European medical world was an understatement. No one, rich or poor, could be smug about typhoid.[4]

Typhoid, also known as "the fever," was commonly spread by polluted water, and because everyone drank water, everyone was vulnerable. Water filtration was far more common in Europe than the United States in 1902, but it was done mainly in the large cities. Neither continent had yet embraced the use of chlorine to kill typhoid bacilli in drinking water. That would not happen in America until 1909. Some of the better-known typhoid victims in history included former first lady Abigail Adams in 1818; Prince Albert, husband of Britain's Queen Victoria, in 1861; President Lincoln's son Willy in 1862; Mark Hanna, President William McKinley's chief political strategist, in 1904; and Wilbur Wright of airplane fame in 1912. There were countless others, real and fictional.

Among the latter were Hanno Buddenbrook, the fifteen-year-old musical prodigy in German author Thomas Mann's 1901 novel and family saga, *Buddenbrooks,* and Molly Malone, a young Irish lass who sold shellfish from a wheelbarrow on the streets of Dublin. In the mournful Irish folk song that memorializes her, Molly's ghost still roams the streets crying, "Cockles and mussels, alive, alive-o." Live cockles, which are similar to scallops, were supposedly safe to eat, but as Molly herself learned, an unwitting diner could end up dead if that cockle, mussel, or oyster came out of typhoid-contaminated waters. Any number of nineteenth-century typhoid outbreaks in Europe and America were linked to shellfish harvested too close to a sewage discharge pipe, although most cases still resulted from drinking contaminated water. It was a dirty age.

In the fall of 1894, for example, twenty-five students at Wesleyan University in Middletown, Connecticut, contracted typhoid, and four of them died. Each had attended one of three fraternity dinners for new members the night of October 12. Raw oysters were the appetizer. They had been harvested in the deep waters of Long Island Sound but then were placed in a pen in the freshwater Quinnipiac River near New Haven, Connecticut, for several days of fattening. This was a common practice at the time. The pen, probably unbeknown to anyone, was three hundred feet downstream from a private sewage discharge pipe leading from a house where a woman lay dying of typhoid. An investigation by Dr. Charles J. Foote of Yale University Medical School found that typhoid bacilli between the shells of oysters taken from the river were still virulent after forty-eight hours. Later research found that the virulent period could be as long as five to nine days.[5]

The 1890 United States census found the worst typhoid fever death rates in Birmingham, Alabama, with 264 deaths per 100,000, and Denver, Colorado, with 217 deaths per 100,000. The 1900 United States census reported 35,379 total deaths from typhoid that year, which meant that roughly 350,000 Americans had contracted the disease. Dr. Edwin O. Jordan, a prominent bacteriologist from Chicago, considered those numbers to be "considerably below" the true figures.[6]

Koch's interest in conquering typhoid derived from all this human suffering but also from the military needs of Germany. For every great power of the early twentieth century, typhoid was a pressing national security issue, capable of turning modern armies into tents of feverish, moaning invalids and killing off 10 percent or more of the soldiers who became infected. As Koch noted at the beginning of his speech in Berlin, some seventy-three thousand German troops contracted typhoid during the Franco-Prussian War in 1870 and nine thousand of them died. Nearly fifty-eight thousand British troops contracted typhoid during the Boer War in South Africa between 1899 and 1902, and more than eight thousand died.[7] The United States lost more troops to typhoid than to Spanish bullets and artillery during the Spanish-American War of 1898.

Even though German Army deaths from typhoid had declined by 25 percent since the 1880s, thanks to cleaner drinking water and better sewer systems in its garrison cities, the smaller towns and vast rural areas of

Germany, including the western border region with France, had not benefited from this new attention to public health. There remained hotbeds of typhoid almost guaranteed to infect the troops if they had to mobilize for another war with their historic foe. By framing typhoid as a national security issue, Koch was more easily able to get funding and facilities from the German government to do the research that needed to be done.[8]

The irony, of course, is that his speech occurred at the very time work on the Six Mile Creek dam was ending for the season and the countdown to the Ithaca epidemic had begun. As momentous as it was for the future of typhoid treatment, the speech had no impact on Ithaca because important medical findings at the beginning of the twentieth century could take months, if not years to cross the Atlantic from Europe. Instead, Koch is our oracle, voicing warnings that were an accurate road map to the Ithaca catastrophe.

"We know that typhoid fever is an illness which spreads mainly, I would like to say, really depends nearly completely, on how one handles sewage," Koch said that night. "Feces is the vehicle by which the typhoid bacilli are spread from the human body to the outside world."[9]

His method of fighting cholera and malaria, which he now adapted to typhoid, had been to find the patients—not always an easy task—then isolate them and disinfect their environment so they could not spread the disease to new hosts. Because cholera and malaria microbes could not live, or at least not for very long, outside of a host organism, a properly contained epidemic expired on its own. Koch believed the same would work with typhoid.

The problem with typhoid was that it was difficult with existing diagnostic methods to quickly confirm a case, leaving a large window of opportunity for ignorance to spread the disease. For example, the test known as the Widal Reaction, based on discoveries by French medical researcher Georges Fernand Isidor Widal in 1896, only gave results beginning around the second week of a typical three-week course of typhoid, by which time the patient could have infected his caregivers and anyone else in the vicinity. If given too early, the Widal test might yield a false negative. Diagnosis by examination of bacterial cultures under a microscope was only a little better, requiring several days to grow the culture to a point in which the typhoid bacilli could possibly be distinguished from their *E. coli* neighbors, which produced somewhat similar symptoms. "If one must wait several days for the diagnosis, then it is not useful for our purposes," Koch told his audience in Berlin.

Aided by his associates, Wilhelm von Drigalski and Hermann Conradi, Koch adapted a method that had provided quick diagnoses of cholera. Nutrients were added to the culture to speed up the growth of typhoid bacilli, while other substances were added to retard the growth of *E. coli* bacilli. Then, taking advantage of the acidic nature of *E. coli* and the alkaline nature of typhoid, they added litmus solution to the culture, turning the typhoid blue and the *E. coli* red. One further step, agglutination, or clumping together, made certain the bacilli were typhoid and not dysentery. The whole process took twenty to twenty-four hours.[10]

Once satisfied that their new diagnostic procedure worked, Koch and his associates examined several typhoid cases in Berlin, looking at the patients and the people around them, just as they would in a cholera outbreak. In some cases, they found typhoid fever bacilli "in humans who had no clinical symptoms," again replicating findings in cholera outbreaks. Such a person was a "carrier," or in German, a *Typhusbazillentrager*, meaning he or she harbored and could spread the disease but displayed no symptoms and appeared to be outwardly healthy. From Berlin, Koch and his assistants moved on to Trier in the German state of Rhineland-Palatinate and then to a group of four villages about twenty-five miles from the Luxembourg border.[11] This region, known as the Hochwald, was in the forward deployment zone of the German Army and was a hotbed of typhoid.

They learned many things in the Hochwald, notably that young people were the most likely victims of typhoid because they "come new to the infection," not yet having had an opportunity to pick up immunity. They found that local physicians knew little about stopping a typhoid outbreak, and even in rules-conscious Germany, could not be counted upon to report all typhoid cases they treated to public health authorities. Typhoid sufferers often did not seek treatment out of fear of the cost but came readily to Koch's clinic once assured there would be no charge. There was a catch, though. Patients were kept "from diagnosis to dismissal," often several weeks, and were not allowed to go home until three bacteriological examinations proved them to be free of the typhoid bacilli.

The new methods worked. Typhoid was exterminated from the four villages after three months and did not return, even though other villages in the Hochwald had their usual annual outbreaks, typically in August or September. He had broken the chain of transmission from one new patient to another, and finally, with nowhere to go, the typhoid had simply expired.

Koch found validation in the Hochwald, too, for his belief that infectious diseases did not spring to life from the miasma. Miasma believers, who in 1902 included surprising numbers of physicians and sanitarians, argued that diseases such as typhoid sprang to life from dirt, filth (i.e., horse manure in the streets—a common problem before the ascendancy of the automobile), and foul gases arising from putrid matter. Even the *Encyclopedia Britannica* wrote in its ninth edition in 1894 that the connection of typhoid "with specific emanations given off from decomposing organic or faeculant matter . . . is now almost universally admitted."[12] But not in Berlin. At the core of the miasma belief was a certain moral smugness, a justification for the well-to-do to blame the poor and their living conditions for diseases that afflicted them. Koch dismissed miasma in his Berlin speech, stating that the results of the Hochwald clinic showed that people and people alone were the sources of typhoid. "If, for instance, the infection could attack humans in some other way, such as from the soil, then despite our efforts we would have had new cases of typhoid fever," he said. Case closed.

But the biggest news that night was of typhoid carriers, Koch's groundbreaking finding that seemingly healthy individuals could harbor the typhoid bacilli and spread it to others for years after apparently recovering from the disease. It didn't happen often, but often enough. "The so-called carriers are the most dangerous," he said during the question-and-answer period that followed. "They are not lying ill in bed, where everything can be disinfected, but they travel around, sometimes make long journeys and carry the bacilli everywhere."[13] Carriers were the answer to why typhoid outbreaks sometimes seemed to occur for no reason, when there was no evident Patient Zero.

Koch was not the only physician to study typhoid. Many had gone before him, back well into the nineteenth century. One famous predecessor was Dr. William Budd of Great Britain. Budd published a pair of articles in the British medical journal *Lancet* in November and December of 1856 outlining his findings on typhoid, nearly all based on observation rather than laboratory work. He was the first to assert that typhoid was transmitted through the excretions of a typhoid patient, usually after they found their way to the local water supply.[14]

Over the years, medical researchers spent considerable time studying how long the typhoid bacilli could live outside a human body. While the estimates varied widely depending upon whether the bacilli were in water, excrement, or ice, the consensus was that at most, typhoid could survive no more than five months in a frozen state, including frozen excrement, and just a few days to a couple of weeks if not frozen. Modern research mentioned in an Indian medical journal in 2001 slightly reduced the survival time of the typhoid bacilli to forty-eight hours to seven days in water, up to a month in ice, and up to seventy days in soil irrigated with sewage.[15]

The outbreak every typhoid researcher remembered before Ithaca occurred in the winter of 1885 in Plymouth, Pennsylvania, a town of eight thousand across the Susquehanna River from Wilkes-Barre. A man who was exposed to typhoid in a distant city arrived in town and fell ill in a house that happened to be on a hillside. We know little about him other than he was nursed by the occupants of the house for several weeks and gradually recovered. The weather was bitterly cold, as cold as twenty-two degrees below zero. His caregivers threw his contaminated excrement out into the snow on the hillside behind the house, where it quickly froze. The hill sloped toward a stream that was Plymouth's water supply. When the spring thaw came on March 26, the melting snow carried the excrement into the stream. The still-live typhoid bacilli caused an explosive outbreak in Plymouth, sickening 1,104 residents and killing 114 of them. The death rate was a whopping 1,368 per 100,000. It was the worst typhoid epidemic in America in percentage terms up to that time, but the victims were mainly miners and their families, and so their deaths were mainly of academic interest, if at all, to the rest of America.[16]

~~~~~~~~~

The Ithaca typhoid epidemic was caused by a fatal combination of human recklessness and bad luck with the weather. The "what-ifs" are many. If William T. Morris, the new owner of Ithaca Water Works, had agreed to Professor Gardner S. Williams's recommendation that he first build a filtration plant, there very likely would have been no typhoid epidemic. It would not have mattered if one or more of the workers was a typhoid carrier or if there was a live case further up the watershed. Similarly, if Morris, his contractors Tucker & Vinton, the engineer Williams, or his assistant, Shirley Clarke Hulse, had enforced sanitary conditions in the camp, as the contract required, we would not be writing this story either. Instead, the typhoid bacilli, aided by the unusual weather, moved remorselessly toward Cornell University and the city of Ithaca.

How do we know one (or more) of the workers at the dam site was a typhoid carrier? Let us examine the evidence. We have already read observations of the grossly unsanitary conditions tolerated at the work camp for those who built the dam. Five witnesses saw significant amounts of human excrement along the banks of Six Mile Creek during the fall of 1902. There was but a single outhouse for the camp, and the workers, being no different from any other workers around the world in 1902, did their business wherever it was convenient. No apparent effort was made to rein in the men and force them to observe the sanitary regulations that were written into the contract.[17]

Why do we suspect one (or more) of the workers was a typhoid carrier? It is not *because* they were immigrants, but rather where they were immigrants *from*. Most had emerged from the river of humanity flowing out of Italy at the beginning of the twentieth century, most often from southern Italy, a hotbed of typhoid. Even today, typhoid has not been fully eradicated there.[18] Italy in 1902 had the highest typhoid rate in Europe, 35.2 deaths per 100,000, and in southern Italy, where many peasants still lived in backward, feudal conditions, the rate was doubtless much higher, with the national rate held down by the relatively cleaner northern regions. One need not look long in nineteenth-century travel and medical literature to find references to the southern Italian typhoid problem. John Murray wrote in 1883 about the effort in Naples to enclose stinking open sewers that ran along city streets, saying, "They are tending to remove the bad name which Naples had not undeservedly acquired for typhoid fever." Dr. J. Burney Yeo wrote in 1889 that "the cities of southern Italy and some even of the more northern ones have laid many a British visitor low by their fever-laden atmosphere."[19] He was referring to typhoid, though also to cholera and malaria.

What this meant is that southern Italian workers were far more likely to have been exposed to typhoid during their lifetime than workers who had grown up in Ithaca, and thus were more likely to be typhoid carriers. Ithaca had been relatively free of typhoid until 1903, with just a handful of deaths each year and no large epidemics. Ithaca City Hospital records show that only twenty-three people were treated for typhoid in all of 1902, with one death. Thirty-six patients were treated in 1901, the year Common Council became concerned about water purity, and six died. On average, about sixteen people annually contracted the disease.[20] Ithaca was not like southern Italy. Had Morris hired Driscoll Brothers of Ithaca (the second-lowest bidder) to build the dam, the likelihood of there being a typhoid carrier among the local workers employed by Driscoll would have dropped dramatically.

The next question we must address is this: If the excrement along Six Mile Creek was first observed in the fall of 1902, and it was indeed virulent, why did it take until the middle of January 1903 for the epidemic to break out?

The most helpful testimony in this regard came much later in reference to a different typhoid outbreak. Olin H. Landreth, a well-known engineer on the faculty of Union College in Schenectady, New York, testified before a New York legislative committee that the absorbent quality of the soil made all the difference in whether rain would wash virulent excrement into lakes, rivers, or streams. "In winter, there is no absorption by the soil of the impure material whatever; that is when the ground is frozen. As a consequence, the accumulation is the same as it is during a drought."[21]

Tucker & Vinton did not bring the Italian immigrants and striking anthracite coal miners from Pennsylvania to the dam site until September, which along with October had close to normal rainfall. Assuming the typhoid carrier was on the job from day one, much of his waste would have been dissolved harmlessly into the absorbent soil by the rains of September and October, according to Landreth's theory. The rains in the first two months of the project were not enough to create a sudden, broad, sweeping action pushing most of the excrement into Six Mile Creek. Even if some survived these normal rainfalls, perhaps it was not virulent or the virulence died with the passage of time.

In November, the weather changed. It was the driest November in Ithaca in a quarter century, with only 0.99 inches of rain recorded by the National Weather Bureau office on the Cornell campus. There was little opportunity for virulent excrement to be dissolved into the soil. Work stopped for the season in late November. While shelf-life issues would have rendered some of the excrement harmless, enough of it could have stayed virulent until an insulating blanket of snow in early December covered, froze, and preserved it. As Rev. William Elliot Griffis, pastor of First Congregational Church in Ithaca, wrote in his journal on December 5, 1902: "Woke up to find the world in white. Shoveled snow."[22]

December's precipitation in Ithaca made up for November. It was the snowiest December in twenty-five years. Some 44.9 inches fell, twice as much as any other December since 1879. The snow piled up across the valley where the reservoir would form once the dam was completed. The Italians had denuded the valley of trees, standard procedure in creating a reservoir but eliminating the brakes on the flow of storm water. A thaw occurred on December 16 but was not accompanied by significant rainfall and the ground stayed frozen. Without enough push from the rain, the contamination stayed out of the water supply. More snow fell.

Matters came to a head on January 2 and 3, 1903, when unseasonably warm temperatures arrived and a heavy rainstorm pelted the Ithaca region. This time the snow on the reservoir site melted and water raced down the frozen, denuded hillsides to Six Mile Creek, sweeping the valley clean. Within two days, the typhoid bacilli entered the Ithaca Water Works intake pipe and the countdown began.

Chapter 9

Denial

CHRISTMAS RECESS ENDED ON TUESDAY, JANUARY 6, but most students returned during the weekend of the rains, emptying out of trains at the Lehigh Valley Station and making their way in carriages or on foot through the slush to their rooms on East Hill. For those who lived in rooming houses with city water instead of a private well, or who patronized downtown restaurants like Theodor Zinck's Hotel Brunswick, a slow waltz with death began.[1] They drank the typhoid water at its most concentrated and virulent.

Not everyone who did became ill, and we will never know with certainty what determined the outcome of this lottery. It may have been as simple as natural defenses. Stomach acid is the enemy of typhoid bacilli. Large numbers must invade the stomach for a few to have a chance to climb over the walls into the intestine and begin to wreak havoc. Drinking a lot of water, on the other hand, can dilute stomach acid, and milk or ice cream can neutralize it. There are so many variables that one can never be sure. As in any epidemic, ill fortune was important in determining who lived or died.[2]

Here and there around town, people fell ill, but not in numbers to arouse suspicion. Some parts of Ithaca received water only from Six Mile Creek, and some received it only from Buttermilk Creek. Cornell University, including Sage College and some fraternity houses, received water from Fall Creek, and some 1,500 private wells served the outlying areas of the city but were not unknown elsewhere. Only Six Mile Creek carried the typhoid bacilli. The student boardinghouse district of East Hill, which received only water from

Six Mile Creek, became the epicenter. Dr. Edwin O. Jordan, the Chicago bacteriologist who investigated the Ithaca epidemic and wrote a four-part series on his findings for the *Journal of the American Medical Association*, was shaken when he realized what had happened: that the typhoid water had flowed first to where it could do the most damage. "It is well known that the greatest susceptibility to this disease is between the ages of 15 and 25, and that consequently a population of college students presents a mass of material of peculiarly inflammable nature."[3]

Typhoid's incubation period is ten to fourteen days. Some physicians might go short on one end or long on the other, but a week and a half to two weeks is about in the middle of medical thinking on the subject.[4] George A. Soper, who was a renowned sanitary engineer but not a medical doctor, and about whom we will hear much more in later chapters, believed that Patient Zero made his way to a physician's office or to City Hospital on January 11. We know little about these first few patients. Two new cases were reported on January 12, one on the following day, four on January 14, five on January 15, and three on January 16. Dr. Jordan believed that the epidemic began "about" January 15.[5] The appearance of the first patients corresponds to an incubation period of about ten days and provides more evidence that the heavy rains of January 2 and 3 triggered the catastrophe. Soper found the typhoid in Ithaca to be "extremely malignant."

Typhoid, as Dr. Jordan noted, is mainly a disease of youth and middle age, with the majority of cases grouped around age twenty-one. There were patients outside that group, but they were rarely under age two or over age fifty. Why the very young weren't affected was a mystery, but the older a person was, the more likely it was that he or she had been exposed to typhoid earlier in life. Data gathered during the 1900 federal census showed that more than a third of typhoid deaths occurred among people aged fifteen to thirty years. Only 10 percent occurred in children under age five.[6]

The symptoms of typhoid were sometimes mistaken for the *grippe*, meaning influenza, but usually not for long. For many physicians, the first clues were a swollen spleen and the characteristic rash of flat, pink spots associated with typhoid.[7] Other symptoms followed in quick succession. Dr. Julius Dreschfield wrote a description of the onset of typhoid for *A System of Medicine*, a multi-volume medical encyclopedia first published in

London and Philadelphia in 1897. He wrote that typhoid patients initially complained "of pain in the limbs, of excessive fatigue, of cold and chilly sensations, of headache often very severe, of loss of appetite, and sleeplessness." Nosebleeds erupted by the second or third day. As the symptoms became more severe, Dreschfield wrote, the patient rarely got out of bed. Body temperature rose steadily, and by about the fourth day reached 103 or 104 degrees Fahrenheit and the patient became thirsty and sleepless. Diarrhea might or might not be present from the start. The patient's skin turned dry, but there could be sudden attacks of profuse perspiration.[8] Such was the first week of typhoid.

One thing Ithaca did not lack was physicians. According to *The Standard Medical Directory of North America* for 1902, Ithaca had forty physicians, which in a town of 13,136 people gave it the highest ratio of physicians-to-population in New York State, higher even than New York City.[9] Of these physicians, eight were homeopaths and one was listed as "eclectic." The allopaths, or what we consider today to be "regular" physicians, had not yet won their war against homeopathy. Although often derided as quackery, homeopathy began with the best of intentions. It sprang from the disgust of its founder, Samuel Hahnemann of Germany, with the brutality of traditional medicine in the eighteenth century. Bloodletting and severe bowel purges appalled him. Hahnemann and his latter-day disciples used natural remedies, including very dilute poisons, to stimulate the body to heal itself. Homeopaths in Ithaca actually had more in the way of medicine to give their typhoid patients than did the allopaths, and as we shall see, claimed some success in curing them.

Most typhoid patients in Ithaca were treated by traditional physicians such as Dr. Alice M. Potter, a member of a large and amazingly accomplished Ithaca family. Unlike five of her ten siblings, Alice Potter had not gone to Cornell University but instead migrated directly from Ithaca High School to the University of Buffalo Medical School, graduating in 1897. She went into practice at 116 W. Seneca St. in Ithaca. (Her sisters, Bina and Jaennette, were also physicians, though not in Ithaca, and her brother, Charles, a veterinarian in Chicago. Two other brothers were lawyers.) Women physicians were still a novelty in 1903, but

their numbers were growing: Cornell Medical College in New York City graduated nine of them (plus forty-four men) in June 1902.

Another Ithaca physician, and one who had a prominent role during
the epidemic, was Dr. Luzerne Coville. He graduated from Cornell in 1887
and from the College of Physicians and Surgeons at Columbia University in
1889, after which he set up practice in Brooklyn. In 1896, he moved his practice to Ithaca, and in 1898, after the founding of the Ithaca branch of Cornell's College of Medicine, Coville joined the faculty as a lecturer in anatomy.
He switched to surgery in 1900. His *Work Book in Surgery*, privately published
in 1902, was a primer for his students. Coville was a determined truth teller,
cautioning his students to be "candid and direct, yet kind. . . . Make the diagnosis what it is, even at the expense of the patient's wishes or preclusions or
his presumptions." He would follow his own advice during the epidemic to
his ultimate sorrow.[10]

But whether Ithaca physicians were men or women, allopaths or homeopaths, the first problem they faced, as Dr. Robert Koch in Germany knew so
well, was making a correct diagnosis. They often looked first for that enlarge-
ment of the spleen and characteristic rash of flat, pink spots, but laboratory
options also existed. Typhoid bacilli were difficult to distinguish under the
microscopes of the day, even when stained bright red with carbol-fuchsin
dye. Physicians could try growing colonies of typhoid, feeding them agar,
a nutrient extracted from Japanese seaweed. Such colonies resembled clus-
ters of tiny rods with rounded ends and whiplike appendages called flagella
that propelled them through fluids.[11] The trick was also to distinguish them
from other bacilli that were of a similar appearance.[12] There was really no
good way to do that with a microscope in 1903, or at least do it quickly.

A better method was using the Widal Reaction. Georges Fernand Isidor
Widal, a French medical researcher, discovered in 1896 that specific agglu-
tins in the blood of typhoid patients could be employed in the laboratory to
cause the typhoid bacilli, and no others, to stop moving and clump together.
The test required drawing blood from the patient, which in 1903 was accomplished either with a sterilized hypodermic syringe, invented in 1853, or a
cupping glass, which used heat or suction to create a vacuum that pulled
blood out of several small incisions in the skin. The blood sample was placed
in a test tube for a period of time to allow the red cells to settle out. Then the

serum was mixed with about the same volume of typhoid bouillon not more than ten to eighteen hours old. Results came almost immediately. "The bacilli will be seen—immediately after the admixture—to become immobile and to collect in clumps of varying size," Dr. Heinrich Curschman wrote in 1901. Through his microscope, he observed the bacilli continue to swarm in a control sample to which no serum had been added.[13]

The problem with the Widal Reaction, as noted earlier, was that it sometimes gave false results. A typhoid patient did not begin producing the agglutinate factor until he had been ill for seven to ten days. So if the physician gave the test too early, it produced a false negative. Or if the patient had been exposed to typhoid earlier in life, it might give a false positive. But in areas like Ithaca, mostly new to typhoid, the Widal Reaction was a valuable tool for diagnosing typhoid. Coville, for example, wrote afterward that he administered Widal tests to about half of the three hundred patients, mainly Cornell students, that he saw during the epidemic.[14]

There was also the Diazo urine test to diagnose typhoid. This actually predated the Widal Reaction, having been discovered by the noted German immunologist Paul Ehrlich in 1883. Physicians could use the Diazo test to diagnose typhoid between the fifth and fourteenth day of the disease. Urine from a suspected typhoid victim was mixed with an equal amount of Diazo solution. Then a few drops of ammonia were added and the mixture was shaken. If the patient had typhoid, the froth at the top of the shaken mixture would be a shade of red. The problem with the Diazo test was that several other diseases, including tuberculosis, could trigger a positive reaction, and so physicians preferred to use it in tandem with the Widal Reaction to be doubly certain of a typhoid diagnosis.[15]

~~~~~~

The first signs that something was wrong in Ithaca appeared during the third week in January. The *Ithaca Daily Journal* reported on January 21 that ninety-six cases of grippe, or flu, were being treated in the city. Rumor had it, though, that these citizens did not have flu, but rather typhoid.

Dr. Edward Hitchcock Jr., the city health officer who had refused to do anything when Holmes Hollister told him about the excrement along Six Mile Creek the previous fall, was quoted in the *Daily Journal* on January

22 ridiculing the idea that a typhoid epidemic had taken hold in the city. Rather, he asserted, what ailed people was "a certain low fever, almost exactly similar to that fever of last year which was termed, 'Ithaca fever.'" Hitchcock, who could have been a character out of the Albert Camus novel *The Plague,* insisted that this supposed low-grade fever was not contagious and that no one had ever died from it.[16]

Ithaca's city government was in a state of uncertainty at the beginning of 1903. The mayoral election of November 1902 had ended in an official tie between Republican Mayor William R. Gunderman and his Democratic challenger, George W. Miller, each with 1,682 votes. The Progressive Party candidate, Edward Spriggs, received 95 votes. Under state law, a tie meant that the incumbent, Gunderman, would stay on until the next general election in 1903. Miller, however, filed a court challenge claiming that in one Ithaca voting district, the Second District of the Third Ward, he had actually received seven more votes than reported. Witnesses said they heard the chairman of the Board of Inspectors call out "140" votes, even though the poll clerks wrote down "133." Tompkins County Supreme Court ordered the voting machine to be opened, and investigators found that Miller had indeed received 140 votes. The court ruled on January 27, 1903, that Miller was the real winner but issued a stay to allow Gunderman an opportunity to appeal. The Republican, however, said he considered the matter settled by the court's ruling and resigned on January 31, as did the city clerk. Miller did not take office as mayor until February 12. Despite Gunderman's resignation, the Republicans did file an appeal that was not resolved until July, when it was dropped. Miller was acting mayor during that five-month period.[17]

At Cornell, final exams for the fall semester began on January 22, the start of a seven-day slogfest of all-nighters that left students tired and drained. The big medical news was of James B. Hopkins, a graduate student in French and Greek who had returned from Christmas break on January 7 and two weeks later went back home to Bath, New York, supposedly ill with smallpox. Hitchcock was all over this one, telling the *Ithaca Daily News* he had "kept a sharp watch for smallpox during the present year, and so far none has appeared in Ithaca." The initial symptoms of smallpox are similar to those of typhoid, and it seems far more likely that Hopkins was one of the early patients in the epidemic.[18]

The first student brought to the Cornell Infirmary with typhoid symptoms was admitted on January 23 and was probably Oliver G. Shumard. The infirmary was housed in a three-story brownstone Victorian mansion at 512 E. State St. that had once been the home of lumber baron Henry W. Sage, a former chairman of the Cornell University Board of Trustees. Sage died in 1897, and his sons donated the house to Cornell for use as a student infirmary, along with a $100,000 endowment to outfit and operate it. It had beds for twenty students and was attended by three homeopathic nurses, one of them a student nurse. Patients were billed $1 a day for room and board, a stiff sum when an average workingman's salary in America was about $543 a year.[19]

One mystery of the Cornell Infirmary was that no physician sat on the three-member committee that ran the facility. Instead, the administrative committee comprised President Schurman; Emmons L. Williams, secretary-treasurer of the Board of Trustees and its Executive Committee; and Roger B. Williams, president of Ithaca Savings Bank and a member of the Board of Trustees and its Executive Committee. None of them were physicians. Local physicians were welcome to have privileges at the infirmary but were not involved in running it. The committee and the nurse matron made those decisions. But why? In their letter to the Executive Committee announcing their gift of their father's mansion and the $100,000 endowment, Sage's sons said only that the infirmary was to be "kept and maintained by the university, under such rules and regulations as may be adopted by its Board of Trustees." The board created the administrative committee about a week later.[20]

The fact that only homeopathic nurses were on the regular infirmary staff suggests that a desire to keep the facility friendly to homeopathic physicians might have played a part in the decision to bar involvement by the medical school, since its staff was all allopaths. But ultimately the odd decision remains a mystery. The lack of physician involvement in running the Cornell Infirmary became a raging controversy after physicians from the medical school criticized the care students received during the epidemic, but we get ahead of ourselves.

Shumard grew up on a dirt farm near Bethany, Missouri, about twenty-five miles south of the Iowa line and nearly as close to Nebraska. He graduated with honors and as class president from the University of Missouri in 1902, receiving his diploma from the hands of Mark Twain himself, the author Samuel L. Clemens. Shumard and his fellows were known ever after as the "Mark Twain Class." The author had come to the University of Missouri to receive an honorary degree after what was to be his final visit to Hannibal, the small Missouri town on the Mississippi River where he grew up and his fiction took root. The white-haired, sixty-six-year-old Clemens was mobbed by well-wishers everywhere his train stopped, and he often became so emotional that he broke down in tears.

Shumard won a $300 scholarship to Cornell, a major award, and planned to study philosophy as a graduate student. He was an admirer of Dr. Frank Thilly, a philosophy professor at Missouri who had begun his teaching career at Cornell in 1892 and would return there in 1906 after two years at Princeton.[21] After spending the summer of 1902 with his family and friends, Shumard set out in September with his family's last $300 in savings—a year's living expenses—on the nearly 1,100-mile rail journey to Ithaca.[22] At Cornell, he enrolled in courses in metaphysics, logic, psychology, and ethics. For financial reasons, the young man couldn't return home over Christmas break, so he was in Ithaca when the death water arrived in the taps. For whatever reason, he was among the first to drink it.

On the evening of Shumard's hospitalization, a full house at the Lyceum Theatre in downtown Ithaca applauded the British actress Lillie Langtry in the play *Cross-Ways*. A legendary beauty, Langtry in 1877 became the mistress of Edward, Prince of Wales, who was crowned King Edward VII on August 9, 1902, and she was linked to many other rich and powerful men throughout her life. By the time she appeared on stage in Ithaca, Langtry was an American citizen. She made it through Ithaca without contracting typhoid (not every actress at the Lyceum Theatre that winter was so fortunate) and to her next performance in Rochester. The following night, Cornell defeated Harvard in basketball at the Armory, 23-9. Life in Ithaca seemed entirely normal as long as one didn't probe too deeply.

Once again, the weather turned bitterly cold. Oliver Shumard was joined in the infirmary by several other students with typhoid symptoms, including Zella Marie Clark, a premed student from Prince Edward Island, whose sister, Clemmie, had died of typhoid in 1899. Their parents had refused to bring the coffin into the house, even with a cold November rain falling, out of misplaced fear of contagion. As it became clear to Zella that she, too, suffered from typhoid, her fear grew, but it was tempered by a deep religious faith and a curiosity about the medical drama going on around her in the infirmary.

At first, both Ithaca newspapers listened to typhoid skeptics like Dr. Hitchcock. On January 26, the *Ithaca Daily News* published a front-page story headlined, "Many Fever Cases Reported in City," but argued that most of these cases were not really typhoid. Rather, echoing Hitchcock, they were a fever "peculiar to this city, caused either by climatic reason or by germs generated in drinking water." The miasma theory seemed alive and well in Ithaca. Yet even Hitchcock was getting the runaround from the water company. The story revealed that Ithaca Water Works had refused to tell Dr. Hitchcock on which dates Six Mile Creek water might have been mixed with Buttermilk Creek water. This was done when the volume of the latter was too low. If this had happened, the Flats of Ithaca, which included the downtown, might also have received contaminated water, not just East Hill. But he refused to be suspicious, at least for the record. "The health officer will neither assert nor deny that the water from Six Mile Creek is responsible for the fever," the *Daily News* said. In an editorial that day, the newspaper urged city officials and the scientists of Cornell to determine what was causing the mystery disease. In the meantime, it warned readers to boil their water.[23] No such warnings were issued from city government. Common Council members were still focused on the perceived threat of the ninety-foot dam on Six Mile Creek that had consumed them since November, and Dr. Hitchcock seemed simply incompetent. It is also possible that he knew what the game was but was under pressure from his main employer, Cornell University, and the Tremans not to confirm there was a typhoid epidemic. Incompetent or spineless, Hitchcock did not carry out his duties as he should have.

No one would be able to deny there was a typhoid epidemic for much longer. Ithaca City Hospital was filling up with fever patients. Housed in the former Burt mansion in the Flats near where North Aurora Street crossed Cascadilla Creek, the hospital opened in 1889 and an operating room annex was added some years later. The *Daily Journal* reported on January 28—again not using the word *typhoid* to describe the illnesses—that City Hospital was full and consideration was being given to moving the nurses into other quarters.[24]

At least one private hospital was also open in Ithaca at the time, operated by Grace Robinson at Linn and Mill Streets. Little is known about the role of Robinson Hospital in the epidemic beyond quick references to this or that patient who had been taken there. Ben Poor, a student who fell ill with typhoid on January 31, was moved to Robinson Hospital by carriage from his boardinghouse at the recommendation of Dr. Coville and stayed until March 5, when he was taken home to Burlington, Iowa, by his mother to complete his convalescence.[25]

Complaints about the quality of care provided by the nurses of Cornell Infirmary were already being heard. Part of the problem was that the nurses had too many typhoid cases to look after, but clearly there were also management and competency problems. Annie Sophia Clark went to visit her sister, Zella, late in January and was surprised when a junior nurse, a Miss Cross, asked her sister to get out of bed and into a chair while she changed the sheets. The hospital matron entered the room while this was going on and became angry, telling Zella that under no circumstances did Dr. Coville want her to get out of bed. On another day, a nurse didn't seem to know how to use a thermometer.[26]

Rumors were beginning to circulate that Ithaca Water Works and the unsanitary work camp at the dam site were responsible for the illnesses. Professor Gardner S. Williams was quoted in the *Journal* on January 29 denying that the water company was in any way to blame for the typhoid outbreak or that the work camp was unsanitary. "Before this sickness appeared, we took every precaution to prevent any contamination of the water. Closets were built on the hills, over deep pit holes, and the place was generally disinfected with lime." The reports by Hollister and others of the ground around Six Mile Creek at the work camp littered with human excrement had not yet surfaced, so he did not have to explain those away. Williams insisted that cases of the "fever" were routine in Ithaca and happened every year.

That morning, Dr. Hitchcock finally advised residents to boil all water used for drinking purposes but strangely refused to say it was a precaution against illness. Simply common sense, he said, rebuffing the obvious follow-up question from the *Ithaca Daily News* reporter. In an *Ithaca Daily Journal* article, Williams heartily seconded Hitchcock's recommendation, adding, "and in fact I have always boiled water since living in Ithaca" and offering helpful hints for making boiled water taste better. He must have assumed people had forgotten that a year earlier, he lied and told them that Six Mile Creek was just fine to drink without filtration.[27]

One suspects the *Ithaca Daily News* would have liked to talk to Williams, too, but the city was dividing into two camps. In one camp was William T. Morris and his friends, including the Tremans, Cornell University, and the *Ithaca Daily Journal*. In the other was nearly everyone else and the *Ithaca Daily News*, which saw its circulation skyrocket. Published by Cornell oratory professor Duncan Campbell Lee, the *Daily News* had decided to abandon the reticence that characterized its initial stories about the typhoid outbreak. Led in the trenches by managing editor Frank E. Gannett, it would aggressively report on and editorialize about nearly every aspect of the epidemic. The *Daily News* became the voice of the people, an oft-misused phrase but quite accurate here. The *Ithaca Daily Journal*, run by George E. Priest and Charles M. Benjamin, and edited by Brainard G. Smith, increasingly became the voice of the embattled Treman family and their friends, especially Morris. President Schurman was in this group, too, although he tried to keep his distance.

<hr />

The two camps met in peace for the last time on the evening of January 30 in a gala at the Masonic Hall in downtown Ithaca. Decorations were pretty, an orchestra performed, potted palms and plants circled the orchestra stand, and couples crowded the dance floor. The story in the *Ithaca Daily Journal* notes that "punch was served at the entrance." Did the ice come from a safe source? One begins to see danger everywhere when writing about an epidemic. Among those present at the "unusually pleasant" event, as the newspaper termed it, was Barbara F. Schurman, but not her husband, the Cornell president.[28]

Jacob Gould Schurman was in New York City, where the previous evening he had delivered a major address to a large audience at Cooper Union containing a plea for the independence of the Filipino people that was reprinted in full in the next day's *New York Times*.[29] Schurman had been on an extended lecture tour through the Midwest, New York, and New England since mid-December, speaking on a variety of topics but especially the Philippines, and spending considerable time away from Ithaca and the university.[30] His speech at Cooper Union was his masterwork as an orator on the Philippine question, delivered on the same stage where, on February 27, 1860, Abraham Lincoln delivered one of his more famous antislavery speeches. Schurman often declared that Lincoln was his role model, so the choice of platforms was probably no accident.[31] As a naturalized citizen, he was ineligible to be president of the United States, but Schurman loved the limelight and considered himself to be doing God's work in bringing the Philippine situation to national attention. He seems to have paid little attention to Cornell and Ithaca during the approach of the epidemic. His eyes were on the world, but the danger was at his feet.

Also at the Masonic gala were Robert H. Treman and his wife, Laura; Charles E. Treman and his wife, Mary; Samuel D. Halliday, chairman of the Cornell University Board of Trustees, and his wife, Jennie; Charles H. Blood, the bachelor district attorney and codeveloper with Jared Treman Newman of Cornell Heights, which needed some of the water that would rise behind the Six Mile Creek dam; and Professor and Mrs. Duncan Campbell Lee.[32] We can only imagine what went through Lee's mind as he walked among the revelers, knowing that the next day his newspaper would publish a story that spared nothing in describing the peril Ithaca faced from typhoid fever. Did he have any doubts about the path he was following? Or did he think back to the sick and dying soldiers in his unit during the Spanish-American War? He counted on Frank E. Gannett, his managing editor, to deliver the aggressive reporting while he wrote most of the bold editorials.

Judging by the editions he put out, Gannett was very much the young Charles Foster Kane, always pushing his reporters to bring back both the daily developments in the epidemic, including long and detailed lists of patients, plus the back story about what was really going on. That was what Lee wanted him to do. At this point we should note that while both men seem to have gotten along fine during this period, and while Lee later wrote Gannett a warm letter of recommendation, nearly forty years later Gannett claimed that Lee was away on sabbatical in England during the typhoid epidemic and that he, Gannett, was entirely in charge of the news coverage and editorials.

The claim first arose in Gannett's 1940 campaign biography, which he commissioned from writer Samuel T. Williamson when he decided to seek the Republican nomination for president in 1940.[33] Not that it did him much good. Gannett placed a distant eighth in first-ballot voting at the 1940 Republican National Convention in Philadelphia. The GOP ultimately picked another businessman, utility executive Wendell Willkie, who went on to lose decisively to President Franklin D. Roosevelt. The claim that Lee was in England during the epidemic is easily debunked. For one thing, Cornell University records show Lee's sabbatical in England to have been during the 1901–02 academic year, not 1902–03. He returned to Ithaca months before the epidemic started. Lee was listed in the Cornell University catalog, *The Record*, as teaching several courses during both semesters of the 1902–03 academic year. There are the mentions of him in the newspaper, such as at the Masonic gala. No, Lee did not leave Ithaca during the epidemic.[34]

After the sun rose on the morning after the gala, Lee made his usual stop at the newspaper office, conferred with Gannett, and determined the story was ready to go. No one who read it could have any illusions about the typhoid fever epidemic in Ithaca.

Epidemic Spreads Throughout City
City Hospital Over-crowded with Sufferers from Fever
Physicians Call it Typhoid
The epidemic of fever which at present is raging in the city is rapidly reaching most serious proportions. Five new cases were taken to the City Hospital yesterday and the building is today so crowded that some of the nurses have been moved to private homes. Only urgent cases are being taken at the hospital and the number of patients being treated at their own homes is very large. Just how many patients there are now in the city is difficult to find out. Nearly all the physicians have from 15 to 20 cases each and it is estimated there are from 150 to 200 cases of typhoid here today.
—*Ithaca Daily News,* January 31, 1903

There was no exaggeration or sensationalism. The *Daily News* was reporting the epidemic as it ought to be reported. There would be no more pretending that the disease in Ithaca was something other than typhoid fever, no more pretending it was not a major catastrophe.

At City Hospital, the arrival of so many desperately ill people quickly filled it beyond the normal capacity of twenty-six. Nurses quarters became patient rooms, and even the reception area on the first floor was turned into a ward. Cots were set up wherever room could be found. Daniel W. Burdick, a druggist who was chief of the hospital as well as president of the Ithaca Business Men's Association, appealed to the public for donations of pillows, sheets, and blankets. Rev. Cyrus W. Heizer, pastor of nearby First Unitarian Church, offered his Sunday school room as an overflow ward.[35] Heizer was concerned about the college students in Ithaca who were away from their families, especially those in the nearby Ithaca Conservatory of Music (today Ithaca College) who sometimes used his church as a rehearsal and performance space. "It is the duty of Ithacans to take care of all such," he said.[36]

The *Ithaca Daily Journal* continued to hold back, even when Mrs. Charles M. Benjamin, wife of one of the two copublishers, became ill with typhoid herself. The *Journal* did not ignore the epidemic completely, but it published fewer column inches and tended to orient its coverage, although not blatantly, toward the interests of the Tremans and Morris. It stressed personal responsibility to avoid the typhoid bacillus rather than assigning fault for the catastrophe that had occurred.[37] Lee's editorials in the *Ithaca Daily News* were clarion calls to action, while Smith's in the *Ithaca Daily Journal* tended to be muted appeals to reason if not defenses of the city elite.

The *Ithaca Daily News* began printing long lists of the names and addresses of people who were ill with typhoid, sometimes adding brief remarks on their condition. These lists, which probably could not be replicated by a newspaper covering an epidemic today, show that typhoid in Ithaca attacked the families of the rich as well as the poor, the intellectuals as well as the day laborers. In the first list on January 31, we see, for example, the name of John Elliot Griffis, ten-year-old son of Rev. William E. Griffis, pastor of First Congregational Church of Ithaca. Rev. Griffis was an Orientalist and a prolific author. John Elliot was ill for a month but survived to become an important American composer of piano and chamber works. His older brother, Stanton, who did not contract typhoid, is perhaps the best-remembered of the family. He became a Wall Street investment banker, acquiring control of Madison Square Garden in 1933 and becoming chairman of Paramount Pictures in 1939. During the early 1950s, he was U.S. ambassador to Argentina during the ascendancy of Juan and Eva Peron. The two boys' older sister, Lillian, who was away at Vassar College, contracted typhoid on a visit to Ithaca early in the epidemic and was now recovering from the illness in Poughkeepsie.

〜〜〜〜〜

Despite the raging typhoid epidemic, many other young women from around the East Coast were about to descend on Ithaca for a major winter social event. Junior Week was a winter revel of long standing, held during the first week of the second term at Cornell after first semester exams were over. It was a big deal. As the editor of the *Cornell Era* magazine complained in 1893, "Junior Ball week is getting rather overdone. What with the Sophomore Cotillion and the Glee Club concert and the Junior Promenade and numerous private and fraternity parties and the entertainment of guests, for a large number of students the entire week is consumed in pleasure."

Conservative faculty members didn't much like it, either. Ever the priggish scold, Professor Burt G. Wilder, who had written a letter to the Board of Trustees in 1902 complaining about Saturday baseball games on the green near his classroom, now wrote to former Cornell president Andrew Dickson White (Schurman was in New York for his Cooper Union speech) complaining about the Junior Prom on hygienic and moral grounds. He said the dances "induce loss of self-control, breaches of decorum, and the use of stimulants." Wilder lamented that behavior rules set by the Board of Trustees might be ignored by the students—he recalled an incident several years earlier when extinguishing the lights to end a dance was foiled by students who brought in portable lamps—but suggested turning the fire hoses on the rowdy youths and expelling them from Cornell if that happened again.[38]

No one, neither Wilder nor anyone else, was publicly stating the obvious: that with a typhoid epidemic in Ithaca that showed no signs of abating, the Junior Week events ought to have been canceled. A typhoid death, possibly the first of the epidemic, had occurred that morning. Emma H. Smith, age thirty-six, a native of Carlisle, Pennsylvania, who had lived in Ithaca for nine years, had died after two weeks of suffering. She left behind a husband, Edgar, and a son, Frank.[39]

Bringing hundreds of young people to a city under attack by a disease with an affinity for young people seems beyond reckless today and clearly left people uneasy in Ithaca in 1903. The *Daily Journal*, in one of its rare expressions of concern about typhoid fever, published an editorial on February 2, "Danger in Junior Week." Brainard Smith, the editor, warned students to be careful and not to overtax their bodies. Then he addressed an issue that must have been lurking in the background: "It is out of the question now to think of postponing or giving up the plans made for the festivities of Junior Week." As with every big Cornell social event, the Junior Prom was as much for the adults of the Ithaca upper crust as it was for the students. Laura Hosie Treman, Robert's wife, didn't miss one for forty years.[40] The *Cornell Daily Sun*, the student newspaper, finally awakening from its normal torpor of that era, reported that twenty-nine students suffering from typhoid were in the infirmary. On February 3, the *Daily News*, after a thorough canvass of local physicians, reported fifty new typhoid cases in the previous day.

The city Board of Health held an emergency meeting on the evening of February 3 to discuss the epidemic. Dr. Veranus A. Moore spoke at length and answered questions from the board about typhoid. He had received a live typhoid fever culture from Boston that morning, which he needed to perform the Widal Reaction test. At the close of the meeting, the board ordered the drinking fountains in the city schools to be turned off immediately.[41]

Already some in Ithaca were becoming nervous and angry about the *Ithaca Daily News*'s reporting of the epidemic. In an editorial, the newspaper acknowledged its critics' point that the news was not good for the city but said that trying to hide the facts would do more harm than good. A majority of physicians called the fever typhoid, the *Daily News* argued, and anyone who doubted it should "see some of the patients who are delirious and close to death's door." It was time for action, not more words. "Ithaca today is not a fit place to live in," the editorial concluded. Two days later, the *Daily News* published another editorial and added these words: "A paper which fails to print the facts when the situation is as serious as it is at present, fails to do its duty; it is cowardly and dishonest to its readers."[42]

Girls began arriving in Ithaca and were met by their beaus at the railroad station. A fleet of horse-drawn omnibuses hired from across the region ferried them from the Lehigh Valley Station to their rooms. The boys were not allowed to ride, but did jog alongside.[43] Both newspapers printed warnings to the out-of-towners. The *Daily News* printed a blunt message in a box, "Guests in Danger," advising student committees in charge of the various Junior Week events to make sure that no city water, unless first boiled, was served to guests. The *Ithaca Daily Journal* did likewise but softened the impact by headlining the warning, "Necessary Precaution." Like the *Daily News*, it worried about the water that would be consumed at the dances. Unless precautions were taken, "there is grave reason to believe that this Junior Week will be followed by even more sickness than now prevails, and that those who come here to participate in the festivities will carry away with them seeds of typhoid that may develop in the most serious way."[44] Cornell University issued no warning of its own, and the festivities moved forward without pause.

At the Cornell Infirmary, Oliver Shumard's condition became critical. He suspected from the start that the typhoid would kill him and telegraphed for his father, William Shumard, to leave his farm in Bethany to come to Ithaca. He arrived by train in time to reach his son's bedside and take down his last good-byes for his mother, brother, and sisters.[45] Then the death watch began. Zella Marie Clark, also in serious condition, had been joined as a patient in the infirmary by her sister, Annie Sophia. By the end of the week, nearly forty students with typhoid were in the Cornell Infirmary.

On the morning of the Junior Prom, the first outside news article about the Ithaca typhoid epidemic appeared in the *New York Sun*, one of the many daily newspapers then published in New York City. Most likely telegraphed in by a student stringer, the small article contained a blunt warning: "There is as yet no check in the typhoid fever epidemic, which is raging in this city." Walter McCormick, acting mayor of Ithaca, and Dr. Hitchcock, the health officer, worried about the impact of the story on Cornell University. They fired back a telegram: "Today's *Sun* contains an article on typhoid fever in Ithaca that is likely to cause anxiety to many parents of students at Cornell. That your readers may know the exact situation from official sources, we desire to say that there do not exceed 100 cases of typhoid fever in Ithaca, of which only forty-five cases are among the students, and that in our opinion there is nothing in the situation which can in any sense be characterized as an epidemic or which should unduly excite the public." It was an amazing and mendacious statement.[46]

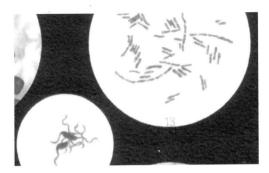

Typhoid bacilli, upper right, and magnified, showing flagella, lower left. *From the article "Bacteriology," in Meyers Konv. Lexicon, 6th edition (Leipzig: Bibliographisches Institut, 1902–08).*

Even as the first student was about to die of typhoid, the Junior Week festivities continued without pause. This advertisement evokes a bygone era. *Cornell Daily Sun*

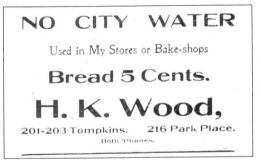

This ad from the H. K. Wood Bakery offered blunt reassurance to customers. *Ithaca Daily News*

Treman, King & Co., the original business of the Treman family in Ithaca, advertised aggressively during the epidemic, such as this ad for a water distiller. Like Ithaca Water Works, the ad stresses the responsibility of individuals to avoid being infected with typhoid. *Ithaca Daily News*

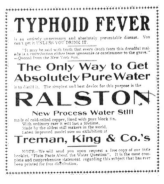

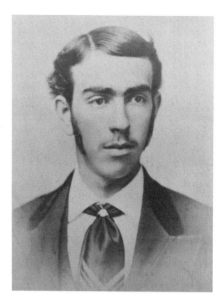

William T. Morris as a Cornell University student, ca. 1873. *Cornell University Rare and Manuscript Collections*

Ebenezer M. Treman as a young *man. Cornell University Rare and Manuscript Collections*

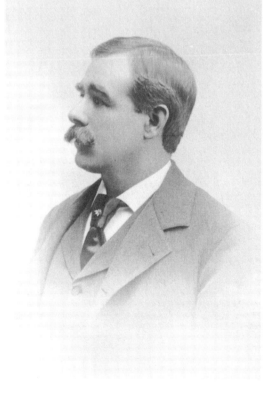

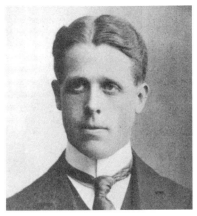

Charles E. Treman, Ithaca business-
man and friend of William T. Morris. *The
History of the Treman, Trumaine, Truman
Family in America, by Ebenezer Mack
Treman, 1901.*

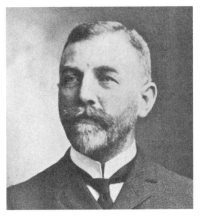

Mynderse Van Cleef was a friend and
critical source of financing for William T.
Morris. He was the brother-in-law of Rob-
ert H. and Charles E. Treman, and like
them a member of the Cornell University
Board of Trustees and the Executive
Committee. *The History of the Treman,
Trumaine, Truman Family in America, by
Ebenezer Mack Treman, 1901.*

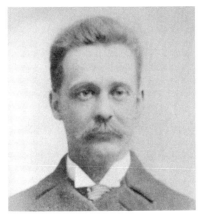

Robert H. Treman was the brother of
Charles E. Treman and a close friend
of William T. Morris. He was a banker
in Ithaca. *The History of the Treman,
Trumaine, Truman Family in America, by
Ebenezer Mack Treman, 1901.*

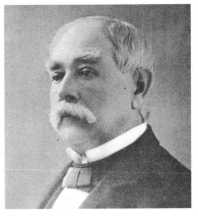

Lafayette L. Treman, patriarch of the Tre-
man family. His death in 1900 was the
first event on the epidemic timeline. *The
History of the Treman, Trumaine, Truman
Family in America, by Ebenezer Mack
Treman, 1901.*

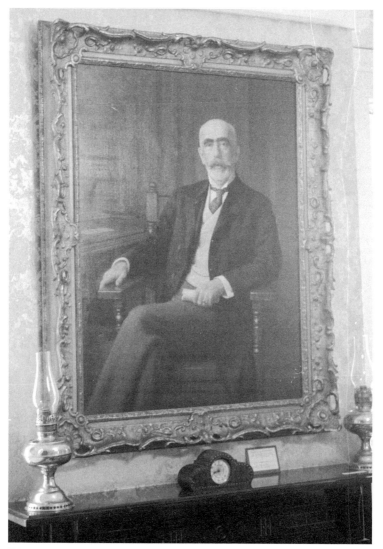

This painting of the older William T. Morris hangs in the Yates County Historical Society in Penn Yan, New York. *Photograph by David DeKok by permission of Yates County Historical Society*

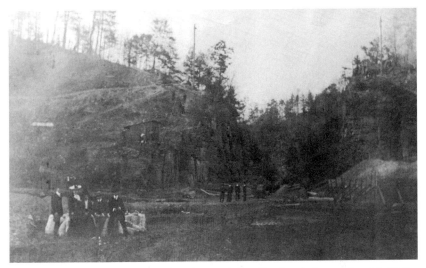

Ithaca residents, most likely Cornell students out for a Sunday stroll, pose for pictures in the future Six Mile Creek reservoir with their backs turned in the direction of Ithaca. The dam will rise in the gorge in the rear. *Marie Paula Geiss Scrapbook, Cornell University Rare and Manuscript Collections*

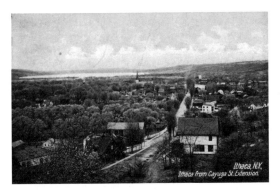

A view of Ithaca, New York in 1908. *Hugh C. Leighton Co.*

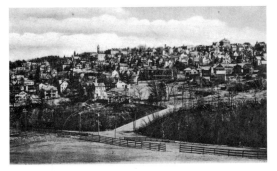

A view of East Hill, Ithaca, in 1905. Many of the people who became ill with typhoid during the epidemic, especially Cornell students, lived on the hill. McGraw Tower can be seen at upper left. *R.C. Osborne & Co., Ithaca, N.Y.*

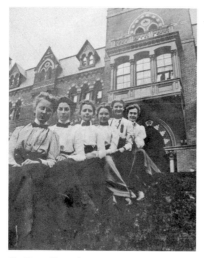

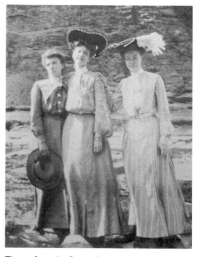

Six Cornell coeds pose on the balustrade in front of Sage College in a happier time. *Marie Paula Geiss Scrapbook, Cornell University Rare and Manuscript Collections*

Three female Cornell students in the gorge of Six Mile Creek near campus, ca. 1902. *Henry Crane Hasbrouck Memorabilia, Cornell University Rare and Manuscript Collections*

This photograph, taken Nov. 20, 1902, shows the valley where the Six Mile Creek reservoir will form after the dam is completed. Note the denuded hillsides, which offer little resistance to torrents of rainwater washing down. *Gardner S. Williams Collection, Bentley Historical Library, University of Michigan*

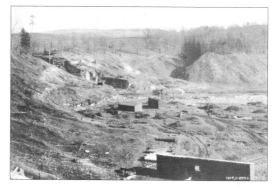

Students root for Cornell football team at Princeton game in the fall of 1902. *Marie Paula Geiss Scrapbook, Cornell University Rare and Manuscript Collections*

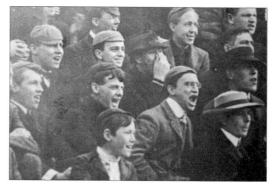

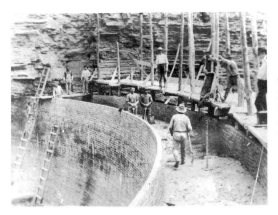

Workmen pour concrete to build the Six Mile Creek Dam in the summer of 1903. *City of Ithaca Department of Public Works*

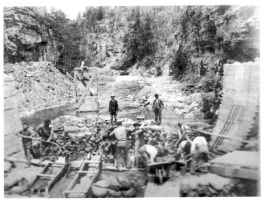

In the spring of 1903, Italian workers open two valves to allow Six Mile Creek to bypass the dam they are building for William T. Morris. *City of Ithaca Department of Public Works*

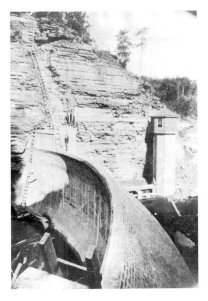

William T. Morris' dam on Six Mile Creek nears completion in the summer of 1903. Although originally planned as a ninety-foot dam, it was reduced to thirty feet to appease public opposition to the project. *City of Ithaca Department of Public Works*

Theodor Zinck ran a popular student tavern in Ithaca. His daughter Louise died in the typhoid epidemic and in despair, he drowned himself in Cayuga Lake. *The History Center of Tompkins County*

Graves of Theodor Zinck, his wife Emelie, and daughter Louise in Lakeview Cemetery, Ithaca, New York. *David DeKok*

By all accounts, the Junior Prom on Friday, February 6, was an event to remember. Carriages pulled up two at a time in front of the Armory to discharge the young men and women, and some not so young. Nearly seven hundred guests came in all. No expense had been spared on food for the sumptuous banquet or the elaborate decorations. Isabel Dolbier Emerson of Brooklyn wrote in her scrapbook, "Oh, that blissful night." Most of the boxes inside the Armory had been purchased by fraternities, but one of the few that wasn't had been purchased by Charles H. Blood. His guests included Rob and Laura Treman, Charlie and Mary Treman, William T. Morris, and some of Laura Treman's relatives from Detroit. Not for anything would they have missed this gala.

There was even a fountain on the center buffet table gushing water and illuminated by colored lights, in what today seems almost a deliberate affront to students dying of typhoid. The revelers danced the night away to the music of Patrick Conway and the Ithaca Band, unmindful of the suffering of their fellow students in the Cornell Infirmary further down East Hill. The scene brought to mind Edgar Allan Poe's story, *The Masque of the Red Death*, about a European prince and a thousand of his closest friends who lock themselves away in his palace and hold a decadent revel, thinking they have escaped the plague raging outside. Death finds them anyway.

At 11 p.m. that Friday night, as dinner was ending and the couples were preparing to move out to the dance floor in the Armory, Oliver Shumard died in the Cornell Infirmary, his father by his side. He was the first student to die in the epidemic, but not the last. The Junior Prom continued until morning, with the last revelers departing around 4 a.m. On Saturday morning, William Shumard paid $87 for a casket and embalming for his son and $15 for a hearse to carry the casket to the station. The fare home to Bethany was $80.74, covering both the father and the casket, plus $2 for a special transfer at Union Station in Chicago. At the funeral service in the unfortunately named Morris Chapel, six miles north of Shumard's home, an "immense audience" gathered. Flowers sent by his teachers and classmates at Cornell and by Dr. Frank Thilly brightened the gloomy chapel. The young man was laid to rest in the church cemetery.[47]

That Sunday, the church bells in Ithaca did not ring so their tolling would not disturb the suffering typhoid patients throughout the city.

They would not be rung again until the end of the epidemic.[48] Anyone who thought the suffering in Ithaca had peaked was wrong. It had barely begun.

Indeed, between January 24 and 29, eight inches of snow fell in the Six Mile Creek watershed and quickly melted, most likely causing a new invasion of typhoid bacilli into the water supply. It seems the most likely explanation for the many new typhoid cases in February that developed long after the original germs in the water supply should have died out.

Contrast the water samples collected by Dr. Emile M. Chamot at East Hill School and City Hall on January 27 with those collected at the same locations by Dr. Veranus A. Moore on February 10. The school sample contained 325 colonies of colonic bacteria per cubic centimeter on January 27 and 12,510 on February 10. For the City Hall samples, the count was 600 colonies per cubic centimeter on the first date and 28,980 on the second. "There are undoubtably fecal bacteria in both specimens," Moore told the Ithaca Board of Health, referring to the February 10 samples. "Bacteriologically, the water is very bad."[49] We don't know for certain there were typhoid bacilli in the February 10 samples, but the presumption is that there were.

Chamot and Moore believed they had found two active typhoid cases in Brookton, New York, further upstream on Six Mile Creek. The cases had been contracted in Ithaca early in the epidemic, and patient excrement was thrown in the snow at creekside.[50] Even if the contaminated excrement of the workers had all been washed downstream during the early January thaw, the sloppy handling of these cases might have been enough to reinvigorate the epidemic when the late January thaw occurred. It was Plymouth, Pennsylvania, all over again.

Some Ithaca residents began to shun the water or boiled it before using it for drinking or cooking. But others ignored the warnings or did not understand them, and so the epidemic lived on, gaining new strength and ferocity.

Chapter 10

Apocalypse

THE TRUE HORROR OF THE ITHACA EPIDEMIC was not in the total number of citizens afflicted with typhoid, but in the percentage of the population who became ill—one in ten by the time it was over. That percentage gave the real picture of how hard the community was being hit. Even in a city with a more favorable doctor-patient ratio than any in New York, the physicians, nurses, and medical facilities in Ithaca were strained to the breaking point and beyond. Typhoid erupted in Ithaca like nothing it had ever encountered or imagined in its worst nightmares.

Newspapers outside of Ithaca did the math and were horrified. The Philadelphia *Press* looked at the numbers early on, when only 342 people in the town of just over thirteen thousand were ill with typhoid, and calculated that one in thirty-eight Ithaca residents were battling the deadly disease. If Philadelphia, then the nation's third-largest city with about 1.3 million people, had been hit by a typhoid epidemic of similar intensity, some thirty-four thousand people would be ill. The New York *Evening World*, which sent two reporters to Ithaca in mid-February, was more sensational: "Confined as this fever pestilence is to so small an area and so limited a population, it is nearly as sweeping in its destruction of life as the 'Black Plague' of India."[1] Actually it wasn't—bubonic plague typically claimed far more victims—but it probably sounded right.

The fact that nine-tenths of typhoid patients recovered in that era was misleading in a couple of senses, because some survivors took months, even more than a year to regain their health and ability to work, and others became semi-invalids. One pioneer of typhoid research, Dr. William Budd of Great Britain, wrote in 1873 how typhoid took a terrible toll on the families of patients as well, since they could do little but wait and worry as their loved ones hovered between life and death. "The dreary and painful night watches—the great length of the period over which the anxiety is extended— the long suspense between hope and fear, and the large number of cases in which hope is disappointed and the worst fear is at last realized, make up a sum of distress that is scarcely to be found in the history of any other acute disorder," he wrote. "Even in the highest class of society, the introduction of this fever into the household is an event that generally long stands out in the record of family afflictions."[2]

From the patient lists published in the *Ithaca Daily News*, and to a lesser extent in the *Ithaca Daily Journal*, we cannot help but be drawn to the unfortunate homes where more than one person was ill with typhoid. One of the worst hit was the Theta Delta Chi fraternity house at 15 South Ave., where eleven of the brothers lay ill, including Ernest H. Greenwood, chairman of the Junior Prom committee. The Phi Delta Theta house at 125 Edgemoor Lane had five ill brothers, and the Chi Phi fraternity at 107 Edgemoor, to which William T. Morris and Ebenezer M. Treman of Ithaca Water Works still belonged, had two cases. The boardinghouse operated by Richard Wallace at 409 Huestis Street had five ill students and went out of business after the epidemic.

The mind reels at the calamity that struck the George family of 308 Lake Ave., where six members of the family were ill. They all survived, but what their lives were like afterward remains an uncomfortable mystery. At 408 N. Aurora St., Misses Claire, Helen, and Margery Chapman were all ill. Misses Alice and Lillian Van Zoil and their Cornell student roomers, Charles A. Williams and William H. Snowden, were bedridden at 101 Eddy St. At least they survived; at 201 Hazen St., student Otto Kohls, who had emigrated from Germany with his parents at age two, died on February 17, while John Vernon, a freshman from the Bushwick section of Brooklyn, died a week later. Their housemate, Austin F. Stillman, contracted typhoid but survived.

In the week following the Junior Prom, deaths occurred almost daily. The earliest patients were approaching the crisis phase of the illness, when their stricken bodies either began to recover or gave up the ghost and died. On February 9, Rev. John Frederick Fitschen Jr. of First Presbyterian Church in Ithaca conducted back-to-back funerals for typhoid victims Dean G. Robinson, twenty-one, and Edna Fulkerson, thirty-five, his own church secretary. A day later, Charlotte E. Spencer of Jasper, New York, became the second Cornell student to die. Her mother was at her side in the Cornell Infirmary when the end came. Two days later, another Cornell student died, Harry C. Francis Jr. of Philadelphia. So did Ithaca High School student Ruia Coon, eighteen. Her mother, Kate Coon, ran a boardinghouse at 142 S. Aurora St. Word of her death brought an abrupt end to the eleventh annual banquet of the Ithaca Cycle Club that night. On February 13, it was George A. Wessman, a Cornell junior from Passaic, New Jersey, who was a Pulitzer Scholar majoring in mechanical engineering. His mother helped with his nursing during the last week of his life. The youngest known victim of the epidemic, five-year-old Esther Howell, whose father, Charles C. Howell, was a member of Ithaca Common Council, died at home that same day after sixteen days of suffering.

Death from typhoid might come from intestinal perforation, intestinal bleeding, or even pneumonia. Perforation was agonizingly painful and led to death from septic poisoning as fecal matter escaped into the peritoneal cavity. Charles E. Helm, forty-six, a former carriage builder who had been a blacksmith on South Aurora Street in Ithaca since 1891, died at City Hospital of perforation. Dr. Robert T. Morris operated, but it was too late. He found a large intestinal perforation and evidence that septicemia had set in.[3] Similarly, if the typhoid bacilli ulcerated their way through an intestinal blood vessel, the victim could bleed to death, expelling half-clotted blood from the rectum. Physicians could sometimes save bleeding typhoid patients if they operated quickly, and nurses tried to be alert for symptoms. There might be a sudden drop in the patient's temperature, or a complaint of faintness or a sinking sensation. But if the bleeding was profuse, the patient might die from shock almost simultaneously with the gush of blood from the rectum.[4]

James C. Vinton, twenty-two, a senior mechanical engineering student from Canal Dover, Ohio, bled out in the early morning hours of February 14. A law student, Henry A. Schoenborn of Hackensack, New Jersey, died that way three days later. He had been the first law student to win a university scholarship. Already displaying symptoms of typhoid during exam week, the last week in January, Schoenborn struggled to complete his tests and then collapsed. He had been at the Cornell Infirmary since around February 3.[5]

~~~~~~~~~

It seemed like a demonic lottery, with the names of 10 percent of the patients picked to die horribly. Physicians in Ithaca and elsewhere had a variety of methods they used to treat typhoid, but there was no cure. Dr. David Stewart wrote in 1893 that "careful nursing is the one great essential" in management of a typhoid case. The nurse's duty was to keep the patient fed and clean and comfortable. Complete bed rest was essential, he wrote, and the patient's diet should be mostly liquid, especially diluted milk, to avoid further irritation to the intestines. Beef broth was highly recommended.[6]

Hattie M. Greaves, a typhoid nurse from Elmira, New York, wrote in 1906 that "the constant attention to all of the little things always gives the best results." Typhoid patients should have a large, well-lighted, and well-ventilated room kept at a cool temperature, clean sheets every day, plenty of cold water to drink, daily sponge baths, and a proper diet that did not irritate their damaged intestines. She stressed the need to always treat the typhoid patient kindly and with patience. "Typhoid patients are frequently in a dreamy state of partial consciousness, from which a harsh word might arouse them to the wildest frenzy." It was important, Greaves wrote, to keep typhoid patients in bed and lying down, especially during the critical third week of the disease when strain on the lower body caused by abruptly sitting up or standing might be enough to tear the damaged intestinal wall.[7]

Physicians had their favorite remedies. Dr. Stewart spoke highly of the "justly celebrated Brand method of baths." Dr. Ernst Brand was a general practitioner in Stettin, Germany, in the middle of the nineteenth century. He did not originate the idea of breaking the high fevers of typhoid with cold baths, but he turned earlier ideas into a system of treatment that became associated with his name. Brand's regimen called for fifteen-minute baths in sixty-five- to seventy-degree water every three hours, especially if the patient's temperature was over 102 degrees. An obituary in the *British Medical Journal* upon his death in 1897 said the baths were responsible for reducing the typhoid death rate in German and Swiss civilian hospitals from 20 percent of patients to between 6 to 13 percent.[8]

Stewart lamented that the Brand method was difficult to use in private practice, where patients were often seen in their homes, because it was simply inconvenient. An attendant was needed to draw the bath, lift the patient in and out of the tub, give the patient a rubdown while in the cold water, and reassure him that he wasn't going to die from the cold. Then there was the problem, he wrote, "of the prejudices of those near the patient, who cannot but look upon the cold bath in cases of illness as barbarous in the extreme, if not actually homicidal." Some physicians scorned the Brand method for this reason. Dr. Luzerne Coville of Cornell University asserted that the cold baths "used up the energies of the patient" and did nothing to eliminate the typhoid bacilli from the intestines. Proponents of cold bath therapy acknowledged all this but pointed to reduced death rates nearly everywhere it was used.[9]

Interestingly, the homeopathic physicians claimed somewhat more success than their allopathic brethren in treating typhoid. An article in the *Hahnemannian Monthly* later in 1903 described the work of Dr. Elma C. Griggs, who is said to have treated forty-two typhoid patients during the Ithaca epidemic without a death. She employed very different medicines from those the allopaths used, prescribing the medicinal herbs baptisia, bryonia, and belladonna, as well as arsenicum, which is derived from arsenic. Used in very diluted form, it is part of the homeopathic bag of tricks even today.

Griggs administered saline enemas to typhoid patients twice a day and credited these for "the escape of [most of her] patients from the prevailing hemorrhages." She gave them tepid baths instead of cold baths. None of her patients contracted pneumonia, the article asserted. "The doctor was careful not to wear out [her] patients, and they all recovered under [her] straight, old-fashioned homeopathic treatment."[10]

Ithaca City Hospital normally housed twenty-six patients but packed in as many as sixty-five during February, of whom about forty-eight were undisputed typhoid cases. Cots were shoved into every available space. The Cornell Infirmary was meant to house twenty patients and had about three times that on February 24, even after the first annex in a house at State and Quarry Streets was opened. A second annex was opened later in the new Stimson

Hall. Major Burdick at City Hospital put out regular appeals during the month for blankets, pillows, linens, flannel wrappers, slippers, men's night-shirts, and screens, which were portable dividers to create privacy around individual beds in the wards. Other appeals went out for food, including oranges and lemons, and chickens to make broth. Many people sent flowers to patients in the hospital, finally prompting a plea from the major that notes of sympathy were far less work for the overburdened nurses. He also asked for cash to pay bills and to pay down the large debt the hospital had incurred, suggesting that not all patients could pay upon discharge.[11]

Many in Ithaca opened their hearts and wallets to the plight of City Hospital and their fellow citizens. Helen M. Baker, a local socialite, organized a euchre party at the Lyceum Theatre to raise funds. Rev. William Elliot Griffis, who had two children of his own ill with typhoid, appealed to the public to drop off cash, linens, or hospital supplies at his First Congregational Church. His own church ladies were busy sewing for the hospital, and so were church ladies all over town. Individual donors, mostly anonymous, gave $3,000 to the hospital. Among the known donors were Franklin C. Cornell of Ithaca Trust Company, who gave $100, and Jared Treman Newman, codeveloper of Cornell Heights, who gave $50. It is impossible to determine whether Morris or the Tremans donated to the hospital. There is no record that they did or didn't.[12]

There were no public appeals to aid the Cornell Infirmary, where sloppy care contributed to a higher death rate among students who sought treatment there as opposed to City Hospital. Dr. Coville calculated that as of February 20, the death rate at the Sage infirmary (but not at the Stimson Hall infirmary annex) was 19 percent, significantly higher than at City Hospital, where it was 6 percent. Coville, who visited the infirmary regularly to treat students, was highly critical of how it was being managed by a three-member university committee that included no physician. Coville believed the terms of the Sage endowment of the facility prohibited the university from using its own medical school physicians to operate the infirmary. The committee did not appoint a medical adviser, Dr. Abram Kerr, a member of the medical school faculty, until February 17, by which point several students had died. Kerr's suggestions for improving care were ignored, and he quit the following day.[13]

Coville painted a stark picture of incompetent nurses and foul conditions in the Cornell Infirmary. On February 24, he wrote, some sixty ill students were crammed into space intended for a third of that. There was little ventilation, and the air was foul. Some nurses could not give proper baths or take a temperature or pulse correctly, a problem witnessed by a woman who visited Zella Marie Clark at her sickbed. Coville heard reports of thermometers being used on multiple patients without sterilization in between. Patients in one ward were bathed from the same bowl and with the same washcloth until one of them complained. Some nurses came back to the infirmary drunk from evenings out. There were no male orderlies, so if a stretcher needed to be carried or a bed moved, whoever happened to be there was drafted, be they physicians, college deans, parents, or students. One day the infirmary ran out of broth. Another day it ran out of clean artesian water, and more than fifty typhoid patients were without water for over five hours, Coville wrote. Desperate thirst is a hallmark of typhoid.[14]

For hundreds of other typhoid patients, home was where the hospital was. Of the approximately 1,350 typhoid cases during the Ithaca epidemic, many were treated at home by visiting physicians and nurses. One physician told the *Ithaca Daily News* that he made seventy-two patient visits on February 10. Medical personnel were bone tired, staggered by both the sheer number of patients and the shortage of trained nurses in Ithaca, which was only partially remedied by the importing of nurses from other cities. "Patients suffer for want of the many attentions which only a professional nurse can give," the newspaper noted.[15]

～～～～～～

But even with regular nursing, some typhoid patients died. Edwin Besemer was one. A widower, he lived with his ten-year-old daughter, Ethel, at 138 Giles St. When he fell ill at the beginning of February, father and daughter moved to the home of his brother, Arthur, who was a homeopathic physician in Dundee, New York. He stayed there until his death on March 3. A nurse attended Besemer during his four-week illness. Because an itemization of the costs of his treatment was filed with his estate in Tompkins County Surrogate Court, we know the methods his brother and a consulting physician, a Dr. Bryan, used to treat him.

Here is the list of purchases: February 4, nightshirt, bedpan, medicine, brandy, package of chloride of lime (a strong disinfectant, probably used to kill the typhoid germs in his excrement, clothing, and linens); February 7, nightshirt; February 11, medicine, brandy; February 12, bottle of grape juice, telephone call to Dr. Bryan, brandy; February 16, extra washing; February 17, bottle of grape juice; February 19, package of lime chloride, twenty yards of cheesecloth, which was probably used to hold the brandy against Besemer's skin in an effort to reduce his fever, and a bottle of some sort of homeopathic remedy; February 22, cheesecloth, brandy; February 23, cheesecloth; and February 24, one package chloride of lime and a bottle of Eucalyptol, a medicine with a variety of uses. After Besemer died on March 3, there were expenses for telegrams and telephone calls, rail fare for taking his remains back to Ithaca, and rail fare for Ethel, his daughter, to return to Ithaca for the funeral. The carpet in his room was burned, according to the itemization, as were four bed quilts, eight new sheets, and the mattress. Everyone seemed aware of the public health dangers of anything that came in contact with him.[16] Young Ethel, now an orphan, lived with her uncle in Dundee for a time and does not appear to have returned to school in Ithaca. She was one of many students in the Ithaca public schools who were hit hard by the epidemic, either through contracting the disease or by losing a loved one or a teacher.

On February 17, Frank David Boynton, the young and dynamic superintendent of schools in Ithaca, taking note of four deaths of students or recent alumni, urged students not to panic but rather to be cautious. He was referring to the deaths of Dean G. Robinson, twenty-one; Ruia Coon, eighteen, Jennie Berber, twenty-one, a 1901 graduate and now a teacher; and Willis J. Dean, seventeen.

Dean's funeral was held at his home at 436 N. Tioga St. Many of his classmates attended. The Ithaca High School Student Congress, of which he had been a member, sent flowers, as did the Philomathean debating society of Newfield, of which he was a member. Among his pallbearers was Stanton Griffis, the future U.S. ambassador to Argentina during the time of the Perons. But for now he was just a high school student doing a final service for a friend on a cold winter day. He and his fellow pallbearers, most of whom were Student Congress members, carried the lavender casket to its final resting place in Brookside Cemetery in Newfield, where graveside services were held.[17]

Four other members of the Student Congress at Ithaca High were ill with typhoid. Five teachers in the public school system were ill and had been replaced by substitutes, one of them Sarah Griffis, wife of Rev. William Elliot Griffis. Despite having two ill children of their own, they did not slack off on their social work.

Superintendent Boynton took immediate action when it became clear the city water was contaminated with typhoid germs. The Board of Health ordered some of these moves, but he required little urging. On February 3, after Professor Chamot's report to the Board of Health on the poor state of the water in East Hill School, Boynton sent a plumber to implement the board's order to cut off city water to all public schools except what was needed to flush toilets. The plumber, at Boynton's direction, even cut the pipes to drinking fountains and wash basins so there would be no accidents. The superintendent arranged for clean artesian well water to be brought in daily in new six-gallon tin pails with faucets.

Despite his precautions, many parents kept their children home from school, which frustrated him to no end. "There is less danger from infection from city water at school, where all fountains are closed, than at home, where a child can get water from any faucet," Boynton pleaded.[18] The *Ithaca Daily Journal* reported, without specifics, that some children were daring others to "drink a few germs" and that those who did were now ill with typhoid.

Parental panic was understandable. Children were still dying of typhoid. Not long after Boynton urged students to return to classes, Katherine Caveney, eleven, a student at the Catholic school, and Cesar Larrinaga, seventeen, an exchange student from Puerto Rico attending Ithaca High School, succumbed to the disease. In the last week of February, an average of ten people contracted typhoid each day, the legacy of that additional infusion of typhoid germs at the end of January. Rev, Griffis wrote in his journal on March 2, "The air is filled with farewells for the dying." They were not his own words—the American poet Henry Wadsworth Longfellow wrote them—but they perfectly captured the mood of Ithaca. No one seemed able to stop the epidemic, neither God nor man.[19]

Among the ill young people in late February was Louise Zinck, twenty-four, daughter of Theodor Zinck, owner of the popular Hotel Brunswick in downtown Ithaca, and his wife, Emelie. Lula as she was known, was their only child, and they idolized her. She was a talented piano player, a skill certain to warm the hearts of any middle-class Franco-German family, as the Zincks were. Lulu was the accompanist for the Ithaca High School choir at graduation ceremonies. She had a wide circle of friends, traveling as far as Syracuse for parties. Zinck's name first appears in the *Ithaca Daily News* as one of 449 typhoid cases on February 18. Her temperature reached 103 degrees on February 20. On February 21, she was "not as well today." Her cousin, Edmond Zinck, was reported critically ill with typhoid on February 23. Lula's condition did not improve and the next day she was dead, dead in the home at 416 E. State St. where she grew up. Theodor Zinck's world fell apart. He and Emelie buried her in Lake View Cemetery, and he went to see about his will. Louise Zinck was little different from many other typhoid sufferers in Ithaca that winter, but she became a symbol of all of them because of her father and his inconsolable grief.[20]

Chapter 11

The Fixer

THE ITHACA BOARD OF HEALTH CONCLUDED THAT the typhoid must have come into the city in the drinking water supplied by Ithaca Water Works. An order went forth the evening of February 3 that all water used for drinking or cooking in the city must first be boiled for five minutes to kill typhoid germs. The board snubbed the optimism of its own hapless health officer, Dr. Edward Hitchcock Jr. He professed to believe that people were already boiling their water and that as a result, the epidemic would soon be over. Joseph Utter, chairman of the Board of Health, did not believe the danger would go away until a water filtration plant was built in the city.[1]

Utter and his board set out to determine the cause (as opposed to the delivery vehicle) of the typhoid epidemic. They had no doubt that water from Six Mile Creek had poisoned the city but wanted evidence of how it became contaminated. One board member, Dr. Walter L. Williams, a professor of veterinary surgery at Cornell, decided to take a walk up Six Mile Creek to the dam site and have a look at the Italian camp. He reported back that the single latrine available to the workers sat on sloping ground barely twenty paces from the edge of Six Mile Creek. It was in filthy condition. After Williams's findings were publicized in both city newspapers, Shirley Clarke Hulse, the twenty-two-year-old engineer who had failed to enforce camp sanitation, flew into a rage and confronted the professor at his home. Hulse claimed in a letter to the *Journal* that Williams retracted his accusations. He hadn't. In a letter to the *Daily News*, Williams said his account was correct in every essential particular and called Hulse "a disgruntled official of the water company." Technically, Hulse wasn't, but he did work for Gardner S. Williams, the architect of the dam, and Tucker & Vinton, the construction firm.

The Board of Health hired two inspectors to patrol the watersheds of Buttermilk Creek and Six Mile Creek and determine if unsanitary conditions were polluting Ithaca's drinking water. They inspected Buttermilk Creek first and brought back an eye-opening report that showed how lackadaisical Ithaca Water Works had been under the Tremans and Morris in policing its watershed, an important duty for any water company. John R. Woodford and R. T. Conover told of farmyards that came to the water's edge, outhouses that drained toward the creek, manure piles by the water, and every other frightening aspect of early-twentieth-century farming. The conditions, which seemed to truly shock Ithaca's citizens, may have explained the mild intestinal disorders experienced by Cornell students when they arrived as freshmen, and Professor Emile M. Chamot said conditions in the Six Mile Creek watershed were as bad or worse. But the barnyards did not explain the typhoid epidemic.[2]

"Now that the conditions have been brought to light, will the citizens do something?" the Ithaca Daily News demanded to know. "The public will never again feel safe in drinking water that has come from such a source. There must be a radical change. . . . The city of Ithaca must take action and prompt action. There should be no halfway business."

The Daily News demanded pure water for Ithaca, preferably from artesian wells. Duncan Campbell Lee gave an impassioned speech at a public meeting against the idea of "filtering sewage," arguing for "a radical change in the source of supply." Lee said the only way to restore public confidence in Ithaca and calm public fears and anger was "to secure pure water and secure this water from the bowels of the earth."[3] This had been one of his crusades since buying the newspaper in 1899.

Ithaca Water Works fought back, beginning an aggressive campaign to persuade the public that the typhoid epidemic was not as bad as the Daily News claimed, and that in any case, the company was not responsible. Thomas W. Summers, who ran the water company for Morris, offered soothing words for the public, telling the Ithaca Daily Journal that the company took the epidemic seriously and was searching hard to find "any possible information that will throw light upon the cause of the epidemic. The investigation will be pursued vigorously until definite information is procured." Morris was not admitting—and never would—that the water he sold to Ithaca residents was killing them. But they would keep searching for the real killer.[4]

Morris sent an Ithaca Water Works agent to the homes of typhoid sufferers and subjected family members to questioning about how their loved ones contracted the disease. Meanwhile, the agent was on the lookout for anything in the house to blame for the sickness, such as water in the basement. The agent claimed that of the forty-eight homes he visited, only twenty-two had "real" typhoid. Ithaca Water Works rushed this spurious finding to the *Daily Journal*, which published it. Given the difficulty trained physicians had in making the typhoid diagnosis, one wonders how an untutored water company agent could do so with such certainty and without conducting any laboratory tests.

Morris also hired a real physician, Dr. John B. Hawes, to debunk the idea that Six Mile Creek water was responsible for the epidemic and to reassure the populace that the search for the real killer continued. Hawes, an Ithaca physician who also claimed to be able to cure diabetes by running electric current along a patient's spine, asserted that the typhoid epidemic sprang from unsanitary conditions in Ithaca remaining from a flood in December 1901. He made that claim even though, as a letter writer to the *Ithaca Daily News* soon pointed out, people had become ill with typhoid and died in a particular city neighborhood untouched by the flood.

Hawes's claim that the typhoid arose from dirt and filth derived from the "miasma" theory of disease, already discredited by many physicians in 1903 but still tenaciously clung to by others and easy for the public to misunderstand. In a letter to the *Daily Journal*, Hawes asserted there was no proof that typhoid germs were in the city water and suggested that Ithaca's epidemic was part of "a great wave of typhoid extending through a large section of Eastern states." Carried on the wind, perhaps? He offered no proof of that hypothesis but then again didn't need to. Hawes was hiding behind a weakness of 1903 science, namely that it was very difficult to *prove* a water sample contained typhoid germs, even if it obviously *did*, judging by the awful results of drinking it. It was not so hard to find typhoid in blood, and Dr. Veranus A. Moore already had through the Widal Reaction, but water was different.[5]

Dr. James Law of the Cornell Veterinary College, a Scot who was one of the professors President Andrew D. White recruited in Europe early in the university's history, tried to debunk the idea that "filth," which typically meant horse droppings, or flood mud in the streets was responsible for the typhoid. Horse manure in the streets was a serious public health problem for every American city and town in the pre-automobile years of the early twentieth century, and while the manure from thousands of horses could make life unpleasant and spread a number of diseases, typhoid was not one of them.[6] Yet it was hard to convince the public of that, conditioned by the miasma theorists for years to believe otherwise.

The discovery of a dead horse near Six Mile Creek by William Couch, who had two children suffering at home with typhoid, caused enormous concern. It was easy to believe, commonsensical really, that diseases like typhoid sprang from the foul decay of horses or their droppings or from odiferous mud carried in by a freshet. Weren't those nasty and foul-smelling things? That it was simply not true was yet a radical notion in 1903, as radical as some in our own century find the notion of global warming to be on days when the mercury plunges and the snow piles against the door. Certain parts of science are easy to slander. The Ithaca Board of Health believed Morris was willing to spend $10,000 to prove the epidemic was not caused by the water, and that made them angry and nervous.[7]

Ithaca Water Works even planted a false story in the *Ithaca Daily Journal* as part of its disinformation effort. The newspaper reported on February 23 that inspector Conover had found an active typhoid case along Six Mile Creek above the water company's intake pipe. Worse, the patient's outhouse stood directly along the creek and emptied directly into it. Case closed. The next day, the *Ithaca Daily News* called the story "a deliberate falsification," noting that Conover had not yet patrolled Six Mile Creek for active typhoid cases and so had made no report to the Board of Health. According to the *Daily News*, the *Daily Journal* reporter was told the story was false, yet wrote it anyway. The *Ithaca Daily Journal* published a retraction the next day, saying it had now learned from the Health Department that, apart from having a somewhat messy house, the patient, a woman, was suffering from nothing more than a bad cold. A finger was pointed at Ithaca Water Works, which the *Daily Journal* said had first reported the supposed typhoid case to the Health Department.[8]

Morris and Summers continued to push "filth in the city" as their explanation for the typhoid epidemic. Margaret Sheehy of 110 Osmun Place found that out when she went to the water company office at Green and Cayuga Streets to pay her bill. Ithaca Water Works had continued to send out advance billings for water during the epidemic, including to people like Edwin Besemer, who had already died of typhoid.[9] She spotted Summers and protested having to pay in advance for water that was unfit to drink. He told her the water was perfectly safe to drink without boiling, that no one had been able to find any germs in it, and that he and his family drank it unboiled in their own home.

Sheehy stormed out in a fury and went to the Board of Health to swear out an affidavit. Summers was hauled before an emergency meeting of the board, where he denied telling Sheehy that the city water was pure or that he and his family drank it unboiled, then admitted he might have said so in "a joking manner." The board was not amused, especially when Summers insisted that while people might assume the water was contaminated with typhoid, no one had proven it. At least partly in response to the incident, the Board of Health passed an ordinance making it illegal to drink unboiled city water or serve it to others. Violations carried a stiff (for 1903) $50 fine or fifty days in jail.[10]

The kicker was that Summers's own son, Richard, lay ill with typhoid in the family home at 122 W. Buffalo St. Perhaps it was corporate policy for him to tell Mrs. Sheehy that he and his family drank the water unboiled. If his family ever truly did that, we can assume or at least hope that they stopped after their son contracted typhoid. Richard Summers was not the only child or close relative of someone in Morris's inner circle to fall ill during the epidemic. Robert H. Treman's four-year-old son, Allen, was ill with typhoid. Charles E. Treman, Rob's brother, fled Ithaca for Europe when the epidemic took hold and did not return until it was over. Presumably his wife, Mary, and two-year-old son, Arthur, went with him. Another typhoid patient was Louisa M. Waterman, fifteen-year-old niece of Ebenezer M. Treman. Her uncle had arranged the sale of Ithaca Water Works to Morris at a price that was good for the Treman family but bad for Ithaca. Louisa lived with her mother, Jeannie Treman Waterman, and grandmother, Eliza Treman, in the latter's mansion at 210 N. Geneva St. Eliza was the widow of Lafayette L.

Treman, whose death in 1900 was the first step on the road to the epidemic. All three children recovered. Thomas W. Summers would not endure the exquisite agony of having a son die young of disease until 1923, when Richard, then twenty-eight, contracted polio on a camping trip in Maryland and died a few days later.[11]

Morris tried to stay in the shadows during the epidemic and operate through Summers, his trusted superintendent. His utility business took some hard knocks apart from the epidemic. Summers was injured and temporarily sidelined in a bizarre accident that occurred while he was standing on the train platform in Canastota, New York, waiting for his Ithaca connection. A large pouch of mail was thrown from a passing train and struck Summers in the head, knocking him to the ground and leaving him with cuts on his face and swollen eyes. Three days later, an explosion rocked Morris's Hornellsville Gas Light Company in Hornellsville, New York. One worker was seriously injured. But these were only temporary distractions. There was no sense that Morris harbored guilt or remorse over what he had done or that he saw any need to spend his own funds, which were depleted in any case, to help Ithaca recover. The typhoid epidemic, like Summers's accident or the Hornellsville explosion, was an inconvenience. It is probably safe to say that Morris wanted it all to go away so he could have his life back because that was the course he seemed to follow.[12]

President Jacob Gould Schurman, that remaining king of Ithaca, found himself in a dilemma that was Homeric in its scope and complexity. A typhoid epidemic was killing his students. The students still on campus (nearly a third, about a thousand, had fled) were increasingly restive and angry, demanding remedies, such as free artesian water delivered to their boardinghouses, that his Board of Trustees and especially the governing Executive Committee were not willing to provide. The Executive Committee was dominated by friends of Morris and in 1901 had arranged for Cornell University to invest $100,000 in Ithaca Water Works bonds so their friend could buy the water company. They showed no signs of backing away from him. And what about the fate of the university itself? Each student death was publicized around the country, and Ithaca was portrayed as a pestilential hellhole. Would any parent ever again agree to send his son or daughter to Cornell?

Schurman needed someone to make an intelligent investigation of how the epidemic came to be if he was to craft a way out of this mess. He wanted to know the present condition of the campus water supply, which came from Fall Creek, and how the campus and city supplies might be kept pure in the future. The Cornell president quietly asked Professors Veranus A. Moore and Emile M. Chamot to carry out the work, which they did forthwith, returning to him a week later with a cogent report that examined all realistic sources of the epidemic.

The two professors believed Six Mile Creek was the source of the epidemic and had been contaminated by the Italian workers on the dam. But they admitted that with the workers gone since mid-November, there was no way to prove the hypothesis conclusively. "The rocks and woods at and near the edge of the stream are reported to have been thickly sprinkled with human excrement and . . . the stream itself received directly much of their excreta. This condition was witnessed by one of us (Chamot) in the fall. At the time of our visit, February 12th, there was still evidence of such a condition." They received a letter from Holmes Hollister, an Ithaca businessman, describing what he saw the previous fall, and collected statements from three Cornell botanists who saw the foul condition of the construction site during plant-collecting hikes along Six Mile Creek around the same time.

They warned Schurman that Fall Creek, which provided the campus water supply, also passed through farming territory and was nearly as dirty as Six Mile Creek. Drinking it unfiltered was a disaster waiting to happen. The thing to do, the professors recommended, was to build a filtration plant for the water from one creek or the other, or to draw all water from artesian wells. Schurman released their findings to the public a few days later.[13]

Earlier in the month, Schurman had directed all professors, assistant professors, instructors, and assistants to read a notice to their students informing them that the typhoid came from the city water but that boiling could make it safe. "President Schurman would ask every student in the university to take this simple precaution and *see that it is enforced in his boarding house* (emphasis added)." Outright class issues are not common in this story, but this is one of them, summoning the image of an eighteen-year-old upper-class student giving a stern lecture to a middle-age, working-class landlady—and she meekly obeying. Just as odd is the assumption of Cornell University that telling landladies to boil water was sufficient to ensure that students did not get sick. As everyone quickly learned, neither wishing nor issuing orders would make it so.

On February 10, Schurman addressed a student meeting that filled Sage Chapel. He tried to minimize the typhoid epidemic, pointing out—as the university would for the next century—that no student who only drank the campus water from Fall Creek had become ill, as if that would make students who mostly lived off campus feel better. He praised coeds who resisted the pleas of their parents to come home and suggested that many students who had left Cornell since the epidemic began did so because they had flunked out or simply wanted some time off. The president, beginning his war against the newspapers, criticized "grossly exaggerated" claims in the press about the number of ill students. He insisted that students were as safe in Ithaca as they would be at home, provided that the water in their boardinghouse was first boiled to kill the typhoid bacillus. Schurman called it "a simple remedy."[14]

Despite the supposed safety of the Fall Creek water, the Executive Committee of the Board of Trustees decided on February 16 to supply artesian well water for drinking to all university buildings. This was done without much explanation, but the reason appears to be a letter Schurman had received from Gardner S. Williams three days earlier warning him that new tests of Fall Creek water showed it had nearly twice the bacteria count as Six Mile Creek. This did not mean typhoid was in the campus water, but it was hardly a clean bill of health. None of this was disclosed at the time. Students living off-campus—all of the men and some of the women—could either come on campus and carry artesian water back to their lodgings in jugs or make sure that their landladies boiled the water at the houses. To that end, the Executive Committee sent two of its members, Emmons L. Williams and Robert H. Treman, to exact signed pledges from the boardinghouse operators not to serve or use unboiled water on pain of being reported to the Board of Health and their student tenants moving elsewhere, assuming they could. Morris attended the meeting, which the *Ithaca Daily Journal* said involved a long discussion of whether Cornell University ought to be closed. The committee ultimately decided that if even one student stayed, the university would remain open, according to the newspaper.[15]

On the following day, unnerved and angered by the continuing illnesses and deaths, the senior class held an emergency gathering in Library Hall to make certain demands of the administration and Board of Trustees. High on their list was getting the same artesian water deal for their boardinghouses that the university had just given itself.

Leading the meeting was class president Floyd L. Carlisle, a debate champion who would go on to head one of New York's largest electric and gas utilities, Niagara Hudson, and be a leading, though principled opponent of President Franklin Roosevelt's utility reform legislation in 1935. Scores of Cornell students had become ill with typhoid and eight had died since the start of the epidemic, including two, Henry A. Schoenborn of Hackensack, New Jersey, and Otto W. Kohls of Rochester, New York, that very morning. A ninth student, Charles J. Schlenker of Batavia, New York, died in the infirmary even as the meeting got under way. Schlenker was a twenty-one-year-old engineering student who had been class president and captain of the football and track teams at his high school. All of Batavia mourned that night.[16]

In their petition, the students painted a grim picture of the apocalypse around them. Alarmed parents had summoned many of their fellow students home, and those remaining in Ithaca were "in a demoralized state." The petition dismissed the university plan to have students enforce the boiling of water in the boardinghouses as an impossible task and demanded that the university supply, at its own expense, artesian water to each of the student boardinghouses. They wanted enough for drinking, washing food and dishes, and brushing teeth. In addition, the students demanded the right to leave the university without penalty until water delivery was under way.

They typed the petition hastily—the version in the Cornell Archives has overstrikes—to get it to Schurman before he left for the day, as they hoped he would bring it to the Executive Committee meeting that night. They might as well have mailed it. The Executive Committee, which that night included Schurman, Samuel Halliday, Burt Lord, Roger B. Williams, Franklin C. Cornell, and Robert H. Treman, thanked the students for their concern, proclaimed that the university was doing its utmost to help them, and then voted it down. In a written response, the trustees said delivering water to student boardinghouses scattered across the city "seems to us well nigh impracticable." They also feared it would cause other, unspecified difficulties, "that would greatly embarrass us in the relief measures we are now pursuing," the meaning of which would become clear a day later. Much faith was placed in the boil-water pledges signed by the boardinghouse keepers.[17]

In an angry report to their fellow students, Carlisle and the other members of the senior class committee said the boardinghouse keepers "could not be trusted with the disinfection of water polluted with virulent disease germs." They said the university policy put student lives at the mercy of their landlords and landladies. "Every student who has lived in a boardinghouse or seen a student eating house kitchen knows the utter folly of expecting careful disinfection of the water, even if the university officials from time to time inspect the conditions."[18]

There had been much more to the February 16 meeting of the Executive Committee than a general discussion of whether the university ought to stay open. What had been hashed out was a plan for Ithaca Water Works, which was nearly broke, to build a filtration plant for the city using a $150,000 loan from the university. The city of Ithaca would need to approve higher water rates—they were already among the highest in the state—to pay for the filtration plant, but would be free to hold another referendum on the city taking over the water system or moving to artesian wells, as many, especially *Ithaca Daily News* publisher Duncan Campbell Lee, had advocated. Loaning more money to Morris seemed to some on the Executive Committee like throwing good money after bad, but Schurman believed there was no other choice if he was to be able to tell students and their parents that clean water would be available by the start of the fall semester.

Morris, whose people were still telling citizens that the city water was fine to drink, had agreed to the deal, in large part because Schurman used the $100,000 in Ithaca Water Works bonds held by the university as leverage to force him to go along. But the *quid pro quo* seems to have been that the university would not deliver artesian water to the student boardinghouses. If we go back to one of the reasons given by the Executive Committee in rejecting the student petition, *that [it] would greatly embarrass us in the relief measures we are now pursuing*, the logical conclusion is that the committee members denied clean artesian water to the students out of fear of antagonizing Morris, the monster they themselves created.

The Cornell president made a dramatic appearance before Ithaca Common Council on February 18 to announce the deal, more or less as a *fait accompli*. Council would have to accept the deal, Schurman believed. What other choice did it have? Because otherwise, Cornell University and all the economic benefit it brought to the city would be doomed.

In his comments to council and the public that night, Schurman ruled out artesian wells or Cayuga Lake as alternative sources of supply for Ithaca. He was not opposed to artesian wells, per se, but questioned whether they could provide the two million gallons per day the city needed. In any case, he doubted they could be ready by September 1, the deadline he imposed. As for Cayuga Lake, well, the lake was fed by streams running through the city, including Six Mile Creek, and was the receptacle of most of Ithaca's untreated sewage. The eyes of the nation were upon Ithaca, Schurman said, waiting for an answer to the question, "Is it safe?"

And now that he had Morris boxed into a corner, Schurman unleashed his rhetoric, holding Ithaca Water Works and its management responsible for bringing the typhoid calamity to Ithaca. Not for nothing did he have national renown as a speaker. "I shall not discuss the cause of the present epidemic nor the parties who may be morally and legally responsible for this disaster," Schurman said and then proceeded to do just that. "There is a general belief that it is caused by the water. I believe it is. It may not be possible to prove the water responsible, yet we believe it to be so. If it is, the officials of the water company are responsible." It was a remarkable speech, but there was more. "So far as the company is concerned," Schurman said, "we have no faith in their management. We insist, first, upon a representation on their board, to have the right to control the plant and patrol the watersheds."

Whatever he said was enough, or perhaps the council members truly believed they had no choice. There was much grumbling, both on council and among members of the public, about an option that forced them to drink "filtered sewage." They eventually focused on the part of the deal that gave them the right to take over Ithaca Water Works by eminent domain. They would fix this later. Council approved the deal that night and set a referendum on municipal water for March 2. Schurman praised the council action as "the salvation of the city" that would ensure that Cornell University would have a full complement of students in the fall.[19]

Schurman had not convinced the *Ithaca Daily News* that his way was the right way. Duke Lee did not abandon his support for moving the city to a supply of artesian water. He did not want filtration and believed most of the public was with him. As he wrote in his editorial the next day, "The point was also well brought out in last night's meeting that, no matter if a hundred chemists or a hundred engineers say that a filtration plant will cleanse the water, it will be impossible to make the public look at the matter in that light. No one will send his boy to Cornell and force him to drink filtered sewage; no one will believe that Ithaca has good water."[20]

~~~~~~~~

Schurman's troubles were far from over. As jubilant as he had a right to feel in fixing the deal for the filtration plant, he still had to win the battle of public perception. Yes, he could tell parents their children would have clean water by September 1, but the suffering and deaths among the students, let alone townspeople like Louise Zinck, had left a public stain not easily washed away. The sins of Ithaca were known to journalists up and down the East Coast, in every city and town that sent students to Cornell. Newspapers around the country were running wire stories about the epidemic. Calling the university to account for its sins was almost a reflexive act for the newspapers. Schurman complained that "among other things from which we have to suffer at the present time are the awfully sensational reports of the newspapers." Most of them were not, but they hurt and the worst was yet to come. Weeks later, he would be railing against "the misrepresentations and lies circulated by a sensational press." While the press made some mistakes, which is true of any big story, much of the coverage and editorials seemed to be accurate and fair.[21]

Schurman's most immediate antagonist in the press was the *Ithaca Daily News*, edited by Gannett and published by Lee. Almost from the very beginning of the epidemic, Duke Lee ordered up aggressive coverage that Gannett was only too happy to provide. The *Daily News* had published casualty lists and patient updates and kept its reporters busy rooting out stories in an unrelenting effort that angered some of Ithaca's downtown merchants. The newspaper even chastised its unnamed business critics ("What Matters the Ten-Cent Sale?") for caring more about profits than the people who provided them. On another occasion, the newspaper issued what we might today call a Schindler-esque statement of regret that it did not do more, did not make the warnings stronger, and was "not able to save the lives of the unfortunate ones for whom today many mourn." There were stories and hard-hitting editorials about the epidemic in the *Daily News* nearly every day. By the time the epidemic was over, daily circulation had climbed by 43 percent over 1902.[22]

A reporter on the *Daily News* staff, Lynn George Wright, who was a senior at Cornell, may also have been one of the stringers, perhaps the most important one, who fed stories about the typhoid epidemic to the Associated Press and to the various New York City dailies.[23] It is not possible to state this with absolute certainty, but the available evidence points in that direction. Wright's obituary in 1919 said he "earned money for his [Cornell] tuition by writing special articles for the city dailies." As a reporter for the *Daily News* and a student to boot, he would have been in a position to know what was going on during the epidemic. Wright was a friend and classmate of George Jean Nathan, who was a reporter that year on the *Cornell Daily Sun*. He gave Nathan his first job as a Broadway critic in 1906 after both had graduated, starting him on a distinguished career. Nathan was then a reporter for the *New York Herald* and Wright the editor of *Outing* and *Bohemian* magazines.[24]

What Schurman seemed to find most unbearable about the *Ithaca Daily News* coverage, though, was that it was done under the editorship of Gannett. Schurman had been a mentor to Gannett when the young editor was a student at Cornell in the late 1890s and hired him as his personal secretary when he went to the Philippines for President McKinley in 1899. He took it as a personal affront that Gannett was running the day-to-day operations of the newspaper that would not let the epidemic story go. On the evening of February 14, he made a remarkable telephone call to Gannett to protest what he claimed to have heard was the plan of the *Daily News* to force the closing of Cornell University.

This sounds like idle bitching among Ithaca's elite, but Schurman took it seriously. Gannett termed it slander and denied it in the strongest terms. After hanging up with Schurman, he gathered his reporters and made them sign a statement denying that they ever said the *Daily News* would "close down the university." Gannett stewed about Schurman's call into the following morning, when he heard the same rumor elsewhere. In his office, he typed out a long letter to Schurman, again denying any intent to close the university and defending, in a proud but wounded tone, the aggressive reporting of the epidemic by his newspaper. "Had we, like the *Ithaca Journal*, tried to cover up the epidemic, tried to make out that there was no great danger in our midst, and tried to defend the existing conditions, then we would have been open to censure, for neglecting our duty." He mailed the letter and included the notarized affidavit from the reporters, signed by A. T. Seaman, whose wife was ill with typhoid, Watson W. Lewis, Lynn George Wright, and Charles A. Stevens.[25]

Looking back more than a century later, the epidemic coverage by the *Ithaca Daily Journal* does not seem quite as starkly one-sided as Gannett sought to portray it. The question of whether the *Journal* would have written the same volume of coverage in the absence of an aggressive competitor can never be answered, but apart from some glaring exceptions, most of the *Journal* coverage was acceptable, and some was first-rate. Those exceptions included the bogus story about the supposed typhoid case on Six Mile Creek and an article, "Fever Stories Exaggerated," which claimed the real number of typhoid cases was less than half that reported by the *Daily News*. For that story, the newspaper had even tried to find physicians willing to debunk the idea that the typhoid came from the water, an effort that largely flopped. Dr. Alice Potter of Ithaca told the reporter that while some past epidemics around the country were supposedly linked to stirring up filth by tearing up streets for paving or laying sewers, all indications here were that the typhoid came from the water. It is very true, however, that on the rare occasions when Morris wanted to say anything to the press, he turned to the *Daily Journal* as a friendly venue.

The *Journal*'s editorials were another matter. Again, they did not entirely ignore the reality of the epidemic but tended to be slanted sharply toward the interests of Ithaca Water Works, Cornell University, and the Treman family. They often stressed the personal responsibility of typhoid patients for their own misfortune, such as one written at the beginning of Lent that stated, "Our people are in grief; mourners go about the streets, we have reason to mourn for our sins of negligence and carelessness, and we know that we have." The editorial was not talking about the Ten Commandments.

Brainard G. Smith, the editor, had written this and other *Journal* editorials. He had been a reporter for Charles Dana's *New York Sun* for nearly fifteen years. It was a good place to learn the trade, known as "the best school of journalism" and "the newspaper man's newspaper."[26] There is no reason to doubt he was a good journalist, but he was working for two owners, George E. Priest and Charles M. Benjamin, who were close to the Treman family. Even when Benjamin's wife contracted typhoid early in the epidemic, the *Daily Journal*'s slant did not noticeably change. That was especially true when the *Cornell Daily Sun*, the student newspaper, and the New York City newspapers began to harshly criticize Cornell University and its Board of Trustees for their mishandling of the epidemic. The *Ithaca Daily Journal* responded in righteous fury, defending Cornell University and the Tremans like a mother bear her cubs.

The anonymous "ALUMNUS" letter published in the student newspaper on February 18 was the first shot in a barrage of harsh criticism of the university. The letter writer, who is unknown, professed to be shocked to learn that Cornell University owned $100,000 worth of Ithaca Water Works bonds and suggested that that investment explained the university's lackadaisical response to the epidemic.[27]

Schurman was livid. In a speech to students the next day in the Armory, he raged, "No statement has stung me more because none was more infinitely criminal." He insisted that a bondholder had no control over a corporation's policy, which was technically true but largely irrelevant given the size of Cornell's debt holdings in Ithaca Water Works and the critical role the university played in making sure Morris had enough money to buy the company from the Treman family in 1901 (one half expects Schurman to grow a Pinocchio nose given the fact he had just used that very leverage to force Morris to build the filtration plant). The *Ithaca Daily Journal* attacked "ALUMNUS" in nearly as strong terms, accusing the letter writer of "foolish" and "silly" utterances and claiming that every educated person should know that a bondholder does not have any control over a corporation. The editorial offered a series of examples that were far removed from the close relationship that existed among the Executive Committee, the Treman family, and Morris.

In the same speech, Schurman partly conceded to the key student demand, saying that, if the students arranged to have artesian water delivered to their boardinghouses, the university would pay for it. He said that the Sage College gymnasium would be converted into a men's dormitory for the duration of the epidemic and that as many as three hundred men could be accommodated there, far fewer than the potential need. And conceding to another student demand, Schurman waived all penalties for students who left campus until the epidemic was over, saying they could make up their classes in the summer.[28]

Now the ball was in the student court. Should they accept the filtration deal, or rather give it their approval? They held their own meeting with their own leaders a day later. The more radical of them, especially Manton M. Wyvell, a law student who had traveled with William Jennings Bryan when he campaigned for president against William McKinley in 1900, did not trust Ithaca Water Works. Wyvell called the water company "an interested party" and doubted that it would carry out its pledge to build a proper filtration plant. But moderation prevailed, and the students in the end voted unanimously to endorse Schurman's plan for filtration. They did urge that the shanty and latrine used by the Italian workers at the dam site be burned but rejected the idea of doing it themselves.[29]

Schurman's press woes were only beginning. The *New York Sun* printed a story on February 19, probably sent in by a student stringer in Ithaca, naming six members of the Cornell Board of Trustees who were "directly or indirectly interested in the Ithaca Water Works Company, which has been furnishing Ithaca with its polluted water." The trustees named were Charles E. Treman, Robert H. Treman, Mynderse Van Cleef, George R. Williams, who was president of First National Bank of Ithaca and Duke Lee's father-in-law, Roger B. Williams, and Charles H. Blood. Someone had been doing his homework.

The *Ithaca Daily Journal* blasted the *Sun* article in "A Dastardly Outrage," and it said the six trustees named were "among the most public-spirited, enterprising, and reputable citizens of Ithaca." Smith's typewriter was on fire as he leveled accusations at his old newspaper. He could not imagine that someone from Ithaca, or even worse, from Cornell University was responsible for filing such a story with the *Sun*. No, it must have been scandal-mongering reporters from New York City who cooked up the story. "The good name of reputable citizens and the honor and reputation of the University are as nothing to such fellows," Smith wrote. "Working in the dark, hiding behind the newspapers that are deceived by them, they do their dirty work and draw their dirty pay."[30] Smith may have had some issues with his old newspaper.

Schurman began to push back and scored an early success. The *New York Tribune,* which the Cornell president considered "staid and conservative," wrote an editorial on February 20 saying that someone in Ithaca was responsible for the epidemic, because "seldom, if ever in the history of this nation has there been a more inexcusable outbreak of pestilence than that which is now decimating the student body of Cornell University." It took the university to task for failing to use all the knowledge possessed by its faculty to head off the calamity. Finally, misreading the *New York Sun* story, the *Tribune* mistakenly called Cornell University "a large and influential *stockholder* in the water company which has been supplying the polluted and deadly water" and thus handed Schurman a tool to divert attention from the facts of the situation. Had the *Tribune* termed Cornell "a large and influential *investor,*" the description would have been accurate.[31]

Who made the first call is unknown, but Schurman met with a *Tribune* reporter later that day and managed to persuade him that the Executive Committee's rejection of the student demand for artesian water for their boardinghouses had nothing to do with the university's ties to Ithaca Water Works. "Dr. Schurman's statements sweep away a flood of misleading dispatches and give cheerful assurance for the future," the *Tribune* wrote the following day in what can only be considered a retraction of the editorial.[32]

Schurman persuaded the Board of Trustees at the February 21 meeting to issue a statement to the media containing the points he made to the *Tribune* reporter. It went more or less like this: 1) no one on the board is a stockholder in Ithaca Water Works; 2) no student who drank only the campus water drawn from Fall Creek developed typhoid; 3) we have provided clean artesian water on campus. Students just need to come and get it, or they can drink city water in their boardinghouses that the proprietors have promised to boil; and 4) students in the infirmary are cared for by fifty professional nurses, and we update parents daily by letter on their conditions.[33]

There was no mention 1) of the $100,000 in bonds of Ithaca Water Works held by the university, or Cornell's critical role in financing Morris's acquisition of the company in 1901; 2) that no one was saying Fall Creek was the source of the typhoid and that only a tiny fraction of students used it as their primary water source; 3) that students didn't trust the boarding-house landlords and landladies to honor their pledges to boil all water; and 4) that many of the nurses working in the infirmary, according to Dr. Luzerne Coville, were not well-trained professionals.[34] Interestingly, the university in its official statement did not claim the students in the infirmary were getting good care, although that claim was made unofficially. Dr. Coville ultimately resigned from the medical school faculty over his differences with the university regarding the management of the infirmary.[35]

At a Cornell University alumni banquet in Buffalo that night, Dean Thomas F. Crane spoke of the "cruel falsehoods and slanders" circulated by the East Coast press. Crew coach Charles Courtney, who had kicked five students off his team in 1897 before the all-important Poughkeepsie Regatta for eating strawberry shortcake, raged that it was the duty of every friend of Cornell to defend the university from the "scandalous attacks" made upon it, especially by a student stringer he did not identify. He called the student leaders who had pushed for the artesian water deliveries "hair-brained," reserving his greatest scorn for "this hair-brained student [Manton M. Wyvell] who went kiting around the country two years ago with the Democratic candidate for president and his head was swollen out of all proportion to his ability." Courtney's rant only stopped when the alumni "jumped to their feet, waved napkins, and cheered themselves hoarse."[36]

~~~~~~~~~~

That day, Henry R. Ickelheimer, a prominent German-Jewish investment banker in New York City and a member of the Cornell Board of Trustees, telegraphed Adolph S. Ochs, publisher of the *New York Times*, and asked him to give the board's statement on the epidemic a good spot in the Sunday edition of the newspaper. Ochs, who had owned the newspaper for only seven years since buying it out of bankruptcy for $75,000, was at a dinner and did not receive the telegram until late Saturday night. According to Ickelheimer's account, Ochs immediately telephoned his newspaper, spoke to the editor in charge, possibly the night editor Carr Van Anda, and arranged for the statement to be run on page one of the second section, guaranteeing it would be seen and read by many.[37] The statement also appeared in many other newspapers around the country, from the *Baltimore Morning Sun* to the *Fort Wayne Morning Journal-Gazette*.

Schurman worried about all the newspaper attacks but seems to have worried most about those from the *New York Times*. While the *Times* did not occupy quite the lofty position in 1903 that it does today, it was moving in that direction and its editorials carried more weight than most. A *Times* editorial on February 18 called the Ithaca epidemic "very much like a crime," and one on February 20 blasted the university for its mismanagement of the Cornell Infirmary and the substandard medical care it provided to students.

Ickelheimer, who in 1905 married Pauline Lehman, granddaughter of the founder of Lehman Brothers, was an 1888 Cornell graduate who may have been the only Jewish member of the Board of Trustees in 1903. It is difficult to make that determination with certainty today, but there is no doubt that Ickelheimer was Jewish and few other trustees were. Partly for that reason, Schurman turned to him for help in dealing with Ochs, who was also Jewish. Whether this was out of practicality or prejudice or both is hard to say. Schurman had not seen the Sunday *Times* on February 22 and wrote to Ickelheimer the following day asking him to pay a call on Ochs and "stop all those unwarranted attacks." Schurman urged Ickelheimer to explain to Ochs that the criticism he was hearing about the Cornell Infirmary had a surprisingly simple explanation: professional jealousy on the part of Ithaca physicians who did not have as many students in their practices as other physicians did. This seems to have been grounded in as much fact as his belief that Gannett was trying to shut down the university. He was certain that if Ochs understood this salient point, "he would probably look at the matter with different eyes."[38]

Ickelheimer wrote back that he telephoned Ochs that afternoon and spoke to him at length. Ochs promised to help Cornell University if he could and asked Schurman to write him a letter if there were any particular facts he wanted brought to the public's attention. The publisher advised Ickelheimer, though, that the information the *Times* had published from Ithaca seemed to have come from reliable sources. Nevertheless, Ochs promised to gladly run corrections if warranted. Ickelheimer wrote to Schurman, "Mr.

Ochs is a fair-minded man, and means to do what is right, and if you have time, when you are in New York again I think it would be well worth your while to pay him a visit."[39]

But nothing seemed to change. The *Times* ran another editorial on February 26 that drove Schurman up a tree, saying that the organization of the Cornell Infirmary was "very inefficient," especially when full of typhoid patients. The editorial criticized the Cornell faculty, especially the medical faculty, for not jumping in to help when the first typhoid case appeared. "If they were afraid of the displeasure of President Schurman and the Trustees, they showed a timidity which brave men cannot respect and frank critics of their course cannot commend." The *Times* even recommended the indictment of Ithaca Water Works for maintaining a public nuisance. Schurman wrote to Ickelheimer two days later complaining that the *Times* had been "atrociously unfair" and again speculated that the newspaper was being deceived by Ithaca physicians with an ax to grind.[40]

James C. Bayles, a journalist and sanitarian with a long and varied career, was probably the author of the *Times* editorials about the Ithaca epidemic. He joined the newspaper as an editorial writer in 1889 after spending two years as president of the New York City Board of Health. He was bothered by the contradictory information he was hearing about the typhoid epidemic and proposed to Ochs that he go to Ithaca, spend a few days there, and write a series of articles about what he found. Ochs was reluctant to send him, fearing that wading into the controversy would result in articles that "gave advice," which he did not want his newspaper to do. Nor did Ochs want the *Times* to be seen as "a meddlesome journal." But Ochs agreed to run the idea past Ickelheimer, whom he then summoned to his office for a meeting with himself and Bayles.

Ickelheimer considered Bayles nearly a hopeless case when it came to the epidemic. He believed the editorial writer was paying too much attention to the opinions of "Dr. Biggs" but did not specify whether he meant Dr. Chauncey P. Biggs, a physician in Ithaca, or his brother, Dr. Hermann M. Biggs, who was the general medical officer of the New York City Board of Health and who had studied with Dr. Robert Koch in Germany many years earlier. More likely it was the latter Biggs. After a long conversation, Ochs decided Bayles could go to Ithaca as long as Schurman invited him.

Ickelheimer, despite his doubts, thought it might be better to have Bayles see conditions for himself rather than continue to write editorials based on what he heard from Dr. Biggs or others. "Mr. Ochs tells me that he is more than favorably disposed towards Cornell, but thought that he was doing his duty by setting forth the facts, as they were presented to him, as it might in the end be in the interests of [Cornell University]," Ickelheimer wrote to Schurman.[41]

Schurman responded to Ochs with alacrity, even inviting Bayles to stay at his home. Ochs telegraphed back thanking him for the invitation, but politely declined, saying Bayles would stay with relatives. Schurman fretted about Bayles's visit, believing he would only write articles that supported his *Times* editorials. But he needn't have worried. Bayles was not a physician and was only as good a reporter as the information people gave him. In Ithaca, Schurman could at least attempt to steer him to the right people.[42]

Almost in spite of himself, President Jacob Gould Schurman had extracted Cornell University from a seemingly impossible situation. He had persuaded Ithaca Common Council to accept a plan for filtration of the town's water that many of the citizens despised, preferring to drill for artesian water, and he had stopped much of the negative commentary in the press that might have killed the university. Yet the disease had not run its course and his students continued to die, often in the homes and home-towns they thought would be a refuge from the calamity in Ithaca.

Chapter 12

Going Home

WHEN THE REALITY OF THE TYPHOID EPIDEMIC HIT HOME in early February 1903, Cornell University students began fleeing Ithaca by train, hoping to escape the plague that was killing their classmates. They arrived by carriage at the downtown station with hastily packed suitcases or trunks, uncertain if they would ever be coming back.

Some, still healthy, acted on their own fears or, more often, those of their parents. A few in this group audited classes at other colleges so as not to fall behind in their studies. Sixteen did so at Columbia University in New York City, where President Nicholas Murray Butler welcomed them, while others landed at the University of Pennsylvania in Philadelphia. Some leaving Ithaca were already ill, sent home by physicians too burdened with typhoid patients who could not leave or wanting to remove them from the horrible student infirmary.[1] For too many, fleeing to the supposed safety of their homes proved to be an appointment in Samarra. Death found them anyway.

Graham B. Wood, the freshman from Camden, New Jersey, who had written to his father in the fall about the thrill of attending his first Cornell football game, contracted what seemed to be a mild- to moderate case of typhoid on February 6. For three weeks, Wood was cared for in his room at 220 Eddy St. by a local physician. His roommate, Charles Worthington Nichols Jr., soon decamped to Camden and escaped the epidemic. When Wood seemed well enough to travel, his mother came to bring him home, and they traveled by train to Camden. He seemed to be okay. His father,

Jarvis A. Wood, an advertising executive with N. W. Ayer & Son, Philadelphia, thought his son's troubles were over. But his seeming recovery turned out to be "but a lull in the battle," the elder Wood wrote to President Schurman. Graham soon developed intestinal complications of typhoid, and surgery became imperative. His father hired one of the best surgeons in Philadelphia, a city famous for them. The surgeon "found his gallbladder full of the poisonous pus" and removed it. The wound seemed to heal, but weeks later, Graham suffered a relapse, bled out his rectum, and died. Jarvis A. Wood, an especially loving father, was prostrated with grief.[2]

For others, the journey home itself could be fraught with peril. Frank A. Mantel, who had been captain of the Auburn High School baseball team and was considered a top prospect to play second base for Cornell that spring, felt the symptoms of typhoid arrive and started for home. He arrived at the Auburn station in a driving snowstorm and could find no carriage to take him to his home on Garden Street. So as weak as he was from the typhoid, Mantel staggered home in the snow, arrived half dead, but in time began to recover. A fellow student, Fred W. Sieder, visited Mantel in Auburn while attending the funeral of Paul Wanke, twenty-two, a graduate student in Germanics who was one of the best handball players at the university. Six Cornell students were pallbearers, and Professor Waterman Thomas Hewett asked Sieder to represent the German Department at the funeral. It cannot have been entirely comforting to Mantel to receive a visit from someone attending the funeral of a fellow typhoid sufferer. But Sieder extended President Schurman's best wishes and reported back to the Cornell president that it appeared "Mantel will pull through." He did but did not play baseball that spring and did not return to Cornell.[3]

Charles S. Langworthy, twenty-two, a young farmer from East Valley outside of Alfred, New York, was at Cornell that winter for an agricultural short course. He developed symptoms of typhoid, as did his Cornell roommate, Edward V. Green of Alfred, and was advised by his physician to go home. Leaving at the beginning of February, Langworthy missed his connection to the Erie Railroad train at Elmira, New York, and was forced to stay overnight, whether in the waiting room of the train station or a hotel, we do not know. In any case, the exertion and cold were not good for him. By the time Langworthy reached home the next morning, his symptoms had worsened. For a time, like Graham Wood, he seemed to be recovering. But his condition abruptly deteriorated, and he bled to death on February 21 in the usual way. Green, his roommate, came home to Alfred on February 11 and eventually recovered from his own case of typhoid.

Word of Langworthy's death was passed from "one to another" in East Valley, according to the obituary in the Alfred *Sun*. He was popular, admired for his character, and his neighbors and friends packed his funeral at the Second Alfred Seventh-Day Baptist Church, where his father was a life deacon. Charles had been one of six children. His only brother died of diphtheria at a young age, and his four sisters eventually married and moved away. With no surviving son to take over the land the Langworthy family had farmed since 1825, his elderly parents sold it in 1928.[4]

Even if students made it home without incident, there was no guarantee their parents would make the right decisions about their medical care. Lewis K. Hubbard went home to Middletown, Connecticut, with symptoms of typhoid that soon developed into a full-blown attack. Instead of calling a regular physician, his father, Robert P. Hubbard, had him treated by Flavia A. Thrall, a renowned clairvoyant healer from Windsor, Connecticut. Her supposed gifts of prophecy and healing first manifested themselves at age fourteen, when she laid her hands on a neighbor's sick child and the youth recovered. Thrall's parents, perhaps not surprisingly, feared she was mentally ill. Thrall would go into a trance, diagnose the disease, and prescribe a cure, usually an herbal medicine concoction. That was what she did for Lewis K. Hubbard, who wasted away and finally died on the day after Thrall left for Florida. There was talk of prosecution, but Thrall continued to practice her unique brand of medicine until her passing in 1910. Hubbard's good friend, Quincy A. Hall, who lived with him in a boardinghouse at 203 Stewart Ave., collapsed upon hearing news of his death and was taken to the infirmary.[5]

~~~~~~~~

President Schurman eventually admitted that the number of students who fled Ithaca was nearly a thousand, or a little over a third of the university's enrollment that spring. Samuel D. Halliday, chairman of the Board of Trustees, said the number was "at least a thousand." There indeed may have been more: The Ithaca Post Office reported on February 17 that more than a thousand change-of-address forms had been filed by students to date, and they were not the last to leave.[6] Many agonized about missing classes, fearing they would fall behind or be penalized, but they were filled with dread over the deadly typhoid.[7] Schurman at first tried to downplay or even criticize the departures, terming many of them grade- or laziness-related and praising the stalwart women of Sage College who seemed especially reluctant to leave.[8] But after a student census conducted on February 13, he conceded that 21 percent of the student body, or about five hundred students, had gone home. That number doubled in the next week as death followed death.

Parents in 1903 proved no less concerned about their children away at college than they are today. The Western Union office in Ithaca was swamped with incoming telegrams, mainly from parents urging their children to leave Cornell and come home at once. Even that relatively new communications technology, the long-distance telephone call, received a workout during the epidemic. New York and Pennsylvania Telephone and Telegraph Company, which eventually became part of AT&T, reported that during the first twenty-three days of February there were more long-distance telephone calls into and out of Ithaca than at any other city in its territory. Long-distance telephone service began in 1885 for AT&T but did not become widely available until 1899, when loading coils were invented, which boosted the signal and allowed construction of longer telephone lines. A call between New York and Chicago cost $9 for the first five minutes, an enormous sum at the time.[9]

Parents wrote frequently to Schurman requesting updates on the epidemic or the condition of their children, and from an examination of the university archives, he must have replied to nearly all of them. Orris B. Dodge, a plow manufacturer in Dixon, Illinois, who had just donated land and money for a public library where a new arrival in town, the nine-year-old Ronald Reagan, would obtain library card #3695 in 1920, wrote to the Cornell president on February 18 after reading in the Chicago papers that morning that the number of typhoid cases in Ithaca was increasing. His son, John O. Dodge, was a junior at Cornell studying mechanical engineering. "While I would regret exceedingly to have his work interrupted, it does not compare with the risk of life that may occur any day," Dodge wrote. "I, therefore, wired him this morning that I thought he better return home at once." He wasn't sure how John's course work or tuition fees would be handled if he came home, so he asked Schurman to send a messenger to his son and ask him to call on the president for a chat. "I am aware that at a time like this you would have a great many calls upon your time but would esteem it a great favor if you will give this matter your personal attention," Dodge concluded.[10]

George B. Rose, a partner in the law firm of Rose, Hemingway & Rose of Little Rock, Arkansas—which became famous as the "Rose Law Firm" during the American far right's obsession with Bill and Hillary Clinton's failed Whitewater land deal in the 1990s—wrote to Schurman on February 24. His son, Clarence E. Rose, was a sophomore at Cornell studying mechanical engineering. Young Clarence had become ill with typhoid earlier in the month and returned home to Little Rock. Rose told Schurman that his son wanted to return to his studies "as soon as his health and the sanitary conditions at Ithaca will permit. Kindly let me know the prospects of an early abatement of the typhoid fever epidemic."[11]

Not every parent who wrote to Schurman was a wealthy executive or lawyer. Hattie E. Cochrane of Newington Junction, Connecticut, was a widow inquiring about the condition of her only child, a son who is not identified in the letter. She asked when he became ill with typhoid, whether he was delirious, if his case was considered serious, and whether she could come to nurse him during the day. "I have had typhoid fever myself and know that much depends on the use of water in nursing. Frequent sponging is a great comfort to the patient, and I could do that as well as a trained nurse," Cochrane wrote. Schurman telegraphed back two days later, reporting that her son had been admitted to the infirmary on March 10 and that his maximum temperature had been 104.2 degrees. "Case rather severe, but responds well to treatment," he wrote. "You may come and assist." There is no record of a Cochrane from Connecticut in the 1908 Cornell alumni directory, suggesting that he never completed his degree.[12]

George G. Cotton, an executive in charge of worker training at the Solvay Process Company in Solvay, New York, a chemical manufacturer, wrote to Schurman to tell him that his son, Donald Reed Cotton, a second-year law student at Cornell, was being treated for typhoid in the Hospital of the Good Shepherd, an Episcopal hospital in Syracuse, New York, then considered the city's best. Donald was a member of the Psi Upsilon fraternity at 1 Central

Ave. Former Cornell president Andrew D. White was a Psi U member, as was his grandson, Andrew White Newberry. Cotton said his son had no idea how he contracted the disease. The fraternity had been paying for artesian water, known as Slaterville water, since the fall. He told Schurman his son thought he might have gotten some city water in his mouth while taking "shower baths" at the fraternity house.

Cotton wrote his letter after hearing from his wife that morning that Donald had spent a comfortable night in the hospital and had been "tubbed"—given an ice bath—every three hours for the past three days. Another second-year law student from Syracuse, Warren S. Barlow, was in the same hospital with typhoid acquired in Ithaca, but he was not doing nearly as well. Barlow, although somewhat improved that morning, was in his third week of the disease and had a severe case. His temperature had soared to nearly 105 and his pulse as high as 150, Cotton wrote. Both young men survived.[13]

A mother of a Sage College coed wondered how her daughter could have contracted typhoid to begin with given the university's bragging about the safety and good health of students who lived in the women's dormitory. Mary D. Huestis, whose husband, George, was a shirt and collar manufacturer in Troy, New York, complained to Schurman that her daughter, Edna, a freshman, had come home from Cornell on February 18 and was soon bedridden with typhoid. Other than three days in the Cornell Infirmary in mid- to late January with tonsillitis, she had consumed only the food and water served to her at Sage College. What was going on, her mother wanted to know.

A week later, Schurman ordered a full-scale investigation, seemingly motivated by a letter he received from Charles S. Francis, editor and publisher of the Troy *Times* and a former United States ambassador to Greece and the Balkans. Francis asked about Edna Huestis and mentioned that his own two daughters had had a rough experience with typhoid when they lived in Athens. Schurman contacted Margaret Harvey, warden of Sage College, and ordered her to investigate how Huestis might have developed typhoid. Whether this was Schurman's intent is unknown, but Harvey, who already believed Huestis to be a problem, set out to pin the blame on the young woman's own behavior over the previous few weeks.[14]

Harvey was in her first year at Cornell, having been hired away from Chestnut Hill Academy in Philadelphia to be the warden, or housemother, of Sage College. Sage, as noted previously, was a dormitory for female students at Cornell and not, like Radcliffe or Barnard at the time, a separate degree-granting institution with a close affiliation to an all-male college. Huestis liked to party, which was no secret, and Harvey interrogated her friends, especially fellow members of the Kappa Kappa Gamma sorority. She looked for evidence to bolster an argument that Huestis's own bad behavior was to blame for her contracting typhoid.

She told Schurman that Huestis had been in a "weak, run-down condition, unable to do her university work or to take her examinations both before and after her stay in the infirmary" for tonsillitis. A premed student in her sorority had even urged her to go home, but Huestis refused, not wanting to miss out on Junior Week. She ate and drank her way through the Sophomore Cotillion and Junior Prom, according to her friends Edward Fernow and Mary Merrit Crawford, the latter a fellow Kappa Kappa Gamma. Harvey had believed Huestis to be physically run-down even before her mother's complaint, and her letter to Schurman recounted a dinner table interrogation of Huestis prior to her going home. Her friend and sorority sister, Olive Morrison, and a third student, Maida Rossiter, who was a library science student and a member of the Kappa Alpha Theta sorority, were also present. Zeroing in like a prosecutor, Harvey demanded to know whether they had consumed any cold drinks at the soda water fountains or confectioners downtown, which the Sage College women had been strictly forbidden to do. Huestis confessed that she had consumed a "chocolate sunday" the day before, perhaps at the Platt & Colt Pharmacy in Ithaca where ice cream sundaes were invented in 1892, although the report doesn't say. Rossiter, who described the interrogation in a separate statement attached to Harvey's report, helpfully explained that a chocolate sundae "is a cold drink" in case Schurman didn't know.

Summing up, Harvey labeled Huestis an "incautious" young woman who was "careless of her health" and who just couldn't stay home during Junior Week. It was meant to be a damning indictment, even if this morality play seems comical today. Huestis may well have contracted typhoid from that "chocolate sunday" but could just as well have picked it up during her stay in the Cornell Infirmary for tonsillitis, which was around the time the first typhoid patients began arriving. As we have seen, sanitary precautions were not always observed in the infirmary. In any event, Huestis survived her case of typhoid, graduated from Cornell in 1905, and went on to become a leading American miniature painter under the name of Edna Simpson.[15]

Margaret Harvey was remembered more fondly by Isabel Dolbier Emerson, the Brooklyn student who had experienced the Junior Prom as a "blissful night." Emerson saved the printed warning distributed by Harvey to the Sage College coeds during the epidemic: "Do not relax care in regard to water used for brushing the teeth, or taken for any purpose in the mouth. Do not eat uncooked oysters. Do not take any cold drinks nor eat ice cream or uncooked food downtown. Do not forget that responsibility rests on you." Emerson pasted it in her scrapbook accompanied by a handwritten note: "She did such a lot."[16]

Some students, in the face of the serious illness and death around them, regretted their past frivolity. Cornell's Chi chapter of the Delta Gamma sorority confessed as much in a report written for the sorority's national magazine, *Anchora*: "In Chi's last letter . . . we were groaning over 'finals' and wondering if life was worth living; but as we look back on these trials, they seem trivial indeed, for now we are in real trouble." More than half the Delta Gamma sisters had fled Ithaca, so the national sorority had given permission to postpone rush. On the other hand, the Alpha Psi fraternity boasted that none of the brothers had become ill and only five had left campus when the epidemic was at its peak. Some fraternity houses had been deserted for much of the semester. "Our perfect immunity is accounted for in the careful precautions taken and our own spring of pure drinking water on the premises," the fraternity secretary wrote.[17]

Winter and spring sports at Cornell sagged during the epidemic. Some teams declined to travel to Ithaca because they feared their players would become ill, such as when Harvard canceled its fencing meet with Cornell. Basketball and baseball were especially hard hit. On February 27, Cornell's cagers lost to Princeton in an away game, 55-18. A story in the *Ithaca Daily News* blamed the loss on demoralization over the typhoid epidemic combined with the loss of star guard Percy L. Lyford, who was ill with the fever. Lyford became ill in New Haven, Connecticut, just before the previous night's game with Yale, and was hospitalized there. Worse was yet to come. On March 12, Robert S. Knapp, a starting forward, died of typhoid.

For the baseball team, the impact of the epidemic was not quite so devastating. Coach Hugh Jennings had two key players out sick with typhoid, but both survived. Nearly half the squad left during the height of the epidemic, which coincided with preseason practice. But by the time competition began at the end of March, most had returned and Jennings and the team finished the season with a respectable 17-9 record. From the description of the season he wrote for that year's *Cornellian*, the student yearbook, Jennings seems to have been a thoughtful and considerate coach, opposite in style to the angry bluster of Charles Courtney, the crew czar.[18]

Some of the worst tragedies occurred when a parent taking care of a sick child caught typhoid and died. There were three known instances of this, and it would not be surprising if more cases had escaped public attention. Ill Cornell students dispersed across the United States during the epidemic, some to distant farms or very small towns in the Midwest and South. These secondary deaths by rights should be added to the grim statistics of the Ithaca epidemic, bringing the known death toll to eighty-five rather than the official figure of eighty-two.

The danger of secondary infections during a typhoid epidemic, especially to physicians and nurses, was well known. Typhoid cannot be spread through the air, like a cold. The danger comes through the hands. A caregiver is continually cleaning up after the patient and coming in contact with things he touched or wore. Dr. Edwin O. Jordan, a prominent Chicago bacteriologist who went to Ithaca to investigate the epidemic for the *Journal of the American Medical Association*, said it took only a tiny drop of patient urine or a speck of excrement to transmit typhoid to a caregiver. "In almost countless ways," Jordan wrote, "typhoid bacilli may find access to the alimentary tract of attendants or associates."[19]

Physicians and nurses were trained in the dangers of typhoid patient care, but most parents were not. We can only imagine the guilt of the sons in the two cases in which they survived and their fathers died. One survivor could not talk about his father's death even as an old man. In the other case, the family tried to deny the father's typhoid was connected to the son's, even though the link was obvious. It was no doubt an attempt to spare him the mental anguish of having been partly responsible for his father's death. In the third case, the son died before the father became ill.

The story of the Pray family of Sherburne, New York, reads like something out of Dickens. Fred J. Pray was a freshman at Cornell in the veterinary school, the only child of James A. Pray. James's wife, Nettie Pray, was Fred's stepmother. His birth mother, Emma Pray, had died in 1887 when Fred was six years old, and his father had subsequently remarried. By all accounts, Fred Pray and his stepmother got along fine. The parents, like other families of modest means who sent a child to Cornell, scrimped and saved to find the money to pay his tuition and expenses. Fred Pray came home on February 17 ill with typhoid fever and was treated by Dr. Lewis A. Van Wagner, a Sherburne physician. His parents, and especially his father, nursed him at home, but James Pray was fated to watch his son die on March 12. He was buried next to his birth mother two days later in Christ Church Cemetery in Sherburne.

To his second wife's horror, James Pray began to exhibit the symptoms of typhoid on March 26, within the standard incubation period of the disease. Within days, he developed a full-blown case of typhoid, and on April 8 he died. Three days later, he was buried in Christ Church Cemetery next to his son and first wife. Nettie Pray barely had him in the ground when her husband's sister, Nellie Pickert, and other family members descended on the house like locusts, began taking things, and demanded she leave. James Pray left no will, and under New York State law of the time, his estate went mainly to his birth family, which clearly was not on good terms with the second wife. They knew what state law allowed, and they were executing their claim. Nettie Pray was turned out of her house, which was then sold and the proceeds applied to the remaining medical and burial expenses of Fred and James Pray. The rest went mainly to Nellie Pickert, and the widow received nothing.[20]

Edwin G. Nourse was a freshman at Cornell who planned to stay for six years and become an engineer. He was on a tight budget in the winter of 1903, trying to make $200 cover his room and board for the remainder of the semester, and so was always hungry. When typhoid symptoms appeared one day, Nourse feared he would never recover if he went to the overcrowded Cornell Infirmary. So he set out by train for his home in Downers Grove, Illinois, a suburb of Chicago. It was a grueling experience. When his sister, Alice, arrived from Evanston, where she was a student at Northwestern University, "he was lying on the couch by the window and looking pale and thin against its red plush." She heard her brother say repeatedly, "I thought I'd never make it." He was sick and exhausted.

Although Nourse had no fever to speak of that first night home, by morning he was too ill to get out of bed. His condition worsened by the day, and soon his life hung in the balance. He became delirious. "His mind was affected and he had no control of himself, making the care of him unnecessarily hard," his stepmother, Alice P. Nourse (both the stepmother and daughter were named Alice), wrote to President Schurman. Both parents struggled together to care for their son. Alice cleaned the soiled bed linens in a washboiler atop the stove and then put them through a wringer. Edwin H. Nourse, who was seventy years old and living on a meager pension after being forced out as director of music education in the Chicago public schools for political reasons, rolled over and lifted his unconscious son as necessary. But they finally had to bring in a nurse, despite their limited resources. Identified only as "Miss Whitcomb," she had done home care for the family during a previous illness and was much loved.

One day, young Alice Nourse found both Miss Whitcomb and her father ill with typhoid. They had caught it from Edwin. Now she and her stepmother had three people to care for. Her brother gradually recovered, but his father died ten days later, blood pouring out his rectum. As with James Pray, his close and loving care of his ill son had led to his own death.[21]

When Edwin G. Nourse finally had the strength to return to Cornell University, he decided for economic reasons to give up engineering and get a bachelor of arts degree, ultimately gravitating to agricultural economics and the Brookings Institution. From 1946 to 1949, he was President Harry S. Truman's chairman of the Council of Economic Advisers. In an oral history conducted by the Truman Presidential Library in 1972, Nourse mentioned Cornell University and his bout with typhoid but not how it led to his father's death. His sister, Alice, was forced by their father's death to drop out of Northwestern University. She did not return. Five years later, she traveled to China to visit her sister, Mary, the third Nourse child, who was a teacher in Hangchow. While there, Alice met and later married Earle Tisdale Hobart, a Standard Oil executive. As Alice Tisdale Hobart she became a best-selling novelist, writing of her China experiences in *Oil for the Lamps of China* and other books. Her 1959 memoir, *Gusty's Child*, contains an account of how her family was devastated by the Ithaca typhoid epidemic.[22]

For the Mudge family in Brooklyn, the tragedy took much the same course. Alfred E. Mudge Jr., a junior at Cornell who seems to have been one of the last students afflicted with typhoid during the epidemic, returned home sick and was ministered to by his father, Alfred Sr. The elder Mudge was a lawyer and the last corporation counsel of Brooklyn before it became a part of New York City in 1898. He contracted typhoid and died on April 28. The family and their physician denied that Alfred Jr. had infected his father, but the chances of any other source for the infection seem remote. The younger Mudge also became a prominent lawyer, a name partner in his firm even after his death in 1945. As Mudge, Rose, Guthrie & Alexander in the 1960s, the law firm became a home for former Vice President Richard M. Nixon before he ran successfully for president in 1968. The firm dissolved in 1995.[23]

In the privacy of correspondence with friends, Schurman sometimes let his guard down and allowed his emotions about the epidemic to show through. "It has been and is a time of terrible affliction and sorrow," he wrote in a March 6 letter to a member of the Board of Trustees, Stewart L. Woodford, a walrus-faced man who was a Civil War general on the Union side and U.S. ambassador to Spain when war broke out in 1898. "But though it is almost too much to hope we shall have no more deaths, I think it is at least safe to say the worst is over. Many homes, however, are sorrow stricken." Schurman was wrong about the worst being past; nine more students died from that point forward.[24]

Throughout the epidemic, clergy and lay people alike prayed for divine intervention to spare Ithaca from further suffering. Rev. William L. O'Hara, president of Mount Saint Mary's College, a Catholic school in Emmitsburg, Maryland, was among those sending spiritual blessings to President

Schurman. O'Hara wrote: "We pray that He who is the author of life and strength may stay the hand of death, drive away the dread disease, and restore the sick to health."[25]

The continuing agonies of Ithaca and Cornell University seemed unstoppable. People were coming down with typhoid long after the original contamination of the water supply at the beginning of January 1903. Even the booster shot in late January should have lost much of its potency by now. "Seldom does any institution of learning meet a foe so mysterious, relentless, and persistent," wrote W. H. P. Farmer, president of Brown University in Providence, Rhode Island, in a letter to Schurman on February 21, 1903. But if Ithaca and Cornell University could not solve their own problems, perhaps an outsider could.

Chapter 13

The Man Who Saved Ithaca

IF THERE WAS ANYONE WHO COULD STOP THE TYPHOID and save Ithaca, it was George A. Soper. A sanitary engineer and a good one, he was an autocratic, driven man, a master of planning who had cleaned up Galveston, Texas, after the hurricane of 1900, the worst natural disaster in United States history. But he was also a difficult man, arrogant, class-driven, and in love with himself and his accomplishments. Soper considered himself part of an aristocratic class—engineers—and looked down upon the lower classes in the cities he was hired to save. But despite his personal qualities, or perhaps because of them, Soper got the job done. He saved people no matter their class deficiencies or the color of their skin. His war was against the great and terrible diseases of the day, and humans were almost an afterthought, pieces on a chessboard.

George Soper was *not* a physician, which he would readily admit. That point is often overlooked. He was called Dr. Soper for his academic degree in engineering. Although his work, in Ithaca and elsewhere, often seemed to call for a person trained in both sanitary engineering and medicine, he was trained only in the former although clearly had read much of the latter. There were gaps in his knowledge. When he tried to understand the causes of the Ithaca epidemic in 1903, for example, he was doing so without any knowledge of Dr. Robert Koch's findings regarding human typhoid carriers.

In fairness, few American physicians had yet read Koch's address to the Kaiser Wilhelm Institute in Berlin of November 28, 1902, but fair or not, this should be kept in mind in considering Soper's beliefs regarding the cause of the Ithaca epidemic, especially his contemptuous dismissal of the possibility that the Italians at the dam site could have triggered the epidemic. Normally he would have been quite ready to ascribe the worst of sins to immigrants or the poor, but to do so here would have cast doubt on the integrity of fellow *engineers* who employed and supervised the Italians, especially Gardner S. Williams, the designer of the Six Mile Creek dam. By the time Soper tracked down Mary Mallon, aka "Typhoid Mary," in New York City in 1907, his most famous case, he did know of and admire Koch's work on typhoid carriers, but it was recently acquired knowledge.[1]

Soper climbed up the academic ladder of the engineering world in late-nineteenth-century America, beginning with his bachelor of science degree from Rensselaer Polytechnic Institute in Troy, New York, in 1895. He earned a master's degree from Columbia University in 1898 and a PhD from Columbia a year later. Then he was off and running, obtaining his first job at the Boston Water Works and then traveling the country as an engineer for the Cumberland Manufacturing Company, which built water filtration plants.

After a hurricane destroyed Galveston, Texas, on September 8, 1900, killing more than 8,000 people, Soper was sent by the Merchants Association and Chamber of Commerce of New York at their expense to take charge of the cleanup. Dead bodies lay everywhere on Galveston Island, and efforts to bury them at sea had resulted in them washing back on the shore. The fear of pestilence was great, and the Galveston Central Relief Committee asked for Soper's help. In his first report to the committee, Soper said bluntly that the city was "very unsanitary." He added much later that Galveston, in the first few weeks after the storm, was "in all probability the most unsanitary city in which the American people or others of the Anglo-Saxon race predominated." He simply couldn't help himself, proclaiming the superiority of the white upper classes and the inferiority of the poor and immigrant classes quite frequently, either directly or by implication.[2]

Surprising the relief committee, Soper said the greater danger to Galveston was pestilence arising among the living, not the dead. He urged the burning of debris at central locations and directed his workers to clear standing water from the streets, unclog sewers, and muck out latrines and stables.

Human and animal remains were cremated upon discovery. Methodically, carefully, Soper cleaned up Galveston. The Texans loved him, and he appeared to love them, far more than he would the people of Ithaca, whom he viewed with his usual arrogant contempt. He was inordinately pleased to have been named an honorary member of the Galveston Central Relief Committee, boasting in a newspaper interview that he and Clara Barton of the American Red Cross were the only out-of-towners to be accorded such an honor.[3] When Soper returned to New York, he was made sanitary engineer of the New York City Board of Health.[4]

On February 5, 1903, after the number of typhoid cases in Ithaca had swelled to several hundred, the New York State Department of Health in Albany sent one of its physicians, Dr. Frederick C. Curtis, to Ithaca to do a quick investigation of what was going on. Curtis was a Civil War veteran, although as a foot soldier rather than a physician, and maintained a medical practice in the Albany area when he was not working for the state Health Department. Curtis spent a day in Ithaca and reported back to the commissioner of health, Dr. Daniel Lewis, what he had observed and heard. To Curtis, there seemed little doubt that the typhoid had come from the excrement of one of the Italian workers, swept into Six Mile Creek and delivered to the faucets of Ithaca.[5]

Lewis, a surgeon and cancer specialist, was appointed to the state Board of Health in 1895 and served three terms as president. When the legislature abolished the Board of Health in 1901, replacing it with the Department of Health, Lewis became New York's first commissioner of health.[6] Although accomplished and well-meaning, Lewis did not have a public health background and made a significant error of judgment in Ithaca. During a meeting with President Schurman on February 24, during which Schurman laid out plans for the university to loan Morris $150,000 to build a water filtration plant, Lewis was persuaded to issue a statement that it was "perfectly safe" for students to return to classes at Cornell. Ten thousand copies of Lewis's remarks, incorporated into a Cornell University press release, were quickly printed, rushed to the Post Office, and mailed out to parents, important prep schools, and prominent newspapers across the country. Here is the wording:

Dr. Daniel Lewis, the State Commissioner of Health, who is here today, after having studied the situation carefully from every side, makes the statement that the plans which are already in operation, and which this day are being extended by the city authorities, make it *perfectly safe* [emphasis added] for anyone to return to Ithaca who so desires.[7]

This was at a moment in the epidemic when, as Samuel Hopkins Adams would note in his muckraking article about typhoid fever and the Ithaca catastrophe in *McClure's Magazine*, some four hundred to five hundred people in the city were suffering from typhoid and new cases were being reported every day. "Every weary and overworked physician in the place knew that never had the disease been under less control," Adams wrote.[8]

Blindsided by Lewis's statement, the Ithaca Board of Health was furious. They telegraphed the health commissioner informing him that his "perfectly safe" remark was subject to serious misinterpretation and asking him, with no little amount of sarcasm, if they should issue a statement urging Cornell students to return to Ithaca. The board could not see students safely returning unless they could obtain board and lodging somewhere that guaranteed that no unboiled city water was served. In addition, the board informed Lewis that it viewed secondary typhoid infections as "a new and serious source of danger," given "the numerous cases of typhoid fever now in the city."

Lewis immediately began walking back his remark, saying that students should not be urged to return unless all the "fever houses"—apparently by this he meant the boardinghouses where cases of typhoid had occurred—were regularly inspected and all physicians were reporting all their typhoid cases to the Board of Health. "I stated that in my judgment the worst of the epidemic was over," Lewis said. "I also said, you may remember, that you still had to face the danger of secondary infection from neglect on the part of attendants and house owners where the sick are domiciled."[9]

Schurman, at least for a day, believed that large numbers of students would return to Cornell in response to Dr. Lewis's statement that it was "perfectly safe" to do so, and in truth some were coming back already. He notified the faculty to begin organizing special classes to enable the students who fled the epidemic to make up their missed course work and advised them to expect double duty for a time. He was certain they would not object in this time of emergency, welcoming an opportunity "of showing their interest in our students, their loyalty to the university, and their readiness to cooperate with the trustees in solving this unexpected educational problem."[10] The medical and veterinary faculties, however, quickly came out in opposition to Schurman's optimistic view of conditions and he backed off, issuing this revised statement:

> A few students are coming back each day, and letters are daily being received from others expressing a desire to come. But the university advises no students to return; each must decide for him-self in view of the facts of the case. All students returning must be careful to observe all the regulations prescribed by the board of health.[11]

Confused by the conflicting statements, only a few students actually returned. A survey taken on March 3 by the *Ithaca Daily Journal* found that of the estimated thousand students who had fled, only about 8 percent, or seventy-five students, had returned. Of the 440 Sibley College mechanical engineering students who had gone home, only fifteen were back. At the law school, fifteen out of 105 had returned. It was a similar story at the other Cornell schools.[12]

Probably realizing the mess he had made of things, Dr. Lewis announced that he was sending an expert from the New York City Board of Health to Ithaca to take charge of the cleanup of Ithaca.[13] In a letter to Schurman on March 3, he said George A. Soper had been in charge of the cleanup of Galveston and "had handled the situation with great skill and success. I hope you will keep him there until all the sanitary work of the Board [of Health] is being thoroughly carried out." Soper had an appointment from the state Department of Health so he could do his work without having to worry about arbitrary municipal boundaries, Lewis said, and was leaving for Ithaca that morning.

The letter strongly suggests that Lewis believed the worst of the epidemic was over and that he was sympathetic to Schurman's desire for a return to normalcy on the Cornell campus. "I judge from the reports, as they have come to us from day to day, that the climax of the trouble was past before I visited Ithaca," he wrote, which means he agreed with Schurman's assessment of the situation when they spoke on February 24. There is also a troubling suggestion that Lewis had agreed not to look too hard at how the epidemic came about. "I am convinced that we should not waste any time or energy trying to attach blame to this party or that for the conditions which simply came upon Ithaca unawares, as has often been the case in other communities," he wrote. Had Schurman pressed him to "move on" and not look backward? Schurman had to know that even a cursory examination of the events leading to the Ithaca catastrophe would eventually shine an unwelcome light on the Board of Trustees's relationship with William T. Morris and the Tremans. Lewis wrote in closing that the epidemic would provide a good lesson to Ithaca to "ensure rigid care of the water supply in the future." The effort to shift the fault for the epidemic from the guilty parties to the community had begun.[14]

Although Schurman believed the campus was safe, he remained distressed that six or more new typhoid cases were being reported every day among nonstudents. He looked at the data from a typhoid epidemic in 1901 at Yale University in New Haven, Connecticut, noting that Yale's epidemic began on March 20 and all but ended on April 15. "According to this showing," he wrote to Dr. Lewis, "new cases in Ithaca should have ceased about the middle or 20th of February. Yet they go on." Indeed they did. Part of the problem was that some Ithaca residents simply did not believe the water could harm them and continued to drink it. Soper came to believe there were as many as several thousand of such people. The New York Sun reported the story of an unnamed woman and her daughter who had just been admitted to City Hospital with symptoms of typhoid after defying the ban against drinking city water.[15]

The other part of the problem, of course, was secondary infections. The Board of Health had hired two nurses from New York City to work as district nurses, going from house to house instructing families of typhoid patients in the proper and safe methods of caring for their loved ones. But it still came down to common sense, and even some nurses working in Ithaca seemed to lack it. Dr. Edward Hitchcock Jr., the city health officer, told a story about a trained nurse who prepared broth for an Ithaca typhoid patient. Because it was too hot to eat, she ran a little cold water from the city water faucet into the broth to cool it, potentially turning the broth into typhoid soup. Fortunately for the patient, someone in the house saw the nurse do it, grabbed the broth, and threw it away before it could be served.[16]

The striking thing about Soper's arrival in Ithaca on March 3 was how immediately he was accepted by the public and assumed control. No one seems to have disputed much, if anything, he told them, because it all made perfect sense. He answered questions ranging from the proper chemical disinfectants to use (lime chloride or mercury chloride) to whether carp or bullheads caught in Cayuga Lake should be eaten (no, because they are bottom feeders who might have ingested pollution). Ithaca needed an authority figure willing to wade in and take charge, and Soper filled that role with vigor. It was in his blood.

From the start, Soper raced to disinfect Ithaca before the end of the bitter New York winter and the arrival of a new crop of houseflies, which would greatly complicate efforts to stamp out the typhoid. He charged into his work the very evening he arrived, meeting with Dr. Hitchcock and two other employees of the Board of Health to go over a map showing the locations of typhoid cases. The next day, he and Hitchcock toured the city and parts of the Six Mile Creek, Buttermilk Creek, and Fall Creek watersheds, paying special attention to homes in the city and, of course, the personal hygiene of their inhabitants. Soper told the press his work "dealt only with present conditions and not with the past," suggesting that he and Dr. Lewis had chatted about the parameters for his efforts. The *Ithaca Daily News* noted that Soper disregarded "the cause of the epidemic" at the Board of Health meeting the next night. "I understand that the popularly accepted cause is the water," he said, waving away the question. "Upon that point I am not now prepared to exercise an opinion." Then he launched into a stern lecture about how improper care of typhoid patients could keep the fever in Ithaca indefinitely, which was certainly true.

Soper's goal was to break the cycle of infection, which meant that certain unsanitary practices simply could not continue. If contaminated excrement was thrown into an outhouse or an open field, for example, houseflies, once they arrived in late spring, would inevitably alight on the excrement. Just as inevitably, provided a kitchen window was close by, the flies would touch down upon food sitting out on the family table. Another human would be infected and the typhoid victimization cycle would go on for more months, unless firm measures were taken.

Aggressive disinfection was the key, especially with so many hundreds of typhoid patients scattered around Ithaca. Everything contaminated with typhoid bacilli, from excrement to urine to clothing to sheets to dishes to hands, needed to be made safe again. Soper recommended hiring a team of twenty workers to distribute two potent disinfectants, milk of lime and bichloride of mercury, by horse and wagon to any resident who needed them. Milk of lime, a.k.a. the "White Fluid," was a suspension of calcium hydroxide and water. Soper said it was to be used for disinfecting excrement and urine from typhoid patients. Bichloride of mercury, a.k.a. the "Blue Fluid," was to be used for disinfecting hands, dishes, clothing, and bedsheets. It was toxic, and hand washing with soap and hot water was recommended after immersion in the "Blue Fluid."[17]

He specified the use of real, full-strength milk of lime, not the weak-sister variety sometimes made with ingredients sold in local stores. The Board of Health bought its own supplies of calcium hydroxide from reliable vendors, had it tested in the laboratories of Cornell University to be sure, mixed it with water to create milk of lime, and distributed it to the public at no cost. Sanitarians loved their lime compounds. The basic one was calcium oxide, also known as quicklime, which became calcium hydroxide, or slaked lime or milk of lime, after it was mixed with water. Unlike carbolic acid, another popular disinfectant of the day, chloride of lime had no strong smell. It was inexpensive, readily available, and could be used to disinfect excrement, urine, sputum, or entire outhouses.

All of this cost money, lots of money, and Soper asked the Board of Health to fund a proper cleanup. He envisioned almost a military campaign with himself as general. The board authorized no more than $50 a day, still a substantial amount in 1903, but Common Council removed the spending ceiling entirely, so eager was it to give Soper what he needed. If it took the city's entire budget and entire credit to wipe out the plague, council was willing to do it.[18]

Soper was also investigating the condition of the Fall Creek watershed that provided drinking water for the Cornell campus. Despite repeated boasts by the university that no one who drank Fall Creek water had become ill with typhoid, Gardner S. Williams had warned President Schurman that the creek's water was a bacteriological time bomb that would eventually claim victims, if not from typhoid then from other intestinal disorders. A crew of workers sent out by the university to "purify" the Fall Creek watershed found seven or eight outhouses right at the water's edge. When called to Soper's attention, he arranged for one of his assistants—the infamous Shirley Clarke Hulse—to take four Italian workers and a team of horses and clean out and disinfect the outhouses.[19]

Hulse was the young assistant to Gardner S. Williams whose negligence had allowed the Italian workers at the Six Mile Creek dam construction site to foul Ithaca's drinking water. One almost wonders if this new assignment was a punishment of sorts for his earlier negligence. Hulse was later put in charge of collecting water samples for Soper in Cayuga Lake to determine if the lake water was safe to drink. Cottagers—Charles H. Blood and Umphville come to mind—had concerns, given that summer was approaching and Six Mile Creek had certainly dumped some of the typhoid bacilli into the big lake after flowing through Ithaca. A bigger problem, and one that did not begin in 1903, was that Ithaca's sewage pipes emptied into the lake. Hulse collected water samples in the lake for Soper until September 1903.[20] Perhaps he fished, too. It was as if Williams and Soper didn't know what to do with him and wanted to keep him on the payroll and quiet, given the injunction from Dr. Lewis against delving too deeply into the real causes of the epidemic.

Even four decades later, Hulse offered no regrets about his negligence in Ithaca, at least none he was willing to talk about publicly. Pressed, he could only recall the personal risks he had faced while working on the Ithaca cleanup. Writing his reminiscences for *Civil Engineering* magazine in 1944, by which time he was primarily a banker in Bedford, Pennsylvania, Hulse quipped that "my personal high spot was the evening I learned that a tap I drank from regularly in the Ithaca Hotel supplied raw water instead of sterilized as I had thought. Anyhow, it didn't take."[21] Everything was a joke to him, even if the typhoid germs did "take" for so many other people in Ithaca.

On March 7, news came that Cornell would build a separate, small filtration plant for its campus water supply costing $18,000 to $20,000 in 1903 money. Andrew Carnegie, one of the wealthiest men in the world and a member of the Cornell University Board of Trustees, wrote to the board from his sister-in-law's mansion, Dungeness, on Cumberland Island off the coast of Georgia on March 13. He asked for the privilege of paying for the campus filtration plant, and did.[22]

There were a million things to do to make Ithaca clean again. Testing private wells was one of them. Soper was convinced, as had been Professor Emile M. Chamot, that too many were polluted with high bacteria counts. These were not typhoid, at least not typically, but rather other intestinal bacteria that could make people miserably ill though usually did not kill them. Soper found sections of the city where all the wells were polluted, while in other sections they all were good. The good wells, he found, were in clay, the bad ones in fissured rock. In all, he tested 946 private wells during the cleanup and found that 30 percent of them were bad.

Then, of course, there was Ithaca Water Works. It had miles of water mains in the city that had carried typhoid-infected water and might still harbor the germs. Soper's plan was to force a device called a "wire devil" through the mains under pressure, then flush the entire system with potassium permanganate to kill any remaining typhoid germs. An estimated one thousand to fifteen hundred pounds of the chemical would be dumped in the existing reservoirs and be drawn through the system by opening many taps at once. The chemical would give the water a pinkish to red tinge but would not be harmful to humans, only to the typhoid germs. Because of the large amount of the chemical needed, plans were made to contact dealers in Germany as well as in New York City to determine how much could be quickly obtained.[23]

Soper worried about physicians and how they might react to his take-charge style and especially his stern directives to report every case under penalty of being fined by the Board of Health. He met with them on March 8 and received their promises of cooperation. When he asked how prevalent typhoid had been in Ithaca, he was told the last big outbreak had been in 1882 and prior to that in 1864.[24] Three days later, any negative thoughts the Ithaca physicians might have harbored toward Soper were swept away when James C. Bayles, the *New York Times* editorial writer turned reporter, came out with the first of his reports from Ithaca. Bayles slammed the physicians, accusing them of refusing to report typhoid cases to the Board of Health.

Some, he said, had even refrained from putting the real cause of death on death certificates if the patient had typhoid. As many as 250 typhoid cases might have gone unreported, Bayles speculated.[25]

He exonerated Ithaca Water Works and Morris from any responsibility for the typhoid epidemic, largely because, like so many in his day, he did not yet know about typhoid carriers. We can forgive him for that, but it is foolish to accord his beliefs and opinions on the causes of the Ithaca epidemic much credibility today. To Bayles, it made no sense to blame the water company. No physician had reported treating any typhoid case on Six Mile Creek, he reported, and none of the Italian workers at the dam site had missed even a single day due to illness of any kind. Voila! "Not one fact has been produced which contains the assumption that this colony brought typhoid fever into the Six Mile Valley or left it there," he concluded with satisfaction.[26] Again, and we cannot say this enough, Bayles had no idea that a seemingly healthy worker could be releasing millions of typhoid bacilli into the environment every time he defecated along the banks of Six Mile Creek.

Bayles seems to have been largely responsible for the start of the "blame Ithaca" movement, accusing the citizens of knowing they had a typhoid problem and doing nothing about it. "Typhoid has been more or less prevalent here for many years, and at no time has Ithaca long been free from it. For at least ten years the cautionary signals have been obvious to anyone who might have chosen to look for them," he wrote. But Bayles, who was not a physician, was confusing intestinal disorders that were not typhoid, the so-called Ithaca Fever, with the disease that was ravaging the community and had come from one or more of the Italian workers.

Dr. H. Burr Besemer told the *Ithaca Daily News* that Bayles was simply wrong, that Ithaca Fever was not typhoid. He and other physicians believed Ithaca Fever was caused by other colonic bacteria in Six Mile Creek that had "grown fat on the sewage of the creek . . . and caused a continued fever of toxaemic, but not typhoid type." Besemer said that in the past true cases of typhoid had been "few and far between" and had all been traced to their true source, and that there was no red flag the local doctors had been ignoring. He said that "any physician," a dig at Bayles, "will by most careful study arrive at the same conclusion. To arrive at any other conclusion is doubly deplorable, both for the intelligence of the physician and the good of Godforsaken

Ithaca."[27] Besemer did not know about typhoid carriers, either, but he was only comfortable with facts, not old and pernicious myths.

The *Ithaca Daily News* responded with blazing cannons, accusing Bayles of giving a copy of his article to Ithaca Water Works and thence to the *Ithaca Daily Journal* before it appeared in the *Times*. The *Daily News* wrote:

> The article is apparently written with the purpose of relieving the water company of the blame which has been heaped upon it by indignant citizens. To accomplish this purpose, the author attempts to show that Ithaca has always had typhoid fever; that the city is a pest hole, and the advent of the present epidemic was discernible a year ago. To be brief, Mr. Bayles knows little about the matter. He is not, we understand, a physician. . . . His opinion on the point as to whether the disease here is typhoid fever or the measles is not then so very important.[28]

Bayles's articles were very different from his editorials for the *Times*, to the point where we must wonder if he felt intimidated by the agreement worked out between Ochs, Ickelheimer, and Schurman to send him to Ithaca, whether or not there was any substance to his fears. Sometimes reporters will write the story they assume their bosses want rather than the one they believe ought to be written.

~~~~~~~~~

Although Soper himself did not yet know what Dr. Robert Koch had discovered about typhoid carriers, namely that they could be healthy yet harbor millions of the bacilli in their gallbladders, releasing fresh batches to the environment with every defecation, he did seem to understand that not all recent typhoid patients were fully disease free. But he thought the risk was from their urine. Soper wrote:

> One of the most important measures adopted, and, it is thought, an innovation in the management of typhoid epidemics, was the use [in Ithaca] of urinary germicides to eliminate bacterial infection from the bladders of convalescents. . . . In the event of the discovery of this germ the patient was held under observation and given urotropin until the bacillus disappeared.[29]

Urotropin, made by combining ammonia and formaldehyde, was recommended by physicians in the early twentieth century as a means of rid-
ding urine of typhoid germs after a patient had recovered from the disease.
It did nothing, however, for the typhoid germs hiding out in the gallbladder. Urotropin, better known today as hexamine, is still used as a urinary
antiseptic.[30]

Acting on his fears about contaminated urine, Soper summoned students who had recovered from typhoid to be examined by a physician on
the Cornell University Medical School faculty. One such letter, which was
actually signed by President Schurman, was received by Walter Stevenson
Finlay Jr., a mechanical engineering student, and went like this: "As a means
of assisting the Board of Health in its endeavor to stamp out all traces of
the recent epidemic, Dr. Soper desires that you, as a former typhoid patient,
present yourself for examination at Dr. [Abram T.] Kerr's office, Stimson
Hall, as soon as possible. I gladly second this request." Chances are Finlay
received the Diazo urine test for typhoid. Soper himself sent the follow-up
letter, which informed the student "that there is no longer danger you may
convey typhoid fever to others."[31] Soper believed that a disproportionately
large number of Cornell students had contracted typhoid and so focused
special attention on them.[32]

Besides the follow-up medical examinations, he arranged for systematic
inspections of the many boarding and rooming houses occupied by students.
Some students normally spent the summer in Ithaca, so it was necessary to
do this now, in the spring, rather than put it off until later in the summer.
The new rule in Ithaca was that no lodger or table boarder was permitted in
a house in which there was a typhoid patient. The owner either had to evict
the sick student and give the house a thorough cleaning and disinfecting or
shut down the house until the patient had recovered. It appears from a letter
in the files of Cornell University that not all owners complied voluntarily,
resulting in the university sending letters to students living in such a house
telling them to move out within twenty-four hours.[33]

One of Soper's next projects was to increase garbage pickup in Ithaca
from one to three times per week. But what to do with the trash? Ithaca
typically dumped its garbage in low-lying areas along the lake, accessible to
flies that could light upon typhoid-contaminated materials and spread the

disease. Soper's solution was to build an incinerator. His first thought was to build it at the end of Renwick Pier along Cayuga Lake, but then he discovered an abandoned tannery that had two fire chambers connected to a seventy-five-foot smokestack. The incinerator stayed in operation for eight months and usually handled about fourteen wagonloads of garbage per day running twenty-four hours a day.[34]

A final, dangerous, and distasteful task was to muck out the city's many private outhouses and carry away the filth to a safe location outside of town. Nearly a thousand typhoid cases (some patients, especially Cornell students, convalesced outside of Ithaca) had left untold millions of typhoid fever germs in the environment. Ithaca had upward of thirteen hundred outhouses, and Soper intended to clean them out and close them down. The city had begun building more sewer lines to eliminate the need for outhouses or direct discharges into Six Mile Creek, so few homeowners could any longer claim a need for alternative solutions. Many of the outhouses contained typhoid germs, and some had mounds of contaminated excrement piled against their exterior walls. "With infected privies close to your kitchens you can have no protection whatsoever; you cannot stop the flies from circulating between the excrement and your food," Soper said in an interview with the Ithaca Daily Journal. The work began on April 11, involved fifteen men and eight horses, and continued through the summer. Ever the record-keeper, Soper reported that 418,193 gallons of excrement were removed from the outhouses, piled in horse-drawn wagons, and driven to a farm in the country, where the excrement was plowed into the soil to decompose. "It is a satisfaction to be able to say that in this extensive and dangerous piece of scavenging work there was no sickness nor accident," he wrote. Most outhouses were shut down after being mucked out, the homeowners directed to connect to the city sewer system.[35]

And so it was through hard work like this that the epidemic in Ithaca was conquered. All the projects carried out by Soper did their part, eventually killing off the typhoid bacilli either with strong disinfectants or by denying them new hosts to infect, causing them to expire of their own accord. He considered Ithaca to be one of America's worst typhoid epidemics in percentage terms.

There had been 965 cases of typhoid in Ithaca, he said, not including students who contracted the disease at Cornell but went home to convalesce—or die. By the time he delivered an address on the Ithaca epidemic to the New England Water Works Association more than a year later, on September 15, 1904, Soper had raised the total to an "estimated" 1,350 cases, which is more likely too low rather than too high. A minimum of 522 homes in Ithaca were touched by typhoid, including more than 150 in which more than two people contracted the disease. Probably the worst of those was the George house at 308 Lake Ave., where six members of one family lay prostrate with the illness.

Soper's estimate of 1,350 cases would have included the original 965 plus about 151 Cornell students who became ill away from Ithaca.[36] The remainder was truly an educated guess: cases never reported to the Board of Health, the ones Bayles of the *New York Times* had mentioned in his inflammatory article of March 11, and adults who were exposed in Ithaca but got sick somewhere else. This latter number included the Broadway musical comedy actress Nellie Follis, who contracted typhoid during an engagement at the Lyceum Theatre in Ithaca that winter and developed symptoms further down the road in Chicago. We know of her case only because she had a degree of celebrity in her day and the New York *Evening World* ran a story.[37]

The grave diggers were busy. Typhoid killed eighty-two Ithaca residents, of whom twenty-nine were Cornell University students. The twenty-ninth and last known student death, that of Leslie S. Atwater, an Ithaca native, occurred on May 6. The total does not include the collateral deaths of James Pray, Edwin H. Nourse, or Albert Mudge Sr., who contracted typhoid while nursing their sons. There were almost certainly more of these that did not come to wide public attention.

Even as students returned to Cornell, especially after Easter Sunday on April 12, members of the university faculty struggled to recover from their own bouts of typhoid.[38] Earl Blough, an assistant in the Chemistry Department, was admitted to the Cornell Infirmary on January 23, making him one of the first fever patients in the facility, and was not discharged until April 1. The next day, he requested a leave of absence from his duties to recover fully from typhoid, which was granted. It appears he returned to his job in the fall.[39] Another chemistry assistant, Walter S. Lenk, spent eight weeks in City Hospital and requested a leave of absence for the remainder of the academic year. "Having had severe complications during my illness, I find myself still weak and unable to take up my work for a number of months," he wrote in a letter to Schurman on March 25. Lenk recovered and spent two more years at Cornell.[40]

John C. Gifford, an assistant professor of forestry, was one of three people living in a rooming house at 109 Summit Ave. to become ill with typhoid, another being Mark V. Slingerland, an entomology professor. Gifford saw the epidemic kill several of his friends and severely damage his own health, so much so that his doctors warned him that another northern winter might kill him. Both ill and out of a job—the New York State Legislature zeroed out the budget for the forestry program at Cornell that year, but that is another controversy—he moved to Coconut Grove in Florida and became an expert on the South Florida natural world.[41] Slingerland stayed at Cornell for many years.

There was still the occasional cockeyed optimist. Professor George Lincoln Burr, a librarian who also taught medieval history, wrote to Andrew Dickson White on March 30 that "our typhoid epidemic seems almost a thing of the past" and that "all those still sick are on the high road to recovery." President Schurman, in an odd comment that seemed almost like boasting, told the Board of Trustees that the 9.3 percent mortality rate among Cornell students with typhoid was better than the 13.3 percent mortality rate among Yale students with typhoid in the 1901 epidemic in New Haven, Connecticut, a much less severe epidemic in real terms.

New Haven in 1900 had 108,027 people, more than eight times the population of Ithaca. The epidemic toll was 465 cases and seventy-three deaths overall, not just at Yale, or about 68 per 100,000. Ithaca, by contrast, had a typhoid death rate of about 525 per 100,000 if Cornell's approximately three thousand students are added to the city population of a little over thirteen thousand. Around the same time, Chicago had a ratio of 45 typhoid deaths per 100,000, Cincinnati was about the same, Cleveland was 110, Philadelphia was 72, and Detroit was 17.[42]

One of the last victims of the Ithaca epidemic, and perhaps the most tragic of all, was Dr. Alice Potter, a pioneering female physician in Ithaca who passed away on May 2 after a three-week battle with typhoid. Like every other physician in Ithaca, she had worked long days and nights ministering to dozens of typhoid sufferers, but unlike any of her colleagues, she came

down with typhoid herself, almost certainly from a secondary infection originating with one of her patients.

Potter was operated on by Dr. Matthew Mann of Buffalo, who may have
believed her intestinal pain was related to appendicitis. Mann was a gynecologist who had performed emergency surgery on President McKinley at
the Pan-American Exposition after the president was shot there in 1901. His
decision to perform the surgery in the park, rather than removing McKinley to Buffalo General Hospital, was widely criticized after McKinley's death
from infection. Dr. Potter was an 1897 graduate of the University of Buffalo
Medical School and probably knew Dr. Mann. The story in the *Ithaca Daily
News* about her death is somewhat confusing but clearly states that she was
suffering from typhoid.

She was unmarried and lived simply. In her will, which she filed in Tompkins County Surrogate Court in 1901, Dr. Potter specified that she did not
want more than $75 spent on her funeral, a modest amount even for 1903. A
resolution passed at a meeting of Ithaca physicians on the day of her death
paid tribute to her "cheerful presence, large hearted helpfulness, her untiring zeal in her work, and her never failing kindness and love for humanity."
It lamented that her "short life had been sacrificed in her untiring efforts to
relieve suffering and to save life."[43]

Eight days after Potter's death, the final typhoid patient was discharged
from the Cornell Infirmary, where so many had suffered and died.[44] President Schurman wrote an epitaph for his dead students that appeared in the
1902–1903 *Cornellian*, the university yearbook:

> Toll for the fallen! Some of our best are no more. In the prime
> of manhood, like flowers of the field, they have been cut off and
> withered. The hearts of fathers and mothers, of brothers and sis-
> ters, of friends and some dearer than friends, have been wrung with
> anguish. Their sorrow is our sorrow. Our friends are no more. Never
> again shall we grasp the warm hand or hear the voice of these com-
> rades we knew and loved. Alas! Alas! To all those whom the ties of
> kinship and affection united to our lost friends, this brotherhood
> of scholars, mourning a common loss, tender deep and sincere sym-
> pathy, though, indeed, tears are nearer than words.[45]

And from the Cornell University Class of 1903, a possibly cynical drinking song:

Here's to 1903
Drink her down, drink her down
Here's to 1903
Drink her down, drink her down
Here's to 1903
She will win the victory
Drink her down, drink her down
Drink her down, down, down

Was it meant to refer to the water they drank that year? Or was it nothing more than a drinking song? Isabel Dolbier Emerson, a member of the Class of 1903, preserved the song lyrics in her scrapbook and caught the irony, intentional or not.

Chapter 14

The Man Who Saved
Cornell University

EVEN BEFORE THE ITHACA EPIDEMIC WAS OVER, the financial toll on Cornell students unlucky enough to be attacked by typhoid was obvious. The same was true for Ithaca residents who were not students, but for now let us look at the situation of the young men and women at Cornell. Health insurance was rare to nonexistent in America in 1903, and if a student did not have wealthy parents, paying typhoid bills from hospitals, doctors, nurses, and pharmacies was a crushing burden. They were victims of a crime, but still they had to pay.

Warren S. Barlow, a student from Marcellus, New York, faced bills of $573.12 for his typhoid case, a little more than the average $543 in wages earned by a steadily employed workingman in a year at that time, and considerably more than the approximately $400 that four years of Cornell tuition then cost. Bills of that size were far from unusual. Howard C. Smith, a junior from Texas, spent six weeks in a private hospital in Ithaca and was delirious for much of that time. He was presented with bills for $555.00 upon discharge. A former member of the Cornell cross-country team, Smith was so weak that he could not walk a mile without stopping to rest.[1]

Letitia R. Odell, of Erie, Pennsylvania, who had borrowed much of her tuition money and then enrolled in Cornell as a freshman after ten years of teaching high school math and German, found herself deeply in debt after she recovered from typhoid. One of the two nurses who had provided her day and night care, Mrs. D. D. Hammond, wrote to President Schurman seeking relief, noting that the university was paying to bring in nurses from other cities to work in the Cornell Infirmary. She said some of Odell's friends had raised twenty or thirty dollars to give to her, but Hammond doubted it would cover more than a small fraction of the total. A professor at the University of Chicago Law School who knew Odell also wrote to Schurman asking that he arrange for her to be helped as a deserving charity case.[2]

More than eight hundred students gathered on March 27 to consider how to help their fellows left destitute by typhoid. Many ill students had exhausted their savings and still owed much more. They had planned on working their way through college but were now too physically weak to work. Some had little clothing left to wear. "They cannot pay their medical expenses, some of them cannot even get home to recuperate. We who have not been sick and who are in more fortunate surroundings can, with difficulty, perhaps, realize the situation of the students now needing assistance," the Cornell Daily Sun wrote in an editorial. At the March 27 meeting, the Students' Hospital Fund collected $178.50 in cash and $521.50 in pledges. But as welcome as the donations were, they covered only a tiny fraction of the unpaid student bills.[3]

Schurman had reason to worry about parental anger, especially if their son or daughter had died. Commander Edward L. Prime, a Navy officer from Huntington, New York, was at sea with the Pacific Squadron when his son and only child, Edward, died on February 15. His son's case appears to have been botched from the get-go. A physician at the Cornell Infirmary first diagnosed his disease as tonsillitis, then as paracolon fever, an imprecise, catchall diagnosis used by physicians who weren't sure their patient had typhoid. But it was typhoid. Edward's mother didn't receive any official notice from Cornell that her son was ill but finally heard about it from an Ithaca friend. She arrived in time to bring Edward's body home. Commander Prime received word of his son's death only when the fleet reached Honolulu eight days later. On March 11, finally back home on Long Island, Prime sent a bitter letter to Schurman, who responded by sending Thomas F. Crane, dean of the university faculty and Edward Bailey, an alumnus who knew Prime, to meet with him on March 18 at the Hoffman House hotel at Madison Square in New York City.

Commander Prime arrived at the meeting with guns blazing, despite being accompanied by a minister, and told Crane he meant every word in his letter to Schurman. "His attitude was that of the Centurion [in the Bible] who told men to go and they went," Crane wrote to Schurman. "He referred everything to the standards of the quarterdeck and felt that the university, having received students, was bound to look out for their health and to supervise even their boardinghouses." Crane was relieved that Prime did not bring up the controversial Cornell Infirmary, where his son died, or "the asserted connection of the university and the water company." He did not think he had changed Prime's mind, and indeed he had not. Nor was Prime the only angry parent.

Crane traveled by train to New York the previous day with a Mr. Gilbert, who was taking his typhoid-stricken son, Harold A. Gilbert, home to Brooklyn. To Crane's shock, Gilbert was nearly as angry as Commander Prime. "Mr. Gilbert seemed to think that the university was a stock company and managed for the pecuniary benefit of the trustees," Crane wrote in despair. "If an intelligent businessman can entertain such notions as he did of the purpose and management of the university, it seems hopeless to attempt to enlighten the general public." Told that Cornell University had already spent $12,000 on student care and other epidemic expenses, Gilbert was politely incredulous. But by the time the train reached Hoboken, Crane wrote, Gilbert had come around and seemed to understand the position of the university. Or perhaps he simply agreed with Crane to be left in peace at the end of a long train ride.[4]

~~~~~~~~

Left unchecked, there is no telling where parental anger over their sick children might have led. Lawsuits over dirty water were rare in 1903 because the courts made them difficult, but they were not unknown. But before that anger could boil over, one of the world's wealthiest men came to Cornell University's rescue. One of the more remarkable episodes in the Ithaca epidemic story was the decision by Andrew Carnegie, a member of the Cornell University Board of Trustees since 1890, to pay or reimburse $86,000 in typhoid medical bills for 381 Cornell students, living or dead, in addition to the $18,000 to 20,000 in 1903 money that he donated for the campus water filtration plant.

Carnegie only rarely attended Board of Trustees meetings in Ithaca and had previously rebuffed Cornell University in the mid-1890s when it sought a major philanthropic gift, despite assiduous courting by Andrew Dickson White and Jacob Gould Schurman. The situation was different now, different because he had been showered with untold riches when he sold his steel company to J. P. Morgan in 1901 for inclusion in the new U.S. Steel. He now was a full-time philanthropist and peace activist. Carnegie donated public libraries to cities and small towns across America. In February, he had announced plans to fund construction of a grand "Peace Palace" in the Netherlands to house the new Permanent Court of Arbitration created by the Hague Peace Conference of 1899. He and President Schurman were one in their opposition to the U.S. war against the Philippine rebels.

But Carnegie also provided charity on occasion to individuals who were down on their luck. In the same month the Peace Palace was announced, Carnegie bestowed a $500 check and a $500 annuity on Samuel Nicholls of Kenesaw, Nebraska, whom he had befriended on the ship when he first came to America from Scotland in 1848. Nicholls had applied to Carnegie for assistance several years earlier but heard nothing back until the check arrived.[5]

The unanswered question is whether Carnegie's action was specifically done to head off more angry parents like Commander Prime. Available documents do not suggest this was the motive behind the decision, but that does not completely settle the matter. Prime, incidentally, in another angry letter to Schurman nearly three years after his son's death, called Carnegie's offer "blood money" and "a sop to keep my mouth shut." It is quite possible that Carnegie had more than one motive for offering to pay the student medical bills: a desire to help the students, but also to help Cornell University out of a jam.

The students' financial problems were driven home to Carnegie by a letter in late March from George G. Cotton of Syracuse, New York, the same parent who had written to Schurman twelve days earlier about his son's typhoid and that of another student, Warren Barlow. Paying his son's medical bills would be tough, Cotton wrote to Carnegie, but he thought he could do it. "But *I am of the opinion* [emphasis in original] that there are many of those who . . . will be seriously distressed to pay their expenses, let alone to provide money for the extra time it will take them to make up," Cotton wrote. He told Carnegie that in addition to paying for the new campus filtration plant, he ought to consider helping Cornell students left destitute by typhoid. "A sum of money placed in the hand of President Schurman," Cotton wrote, "might relieve many a case of actual distress." He mentioned Warren Barlow, who had been hospitalized for four weeks, survived hemorrhages, and needed special nurses in constant attendance. His father was superintendent at a livestock farm in South Onondaga, New York, and didn't make much money. For Barlow's father, Cotton wrote, it would be "hard sledding for some time."[6]

Was this all a setup? Are we too cynical if we wonder how Cotton knew Carnegie well enough to send such a chatty, personal letter? He was a mid-level executive in charge of worker training for the Solvay Process Company, a chemical manufacturer in Solvay, New York, and not of Carnegie's social rank. The philanthropist's only known connection with the town of Solvay was a $10,000 grant to build a public library, which was announced on January 14, 1903. Frederick Warren, president of the Solvay Process Company, was another big donor to the library and most likely would have been the company executive to have had dealings, if any, with Carnegie. Did Schurman put Cotton up to it? We don't know, but in any case Carnegie took the hint. He wrote on the back of Cotton's letter, "Dear President, Should be glad to relieve necessitous cases of this kind if any, A.C.," and sent it to Schurman.

Carnegie certainly knew the horror of typhoid. He nearly died of the disease in 1886 at his home in Cresson, Pennsylvania. During his convalescence, he lost first his brother and then his mother, suffering a relapse upon hearing of the former's death. When his mother died, his caregivers kept the news from him, even lowering Margaret Carnegie's coffin out a window so he would not see it pass his bedroom door. Five years later, his wife, Louise, suffered a severe attack of typhoid and a long convalescence that left him shaken and scared. Even one of the wealthiest men in the world had no defense against typhoid.[7] So perhaps it is not so surprising that Carnegie chose to become the health insurer of last resort for the students of Cornell University. Still, questions linger.

Schurman wrote back to Carnegie on April 1 to thank him for the "beautiful and most helpful act of beneficence you propose." He promised to carefully investigate the finances of the ill students, in Ithaca and elsewhere, and let him know the findings. Meanwhile, Schurman took Carnegie's offer to the Executive Committee of the Board of Trustees, which accepted it with thanks on April 6. News of Carnegie's offer broke in the *New York Sun* the following day, and requests for aid from parents and students poured in. Students—or their parents, if the student was deceased—were notified by letter to send Schurman an itemized statement of expenses related to their illness. Carnegie asked that donations or pledges to the Students' Hospital Fund be returned to those who gave them, which suggested that the university might have been embarrassed by the student action on the medical bills. Carnegie instructed his bankers to turn over an initial $59,000 to the university on April 25.[8]

Cornell students on May 8 adopted a resolution thanking Carnegie for helping them. "We wish to express to Mr. Carnegie our deep sense of gratitude and appreciation for the thoughtful and noble gift to those of our number who were stricken with the fever, a gift which enabled many of them to continue their work in the university, and has lifted a heavy burden from scores of others."[9] And students being students, the wags on the *Cornellian* staff came up with a bit of verse, "The ABC of Cornell," expressing the same sentiment in more vulgar language:

> A is Andy of Pittsburgh fame;
> Carnegie is his other name.
> To cure us of financial ills
> He paid up all our fever bills.

The letters sent to Schurman requesting help from Carnegie provide an often raw and searing look at the impact of the epidemic on students and their families. Many writers struggled with accepting the billionaire's money, but ultimately nearly all did. Homer S. Sackett, a student who admitted that his father "is a poor man," opened his letter to Schurman by telling the Cornell president how the "spirit of independence and a sense of right" had battled within him:

> At first, the independent spirit had resolved me not to send in any bills incurred during my late sickness, but later, after due

consideration of the question, and after consultation with my father, I have decided, in as much as my father is a poor man and, as I am helping myself through college to a great extent, to avail myself of Mr. Carnegie's most generous offer."[10]

Parents often argued their moral worthiness for assistance, offering proof that they were not poor managers of their money but rather good people in an impossible situation. Hannah Spencer, mother of Charlotte Elizabeth Spencer, the second Cornell student to die of typhoid, laid out her life story, and an interesting story it was for a woman of her day. She told Schurman how she worked as a young woman to get her father out of debt from a business failure, becoming a teacher at age fifteen and turning over her money to her father after sleeping with it under her pillow for a night. She attended Alfred University in Alfred, New York, married a farmer, and had six children, five boys and a girl, Charlotte. They had a successful farm, of which she was the formal half-owner. Her goal was to put her children through college and she did, even cosigning student loans for them despite the fact that her husband "did not see the necessity for much school." Her youngest boy, Alfred, was at Yale, winning scholarships for his tuition and waiting tables for his board, and Charlotte was in her second year at Cornell when her death from typhoid made all her mother's hard work seem like a cosmic bad joke. Her husband, she wrote to Schurman, placed the blame for Charlotte's death on her, saying, "If [you] had not been so anxious for the children to go to school she would be living now."[11]

Jarvis A. Wood, the Philadelphia advertising executive whose son, Graham, was one of the last Cornell students to die in the epidemic, expressed deep gratitude to Carnegie in his letters to Schurman. He acknowledged that the medical and funeral expenses were a burden but politely rejected any help. "I would not like to do without the satisfaction of paying these last expenses of my boy, and yet I consider Mr. Carnegie's spirit in this matter most beautiful. He seems to me by this act to say that the Alma Mater will go beyond what has hitherto been known, and will do this toward carrying the burden and allaying the grief for those of her sons who have prematurely fallen."[12]

The praise for Carnegie was accompanied by the occasional skeptical note, such as this editorial in the *Oakland Tribune* in California:

The typhoid epidemic at Cornell University has one compensating feature. It has enabled Andrew Carnegie to announce that he will pay the medical expenses of all the students who contracted the disease including those who died. The latter can fully appreciate Mr. Carnegie's kindness. It is a pity a man with such beneficent inclinations must accompany his good deeds with circus poster advertising. The old adage says, "Never look a gift horse in the mouth," but Mr. Carnegie compels you to look. He cannot give a ragged urchin a nickel without having the pipes swirl in his honor. But there are spots on the sun, even.[13]

Carnegie's offer did not extend to Ithaca residents who were not Cornell students. The financial impact on them was no less than on the students, and many families delayed payment to their physicians. The problem was such that the *Ithaca Daily News* published an editorial, "Pay the Doctor Bills," on May 20 urging all Ithaca residents to do the right thing:

Remember how hard he worked, how earnestly he threw himself into the task of saving those who had not yet been stricken and of cleansing the home of the dangers which lurked all about. If you do not know from your own experience that people watched eagerly for his mandates and observed them carefully, frightened lest failure to obey should make conditions worse, take the word of all who were engaged in that work. The people needed help.[14]

Two years after the epidemic, the Cornell University Executive Committee took up the case of Bernard Reilly, an employee of the university, apparently of the grounds crew, who was killed in an accident on the job. Reilly's family, who lived at 129 Hazen St., was left deeply in debt by medical bills and funeral expenses from his injury and death. They still had unpaid medical bills from the typhoid epidemic, when Reilly and two members of his family were stricken with the fever. The Executive Committee did not accept any responsibility for the accident—few employers did before state workers' compensation laws began being adopted in the second decade of the twentieth century—but agreed to pay $405 to Reilly's family, "in recognition of his long and faithful service," to defray his medical expenses, both from the injury and the typhoid epidemic.[15]

Remarkably, there is no record of any lawsuits seeking damages for the epidemic being filed in Tompkins County, New York, the most likely venue for any such lawsuits. Cornell families who had the means to sue were perhaps influenced by Carnegie's generosity to quiet their anger, and for many Ithaca residents, a lawsuit was simply beyond their means in an era before the widespread use of the contingency fee method of financing litigation. People just didn't sue as much back then, even if they had been harmed beyond all reason. Or perhaps they feared retaliation from the people who controlled their livelihoods if they sued William T. Morris.

Chapter 15

Retribution

WILLIAM T. MORRIS LET THOMAS W. SUMMERS be the public face of Ithaca Water Works during the epidemic, so the burning question in Ithaca in the late spring of 1903 was less what to do about him than what to do about the water company. But city officials and public water advocates had no illusions about who was in charge. Can any man responsible for the deaths of people, the deaths of children, expect no retribution? After the Ithaca epidemic, though, the anger flowed in both directions.

The deal announced by President Schurman on February 18 for Morris to build a filtration plant for Ithaca in exchange for higher water rates explicitly authorized the city to hold another referendum on creating its own water system, an act that implied taking over Ithaca Water Works by condemnation. Schurman didn't much care what happened to Morris, blaming his incompetent management for the catastrophe that had overwhelmed the city and university. He wanted to be able to tell parents that their children would have safe water to drink when they arrived in Ithaca for the fall semester in 1903.

Ithaca Common Council members acted quickly to schedule the referendum for March 2. This time there would be no funny business as there was in the 1902 referendum, no landlord agents casting ten to thirty-seven votes because the rules said people could vote as many times as the number of properties they owned and didn't have to go in person. It was widely believed that the landlord agents had given Morris his margin of victory in 1902.[1]

And unlike last time, women who were taxpayers would be allowed to vote in the referendum.

There were things that had influenced the voters in 1902 that would not be repeated this time. Francis Miles Finch, respected dean of the Cornell Law School (but more importantly, an officer of Ithaca Trust Company, which had financed Morris's acquisition of the gas and water companies from the Tremans), had publicly denounced a municipal takeover as "socialism." Morris had hired "opposition talkers" to buttonhole voters and urge them to vote against a takeover and had paid for carriages to haul his supporters to the polls. He won the 1902 referendum, 718 to 583.

During the run-up to the new referendum on March 2, 1903, the *Ithaca Daily News* accused Morris of again trying to influence the outcome of voting, but he protested in a letter to the *Ithaca Daily Journal* that he had not hired canvassers and would stay neutral in the campaign. Nevertheless, Morris used the letter to release information aimed at disarming some of his most vocal critics, namely those who feared the ninety-foot dam he was building on Six Mile Creek, the one they suspected would unleash a Johnstown-like flood upon Ithaca if it broke. He said that "in deference to public opinion and the recommendation of Dr. Daniel Lewis, Commissioner of Health of the State of New York," he had abandoned the dam and would instead construct a steam-powered pump to lift water up to East Hill "and other high levels." That may have been a reference to the Cornell Heights real estate development being promoted by his friends Charles H. Blood and Jared Treman Newman. Trouble is, none of this was true, but the facts would come out only after the election.[2]

Taking no chances this time, public water advocates in Ithaca organized under the banner of the "Committee of 100" and pushed hard for a "yes" vote. They did not simply assume the rightness of their cause would carry the day against entrenched supporters of the water company. Public attitudes had shifted markedly, though, in the wake of the epidemic, and a poll taken by the Ithaca Business Men's Association a few days before the election predicted a five-to-one victory margin for municipal water.

This may have been one of the first elections in New York State open to women voters who were taxpayers, a right not granted statewide in all elections until 1917. Women had borne the brunt of caring for typhoid victims,

and both Ithaca newspapers made much of their participation in the referendum. The *Daily News* commented on how early in the afternoon, "many
women taxpayers" were brought to the Ithaca police station in carriages, got
out, and went inside to cast their votes. The *Ithaca Daily Journal* observed
that the polling place was quieter than usual, which it attributed to the presence of women voters. Several voters of both sexes who were well on in years
and feeble were helped to the ballot box to cast their votes. In the end, Ithaca's anger turned into 1,330 votes—oddly, almost the same number as had
typhoid—in favor of the city owning its own water system. Just thirty voters were opposed. The total number of taxpayers who could vote was about
2,600, so turnout was just over 50 percent. "The people have achieved a great
victory and everyone who has the welfare of the city at heart can well rejoice
over the result," the *Daily News* exulted in an editorial.[3]

In early February, before the vote, Ithaca Business Men's Association
had released a new proposal for the city to take over the water company,
prompting an appeal from President Schurman to hold off until the cause
of the epidemic was determined. As the epidemic progressed, though, he
became obsessed with obtaining clean water for students by the start of the
fall semester. Schurman told one correspondent that while he preferred to
drink pure artesian water, he doubted any water source other than Six Mile
Creek was practical for Ithaca. In any case, he did not believe artesian water
in sufficient volume could be obtained by September 1. Now, in the wake of
the vote, he told Henry R. Ickelheimer that while there might be "difficulties" between the city and Ithaca Water Works, he had no doubt the former
would eventually take over the latter, given the "relentless campaign" pursued by the public water advocates. If in the "chaotic interval," Ithaca Water
Works could supply pure water, perhaps with the help of the Board of Trustees, "the university will at least be safe," Schurman wrote.[4]

For the true believers among the public water revolutionaries, the citizens of Ithaca had come out of the wilderness and reached the promised
land. Many of them, including publisher Duncan Campbell Lee, believed
that vast supplies of pure artesian water—pockets of groundwater trapped
under pressure—lay beneath Ithaca and could be quickly tapped and connected to the existing water system. "The present poisonous supply can be
shut off, the mains and pipes of the city can be cleansed by disinfectants,

and the most delicious, wholesome, and pure water can be supplied the city," the *Ithaca Daily News* wrote in an editorial "Even the thought of it alone is refreshing."

Much artesian water lay deep beneath Ithaca, trapped in ancient gravel deposits and replenished by the streams plunging down from the hills around Cayuga Lake as well as by rainwater. Illston Artesian Water Company, which had done a brisk business supplying jugs of clean artesian water during the epidemic, drew from this source. The company's well yielded 300,000 gallons per day. Robert H. Thurston, dean of the mechanical engineering faculty at Cornell, told Schurman that all the signs pointed to a bountiful supply.[5] The question was whether there was enough to supply a growing city, and whether it could be tapped quickly enough to meet Schurman's September 1 deadline for clean water. The Cornell president obviously didn't think so.

But assuming there was enough artesian water, what if Ithaca Water Works resisted an immediate surrender of its mains? The network of mains would be horribly expensive to duplicate, and the city could not realistically expect to operate its own water system without them. One of the more radical members of the Committee of 100, Marcus E. Calkins, president of the Cayuga Lake Cement Company, advocated confiscation of the water mains if necessary. That is what any large corporation would do, Calkins said—act first and fight it out in court later. Seeking to halt this Jacobin fervor, the *Ithaca Daily Journal* rejoined, "Let us consider this matter calmly. Wild talk of seizing the Water Works Company's plant by force only does us injury."[6]

Before the city of Ithaca could set up a municipal water company, with or without the Ithaca Water Works system, it needed a bill passed by the New York State Legislature to allow it to do so. A twelve-member committee led by city attorney Randolph Horton, whose members came from Common Council, the Board of Health, the Committee of 100, and Cornell University, began drafting a bill. Among the members were Alderman Charles C. Howell, whose five-year-old daughter, Esther, had died of typhoid on February 13, and Jared Treman Newman, a member of the Cornell University Board of Trustees and Executive Committee and codeveloper of Cornell Heights.

Newman and his partner, Charles H. Blood, needed the water that would rise behind the Six Mile Creek dam to serve lot buyers in the new development.

Newman reported back to Schurman on March 4 that the first meeting of the committee had been contentious, especially when he argued for naming the members of the new Water Board in the legislation, rather than giving the Democratic mayor George W. Miller the power to appoint them. He was also opposed to giving the Water Board "unlimited powers without check," although he never explained publicly what he meant by that. The bill as drawn up by Horton gave the Water Board the power to acquire and condemn property, notably the property of Ithaca Water Works, and to incur almost unlimited debt to do so. Some committee members believed Newman was trying to kill the bill entirely for Cornell University. "It required a very free use of my conciliatory 'oil can' to restore my status as a persona grata to act with the [committee] at all," he wrote to Schurman.

The committee agreed to defer action on the draft bill until the following night, by which time Samuel D. Halliday, chairman of the Cornell Board of Trustees and its Executive Committee, was expected to return. Newman proposed a compromise he hoped would ensure that Cornell students had clean water to drink by September 1. "It eliminates the water company as a factor in the situation, and will allay the intense feeling that prevails in respect to anything affecting the company and which prevents dispassionate and disinterested consideration of what is best for the whole city," he wrote.[7] The compromise, hammered out after Halliday's return, provided the mayor with the power to appoint members of the Water Board with Common Council consent, set limits on spending, and most importantly, did not permit the Water Board to mount an immediate takeover of Ithaca Water Works' facilities. The board would first have to negotiate a price with Ithaca Water Works and Morris, but if that effort failed, it could resort to condemnation.

In a letter to Schurman, Newman credited Halliday for the outcome, saying that his "uncompromising vigorous policy" and "occasional sledgehammer blows" had made clear to the rest of the committee the sort of resistance they would face from Cornell University and Ithaca Water Works if the legislation was not modified. He wrote that some of the "rabid artesian men" were disconsolate and had accused the rest of the committee with "absolute surrender."[8]

Now the proposed bill went to state senator Edwin Stewart of Ithaca, who needed little encouragement to run with it. His wife lay seriously ill with typhoid, but he continued to commute to Albany to do his job. Stewart had introduced legislation on February 5 to give the state health commissioner new powers to regulate discharges of sewage and other waste into public waterways, requiring revocable permits and disclosure of what was being discharged. The commissioner was also given authority to order municipalities to improve sanitary facilities, even if it meant raising taxes, and authority to regulate construction of new water and sewerage facilities.[9] He introduced the Ithaca Water Board bill on March 11, and it was signed into law on April 15 by Governor Benjamin Odell, who himself was disturbed by the relentless severity of the Ithaca epidemic.

Buried in the details of the legislation was a startling revelation: the Six Mile Creek dam was back, albeit reduced in height from ninety feet to thirty feet, "for the use of the said filtration plant." The water company's engineers believed that at least a small dam was necessary if the filtration plant was to work properly. And what of the February 26 letter from Morris to the *Ithaca Daily Journal,* the one in which he said he was bowing to public opinion and abandoning the dam? Gardner S. Williams, the architect of the dam, testified in 1906 that the reduction in height was done only because of the passage of the Water Board bill and "not because of public opposition."[10] It is hard to view the letter as other than willful prevarication aimed at influencing the election, but in fairness to Morris, perhaps the need for a dam and reservoir only became evident when he began looking seriously at what a filtration plant would entail.

Although the original plan that Schurman had outlined to Ithaca Common Council called for the university to loan Ithaca Water Works $150,000, the actual cost of the filtration plant turned out to be only about $80,000. Because the start of construction could not be delayed until Ithaca Water Works obtained financing through a bond sale, at least not if the filtration plant was to be online by September 1, Morris approached the Cornell Board of Trustees on April 15 seeking a short-term, $40,000 loan carrying his personal guarantee. The other $40,000 would be loaned by "certain financial interests in Ithaca." Who that was is unknown. Morris complained in his letter to the board that his plans for financing extensions and improvements to the water system had been upset by "the recent epidemic," as well as "this agitation for municipal ownership."[11]

Four days later, the trustees held their noses and approved the loan. The university demanded $70,000 in bonds of Ithaca Water Works' parent company, Ithaca Light & Water Company, as security. Eleven board members voted for the loan, among them Charles E. Treman, back in town now that the epidemic was all but over. George R. Williams, Duncan Campbell Lee's father-in-law, and Alonzo B. Cornell, a son of the university founder, voted against it, and there was one abstention. No one at the meeting was under any illusion that this was a quality investment. The minutes noted:

> It is understood by every member present that the quality and security of this loan are not in accordance with our university standards of investments, but is deemed necessary and warranted by the existing exigencies of the local sanitary situation, and in the interest of this university.[12]

With the money in hand, work on the dam and filtration plant began in earnest. This time nearly 250 Italian workers were on the job, and we can only assume sanitation was enforced this time. No further issue in that regard seems to have arisen. In deference to Schurman's desires, Morris was building a mechanical filtration plant, which included a sand filter but added a coagulant chemical, aluminum sulfate, to speed up the filtration process. The Cornell president believed a mechanical filter could be built more swiftly than a traditional sand filter, and nothing could stand in the way of having clean water available by September 1. Morris hired Allen Hazen, the foremost American authority on water filtration who had designed the filtration plant at Albany, to design the Ithaca facility.[13]

Almost in a parallel universe, the Ithaca Water Board pressed forward with its righteous cause of bringing clean artesian water to the city. The Committee of 100 hired Cornelius Vermeule, a prominent consulting engineer from New York City who specialized in water system design, to investigate the prospects. He tramped the valleys of Fall Creek and Cascadilla Creek from Ithaca to Dryden and Freeville, studying the geology and examining existing artesian wells. What he saw amazed him, especially the Illston well, where the underground pressure was such that it pushed water thirty feet above the ground in a tube and the volume was tremendous. "I have seen no region in my experience which is more promising as a field for artesian wells than this about Ithaca," Vermeule wrote in a letter to the Committee of 100. "This water could be delivered by gravity into the highest reservoir in Ithaca, namely the one on the grounds of Cornell University."[14]

The battle was soon joined. On April 28, Mayor George Miller, acting on behalf of the Water Board, demanded that Morris open the books of Ithaca Water Works so the Water Board could obtain the information it needed to carry out a purchase of the water system. In addition, Miller directed Morris to either attend the next meeting of the Water Board to answer questions, including the price he wanted for the system, or send a knowledgeable representative.

Morris arrived at the May 5 meeting with his posse, Ebenezer M. Treman, Thomas W. Summers, and Mynderse Van Cleef, and told the Water Board that if it wanted to avoid a lengthy court fight, it would have to pay $650,000 for the water system. It was an eye-popping price for a company Morris had owned for just over seventeen months. He had paid the Tremans $100,000 and assumed $250,000 in existing debt, so his sale price represented an 85 percent premium over what he had paid for the company originally. It was hard to justify on business grounds, let alone moral ones: His incompetent management of the company had unleashed a catastrophe that killed more than eighty-two people and sickened hundreds more. We can only imagine the stunned anger that must have greeted his demand. At the conclusion of the two-hour meeting, the board met privately and concluded that it would need to hire experts to examine the water company from top to bottom to determine what it was really worth.[15] A court fight seemed inevitable.

In the meantime, work on the dam and filtration plant continued day and night. The *Ithaca Daily News* speculated that Morris was trying to finish them before the Ithaca Water Board could bring artesian water online, forcing the city to buy both the dam and filtration plant. "Sections of the great dam about 12 feet high and 20 feet long have been built from both sides," the *Daily News* reported. "The work of installing the five-foot outlet pipe and the mains in the section on the north side of the creek has been finished, and the creek channel has been turned so that all the water is now running through the outlet pipe." It seemed the hated dam and filtration plant would be finished in no time, and the reaction among public water advocates was dark anger.

At the council meeting on May 20, Alderman Charles C. Howell, "who was greatly agitated," according to the *Ithaca Daily Journal*, raged against the dam, the dam that had claimed his five-year-old daughter Esther's life by bringing typhoid to Ithaca. He did not mention her that night—everyone knew his sorrow—but cast his opposition as a safety issue, saying that Cornelius Vermeule, the engineer hired by the Committee of 100, had told him the sand used in the concrete was not the proper kind and the concrete itself had not been mixed properly. "Behind this structure will lie a quantity of water so great that it would if released cause damage beyond the conception of the people of Ithaca, and a probable loss of life," Howell said angrily, demanding that council do something to stop the dam. A week later, council directed city attorney Randolph Horton to seek an injunction to stop construction. But the effort went nowhere, and work on the dam continued.[16]

As it sank in that Cornell University and Morris were winning, the editorials in the *Ithaca Daily News* became angry and bitter, even vituperative. In "An Insult to Public Intelligence" on April 29, the *Daily News* attacked its rival, the *Ithaca Daily Journal*, for not daring to print news about the epidemic "without the approval of a certain clique," meaning the Tremans and Cornell University. The *Journal*, which was strongly in favor of the filtration plant, had attacked artesian water as dangerous. "The public understands the *Journal*'s motives," the *Daily News* wrote. "Its object in talking in favor of filtered sewage is too evident to need comment. But it does disgust the people to see published such diabolical rot."[17]

In "Will the Water Company Be Fair" on May 2, the *Daily News* criticized Ithaca Water Works for sending out bills demanding six months' advance payment for water "which is still under the ban of the board of health and unfit for use." It noted that the water company had violated the clause in its 1902 contract with the city of Ithaca requiring it to provide pure water and appealed to Morris not to squeeze Ithaca citizens to pay for water they could not use:

> The water company has violated its sacred contract; it has shown the utmost indifference for the welfare of the people; it has shown

no sympathy for the hundreds who have suffered from the fever, or for the hundreds who mourn the loss of dear ones; it has shown no desire to remedy existing conditions; it has shown no regard for the business welfare of the city. In short, it has done everything to arouse the indignation of a public which has been disgracefully wronged.[18]

When the water company persisted, sending second notices to the apparently large number of Ithaca residents who had not paid the first bill, the *Daily News* wrote on May 26 in "Water Company's Unlimited Gall" that Six Mile Creek water was "dangerous and wholly unfit for use except for flushing closets [toilets]."

But it was the May 28 editorial, "Nothing Less Than an Outrage," that finally triggered a libel suit. The editorial, most likely written by publisher Duncan Campbell Lee, but possibly by managing editor Frank E. Gannett, continued the newspaper's campaign against the dam. It accused the contractor, Tucker & Vinton, of deliberately inflating the cost of the dam because it was paid on a percentage basis. Then it implied that the contractor was paying high prices for poor quality materials and that the concrete was not being properly mixed. And finally this:

> Expert engineers say that the dam is not being built well. The fact that it is proposed to make the city pay an enormous price for the big piece of jobbery does not alter the case. The dam might cost a million dollars and still crumble away in six months time. The people will not trust the water company to build this dam to sell to the city. If we must have a dam we should have the right to build it ourselves. It is an outrage on the community to allow this company to proceed as it has been doing.[19]

Making a direct accusation or even implying that Tucker & Vinton might have been guilty of fraud, incompetence, and professional malfeasance might have triggered a libel suit even under today's much more press-friendly libel laws. In 1903, it was seemingly a plaintiff lawyer's dream, with truth being almost the only defense. "The general rule is that it is libelous *per se* to impute to a person in his official capacity, profession, trade or business any kind of fraud, dishonesty, misconduct, incapacity or unfitness." Those words were written by Henry W. Sackett, a member of the Cornell University Board of Trustees and longtime libel lawyer for the *New York Tribune*.[20] As much as Lee might have believed what he wrote, he was in trouble if he did not have hard facts to back it up. He was writing in anger, writing in memory of the many new graves in Ithaca and the suffering all around him. He let his emotions get the better of him.

Tucker & Vinton sued for libel, naming Ithaca Publishing Company and Frank E. Gannett, managing editor as defendants. The contractor demanded $50,000 in damages for "false and malicious statements" and denied all the allegations in the May 28 editorial. Duncan Campbell Lee did not back down. "The *News* feels that it can do no better public service than to bring out before the courts expert evidence in the matter," he wrote in a new editorial. "If there is not one way of stopping the dam, there may be another. And if we succeed in protecting the lives of Ithacans we will not regret the trouble and cost of a fifty-thousand-dollar libel suit."[21]

Morris, meanwhile, hired Sackett as his own libel lawyer to pursue a case on behalf of himself and Ithaca Water Works against the *Daily News*. Morris sent Sackett clips of articles he found offensive; Sackett selected six for the water company libel complaint and four for that of Morris. "I have been careful to eliminate the publications that would raise issues of privilege or as to the quality of the water, leaving the question to be decided whether the defendants were justified in attacking the integrity and honesty of purpose of the plaintiffs," Sackett wrote. "That I am satisfied is the issue for you to fight on."

What Sackett hoped to do was convince a jury that Lee and the newspaper had made unjustified attacks on the reputation of Ithaca Water Works and Morris for honesty and fair dealing, while avoiding the question of whether Morris had provided contaminated water to his customers. Sackett seemed decidedly ambivalent about Morris's case, telling Mynderse Van Cleef that perhaps Morris ought to reduce his demand for damages from $50,000 to $25,000 or "even less." Nor did he seem to care in which county the case was filed, Tompkins around Ithaca or Chemung around Elmira. There was no telling what an Ithaca jury might do if Morris presented himself as a businessman of good reputation, unjustly libeled by the *Daily News*, because that jury would learn quickly enough who he was and what he had done.[22]

In the end, neither the Tucker & Vinton nor the Morris/Ithaca Water Works libel suits went forward. Those of Morris and the company did not even get to the complaint stage. While we do not know the exact reasons the lawsuits were not pursued, it seems likely that the builders of the dam and the deliverer of the epidemic were finally made to understand that their chances in front of an Ithaca jury were not promising.

Morris suffered a blow on May 18 when the luxurious, four-story Chi Phi fraternity house at 107 Edgemoor Lane caught fire from a carelessly discarded cigarette and was extensively damaged. Morris, who was an alumni member of Chi Phi, happened to be visiting the house at the time, a fact reported by the *Ithaca Daily News* but not the *Daily Journal*. He and one of the young fraternity members discovered the blaze and called in the alarm while two other students tried without success to beat down the flames with a portable extinguisher. Firemen arrived in their horse-drawn equipment but had little success against the fire, in part because of low water pressure but also because it was burning mainly in the attic. They had trouble directing water to the flames. Finally the roof caved in and gave them access. Students threw personal belongings from windows and carried out much of the furniture, but some of the more expensive pieces in the dining room were ruined by water.[23] The following day, Chi Phi alumni met at Morris's office at Ithaca Water Works and vowed to rebuild the house by September 1. The fraternity brothers were greatly inconvenienced, forced to abandon an elaborate reception that was to be held in the house during Senior Week, the last week of school. Morris, though, provided temporary lodging for many of them at his home on Green Street until the end of the school year. When he cared about something, he could move heaven and earth to make it happen.[24]

Morris had resumed an active social life, refusing to be held down by the depression and gloom in the city from the epidemic. After bringing his yacht from Penn Yan to Ithaca via the interconnected Finger Lakes, he invited Charlie, Rob, and Eben Treman and their wives, Mynderse Van Cleef and his wife, and the bachelor Charles H. Blood to join him to watch the Memorial Day regatta on Cayuga Lake. They partied on the dark water as they sipped cocktails and watched Cornell emerge victorious over rowers from Harvard and the University of Pennsylvania.[25]

The Cornell University Board of Trustees had a score to settle now that the epidemic was over. Duncan Campbell Lee, who had turned the oratory and debate program at Cornell into one of America's best, and who, by the by, published the muckraking *Ithaca Daily News*, applied to the Board of Trustees on May 12 seeking promotion to the full professorship that was his due. And at its June meeting, without comment, the board rejected his application. It was a humiliating and career-ending action, and we can assume the board intended it to be so. A year later, Lee resigned from the Cornell faculty.

No documents explaining the board's action have ever been unearthed. We know who was there that day but not how they voted. Among those present were President Schurman, Charles H. Blood, Samuel D. Halliday, Jared Treman Newman, Henry W. Sackett, Rob Treman, Charlie Treman, Franklin C. Cornell, and Mynderse Van Cleef. They all had reasons to stick a knife in Lee. His father-in-law, George R. Williams, was absent from the meeting.[26]

Samuel Hopkins Adams revealed in *McClure's Magazine* in 1905 that Lee had been warned he was jeopardizing his teaching position (this was before universities had tenure policies) by having his newspaper aggressively report and comment on the typhoid epidemic. Lee told university officials, according to Adams, that the policy of his newspaper was "to tell the truth as it appeared." Adams wrote:

> After the scourge had passed, this man found himself persona non grata with the controlling interests of the institution. Owing to the unusual success of his department he was in line for a full professorship. Now he learned that as long as he remained at the head of the department, it would continue to be merely an assistant professor's department.[27]

Adams lamented that Lee, a fellow muckraker, was punished for telling the truth but that Morris was not punished for poisoning the water.

Under the university's governing structure, President Schurman had no veto over board actions. Punishing Lee violated everything he stood for. In 1898, Schurman wrote that if universities are to do their work well, "the teacher must be absolutely free. Knowledge is a thing which cannot be commanded. The truth of propositions cannot be established by councils or tyrants." He wrote again in 1905, "The university is an organ of truth and knowledge. It must be free and unhampered, or it is useless if not pernicious. University authorities must guard jealously the right of freedom of inquiry, freedom of thought, and freedom of speech." But at Cornell, that did not happen. The Board of Trustees trampled on academic freedom in its zeal to punish a critic.[28]

On the morning of June 16, as he set out on his final walk to Van Order's boatyard, did Theodor Zinck comprehend the full injustice of what he and the other parents of dead children had endured? As he rowed out onto the dark water, as he placed his derby hat, pocketknife, and matchbox on the seat in front of him, did he forgive Lula's killers? Zinck stood up, steadied himself, and looked back at Ithaca. The thought of cold water and drowning may have given him pause, but his beloved daughter was calling to him from the hillside. There was a splash and he was gone, sinking to the bottom of Cayuga Lake.

Epilogue
Getting Away with Murder

THE SURPRISE WAS HOW QUICKLY CORNELL UNIVERSITY returned to normal that
fall and put the epidemic behind it. Enrollment actually showed a healthy
increase. In the issues of the *Cornell Daily Sun* from the autumn of 1903, only
one brief mention of the epidemic occurs, in a story about President Schurman's opening address to students on September 25. Then it slipped down
the memory hole, and the *Sun* resumed its regular diet of sports and campus
activities. A student mass meeting called for October 6 turned out to be an
urgent appeal for greater support of the football team. We will never know
what the survivors held in their hearts, but it seems to have been a private
grief, confided only to friends.[1]

Dormitories, or "Halls of Residence" as Schurman insisted upon calling them, for male students were authorized at the April 18 meeting of the
Board of Trustees. No longer would students be forced to live in substandard boardinghouses on East Hill. Schurman insisted the new lodgings all
be "plain, substantial, and convenient" and offer the exact same accommo-
dations to rich students as to poor. "It is unnatural to disturb the free and
generous intercourse of youth by reminders of artificial distinction; and it is
little less than criminal for a university to encourage or permit the classifi-
cation of students according to their money," he wrote.[2] The former Prince
Edward Island farm boy who had gone through university on scholarship no
doubt knew what those classifications meant to students of modest means.

Construction of the first dormitory for men, Sheldon Court, began in the summer of 1903.

As promised, students had clean water to drink on campus and off. Andrew Carnegie's filtration plant for the campus water supply drawn from Fall Creek was completed and put into service in May 1903, even before the academic year ended. Built on the site of an old reservoir, it could handle forty-two thousand gallons of water at a time. Raw water flowed into the first tank and was mixed with an aluminum sulfate solution. That chemical reacted with natural lime and magnesium in the water to magically form a gel that entangled 50 percent of the fine particles and bacteria in the water. Much of this gel sank to the bottom of the first tank, and the rest was captured when the water was moved into the second tank for traditional sand filtration. The water percolated through the sand and emerged "clear and colorless and practically free from bacteria."[3]

The water treatment plant that Morris built for the rest of Ithaca went into service on August 23, 1903. It was much larger than the Carnegie plant, able to process three million gallons of water per day, but worked by the same process. Residents noticed the change immediately, the *New York Tribune* reported. They looked at the water and for once it was clear, not dirty. Tests taken by Professor Emile M. Chamot for Ithaca Water Works in the fall revealed that the filters were working with greater than 99 percent efficiency. Tests of the raw water inevitably showed the presence of fecal bacteria; tests of the filtered water found none. People returned the handles to faucets they had removed in February to keep children from drinking the contaminated water. Warning signs came down. Life returned to normal.[4]

Yet the dream of providing clean, unfiltered, artesian water to Ithaca died hard. The Water Board drilled thirteen wells (average depth: three hundred feet) along West Clinton Street near the Cayuga Lake Inlet in 1904, of which nine yielded water, and built a new pumping station. The work was done under the supervision of the engineer hired by the Committee of 100, Cornelius C. Vermeule. On the day the Water Board took over the water system by condemnation, on December 31, 1904, it shut down the filtration plant and diverted artesian water from the nine wells into the mains instead. The proponents of artesian water had won, or so they thought. The wells yielded two million gallons per day but eventually began pulling water from nearby private wells. Litigation resulted, and in 1907, the Water Board sealed the artesian wells and went back to filtering Six Mile Creek water for the city's use. It was surely a bitter blow for those, like Duncan Campbell Lee, who had dreamed of clean artesian water for Ithaca. Six Mile Creek water is used in Ithaca to this day.[5]

But Morris's last laugh was still to come. The Water Board, even though it took over the Ithaca Water Works system, had been unable to come to terms with Morris over the price it would pay. He demanded $660,000, and the board would not pay a dime more than $436,000, less than the company's bonded indebtedness of about $600,000. Morris told Mynderse Van Cleef he would not give any consideration to the offer. "Evidently, the Water Board do not care to be fair and decent in the matter, and it is apparent to me that the only thing there is left to do is to prepare for a good, strong fight," he wrote. Morris vowed to protect his bondholders, telling the Water Board that they "are largely your own fellow citizens," but his protests fell on deaf ears. The Water Board had no sympathy for Morris or his bondholders. The two sides plunged into lengthy and costly litigation that lasted through 1905 and 1906.[6]

Morris's lawyers were led by Nathan Mathews Jr., a prominent real estate attorney from an aristocratic Yankee family in Massachusetts, who had been the Democratic mayor of Boston from 1891 to 1895. Mathews knew winning would be difficult. The $600,000 in bonded indebtedness was far more than Morris paid for Ithaca Water Works, and no estimate of the reproduction cost of the company could be made to exceed $550,000. Moreover, the net income of Ithaca Water Works had never topped about $20,000. Only if the lawyers and expert witnesses could make a plausible case for a doubling of net income in the near future, and for assigning a higher value to the company's water sources, was there any hope of a valuation above $600,000.[7] The litigation cost Morris a fortune in up-front money; by the time it was over, he had outstanding loans of more than $41,000 from Tompkins County National Bank, of which his friend Robert H. Treman was the president. The loans drew the skeptical attention of a federal bank examiner, who was assured by Treman that most of them were made in connection with the water litigation and that Morris would pay them back when he won.[8]

Three outside judges appointed by Tompkins County Supreme Court heard the case. Testimony began on May 25, 1905, and concluded on December 14, 1906. Thirteen days later, the Commission of Appraisal ruled that Morris was entitled to nearly all of the $660,000 he had demanded, minus only $2,000 for two vacant lots in downtown Ithaca that the company wanted to retain. With interest and court costs, the total amount came to $900,000. There was no nod to morality in the ruling, only the cold application of the law. That Morris killed more than eighty-two people with the water system was irrelevant. It was as if the epidemic had never happened. Even Mathews seemed surprised, calling it the most difficult case he had ever handled. He was amazed that the Commission of Appraisal had not cut the value assigned to Six Mile Creek. After all, the Water Board had introduced a valid, competing water source—the artesian wells—before the litigation began, and competition is supposed to drive down prices.[9]

The ruling shocked the Ithaca Water Board. "At first I think they were stunned and did not know what to do," President Schurman wrote to Samuel D. Halliday, chairman of the Board of Trustees, who was vacationing in the south of France. "Now, however, they are unanimously in favor of appealing and, what is worse, their attorneys are urging them to do so."[10]

Jared Treman Newman, who had resigned from the Board of Trustees in May 1903 and been elected mayor of Ithaca in November 1906, went to work with his famous "oil can" to broker a settlement that would avoid an appeal. He succeeded; after much negotiation, he got the Water Board to agree to drop its appeal in exchange for Ithaca Light & Water Company foregoing interest on the judgment and making certain other concessions. The final deal was for $663,570, with the Water Board agreeing to give back to Morris property around Enfield Falls and Buttermilk Falls plus the two vacant lots in downtown Ithaca. The waterfall properties later passed from Morris to his friend Robert H. Treman, who donated them to the State of New York in 1920 and 1923, respectively, and which today are Robert H. Treman State Park and Buttermilk Falls State Park. The Ithaca Water Board raised the money to pay Morris with a $666,000 bond issue.[11]

Newman and his business partner Charles H. Blood had worked closely with Morris since the day the dam was announced to obtain water service for their Cornell Heights real estate development. Water for Cornell Heights, as we have noted, may have been a contributing factor to the university Board of Trustees deciding in 1901 to loan Morris the money he needed to buy the water company. Blood's correspondence shows him in talks with Morris in April 1903 over the purchase of new water mains to serve Cornell Heights. "I am anxious, of course, to do anything that you or Eb [Treman] want in the proposition," Blood wrote on April 29. But that was as far as things got before Morris became absorbed in his fight with the Water Board.

On December 13, 1904, two weeks before the Water Board took over the system, Newman wrote to the Executive Committee of the Board of Trustees lamenting the time he expected it would take the Water Board to complete its plans for serving Cornell Heights after taking over the system. He asked whether his development could use any of the campus water, which now was filtered, but the board turned him down. Cornell Heights finally got a connection to the city water system in 1907 after Newman became mayor. Once it had a reliable water supply, lot sales took off and Cornell Heights became one of the premier neighborhoods of Ithaca, home to many Cornell professors.[12]

~~~~~~~

Many people weighed in with their thoughts on the Ithaca epidemic. One of the more devastating commentaries was published in the *Journal of the American Medical Association* on March 28, 1903, even as students and townspeople were still dying. The magazine had sent the great Chicago bacteriologist Dr. Edwin O. Jordan to Ithaca to investigate and write about what was going on, and the editorial grew out of his reporting. It began:

> There was a time when the epidemic of typhoid fever at Ithaca would have been looked on as a visitation of God; at the present time, it must be recognized as a failure on the part of some persons to do their duty.

JAMA let no party escape censure for their conduct and performance during the epidemic, not Ithaca Water Works, not Ithaca city officials, and most certainly not Cornell University. It demolished one of the excuses proffered by the university to absolve itself, namely that it had no more control over the water supply in Ithaca than Columbia University did in New York City or the University of Pennsylvania in Philadelphia:

It cannot be said that the responsibility of a university in a great city is at all in the same category with the responsibility of a university in a small town, which it can largely influence or even, if necessary, dominate.[13]

Even before the epidemic was over, Cornell University sought to spin what had happened, to subtly shift attention from what the university had not done to the actions of the students themselves. This largely successful effort has affected some local beliefs about the epidemic to the present day. An important component of this spin, repeated endlessly, was what we will call the "Fall Creek Fallacy," namely that no student who drank only the campus water from Fall Creek became ill with typhoid. Schurman said it many times, including in an official statement on February 14 and in his annual report to the Board of Trustees for the 1902–03 school year. "Fortunately, Fall Creek, which supplies the university, is all right; that is to say, not a single case of typhoid has been found among persons using this water exclusively," he wrote. Professor Waterman T. Hewett, in his 1905 book, *Cornell University: A History*, called it "a striking fact." It is heard on rare occasions at the university even today.

As a defense, the Fall Creek Fallacy made no sense. The problem, which Schurman of course knew, was that the vast majority of Cornell students lived off-campus in Ithaca and drank the city water because that was what was available in their boardinghouses. Was that their fault? Many were exposed even before the first "boil notice" went out or were at the mercy of careless landladies. Schurman and the Board of Trustees seemed determined to impose rugged individualism and personal responsibility on young men and women whose parents expected and demanded a far higher standard of care.

Another person critical to shaping public perception of the Ithaca epidemic was George A. Soper. A year after his energetic and critical cleanup work in Ithaca wiped out the last vestiges of typhoid, he wrote, "The Epidemic of Typhoid Fever at Ithaca, N.Y.," for the *Journal of the New England Water Works Association*. The article was accurate in many respects but woefully wrong in others. The wrong parts reflected the fact that Soper had not yet discovered or come to terms with the findings of German bacteriologist

Robert Koch and his associates. Put simply, Soper believed that typhoid carriers existed but could only spread their deadly bacilli via urination, not defecation. Because of that, he totally missed the significance of the filth along the banks of Six Mile Creek observed by at least five witnesses during the dam construction work in the fall of 1902. When you match that with his class-based assumptions and personal arrogance, it does not make for entirely enlightening reading.

Soper airily dismissed the possibility that the typhoid had originated with one or more of the Italian workers at the dam site, on the grounds that there was no record of any of them being ill with typhoid while doing hard physical construction work, an unlikely possibility in any case. Nor did he have any truck with the assertion of witnesses that the valley around the dam was a sanitary nightmare, because professional engineers like himself simply would not allow that to happen. "The work was in charge of professional engineers of high standing, and precautions were apparently taken to prevent any polluting matter from entering the stream. A young man [Shirley Clarke Hulse] who had recently graduated in engineering at Cornell was especially detailed to look after this matter." Case closed. He blamed bad feelings between the citizens and the water company over the dam "for the mental attitude of some citizens on this point."

Then Soper pulled out his trump cards, "Toothless Ben" and "Dirty Baker," two country characters who seemed to encompass all of his worst nightmares about the unwashed and dangerous working class. Toothless Ben was part of "a gang of laborers of mixed nationality but common bad character" who were building a railroad culvert over a tributary of Six Mile Creek about three miles from the Ithaca Water Works intake pipe. He supposedly developed typhoid and went home to be nursed. Soper says there was human filth along the stream banks at the work site but admits not knowing whether Ben contaminated the stream. The culvert project was carried out in the late summer and early fall, and Olin Landreth's observations on the ability of the ground to absorb rain-dissolved feces during the warm months have been previously noted.[14] And if Toothless Ben's feces *were* contaminated and *had* managed to reach the stream during that time period, the epidemic would have broken out months earlier, not in January.

Dirty Baker, who posed for a photograph for Soper in all his ragged glory, looked like Gabby Johnson, the loony frontiersman in the film comedy *Blazing Saddles*. He lived in a ramshackle dwelling in the Buttermilk Creek drainage area, which had no typhoid in its waters, thus excluding him as a possible source of the epidemic. Soper's inclusion of these men in his report seems to have been intended less to enlighten the public than to horrify his fellow engineers and divert attention from the pathetic state and inadequate supervision of the Tucker & Vinton work camp.[15]

It remained for *McClure's Magazine*, a prominent muckraking journal of the time, to bring the nation's attention back to the dark side of the epidemic, including the university's punishment of Duncan Campbell Lee. The writer, Samuel Hopkins Adams, sent an advance typescript of the Cornell section of his article—it was about typhoid in general, not just the Ithaca epidemic—to President Schurman on April 1, 1905, asking for suggestions or corrections. His letter received a frosty reply from Emmons L. Williams, the secretary/treasurer of the Board of Trustees, who said that Schurman was out of the country and the university would have no comment. But then he added:

> We will simply say that we regard the article as inaccurate, partisan, and unjust. The university will not under any circumstances permit itself to be drawn into a controversy and we say this much solely because we do not wish it to be understood or inferred that by silence we in any way acquiesce in the accuracy of the facts stated in that article or in the fairness and justness of its conclusions.[16]

Perhaps understandably, Cornell professors, students, and graduate students shied away from exploring the darker aspects of the epidemic, at least in depth, for many decades. Word gets around, and after what happened to Duncan Campbell Lee, any faculty member looking for advancement or graduate student wanting an advanced degree might think twice about antagonizing the Cornell administration. Waterman T. Hewett did write a brief account in his book, *Cornell University: A History*, also published in 1905, mentioning the suffering and deaths but dwelling upon the Fall Creek Fallacy and in general being uncritical of the university where he was a professor. Romeyn Berry, a member of the Class of 1904 who, like Hewitt, had lived through the epidemic, wrote briefly and passionately about it in his book, *Behind the Ivy*, published in 1950. Twelve years later, Morris Bishop offered a brief, bland, and pro-university snapshot of the epidemic in his book, *A History of Cornell*. The first known student paper was written by David L. Schiller for an undergraduate history class at Cornell in 1973. Schiller's paper, "The Social History of the 1903 Ithaca Typhoid Fever Epidemic: A Study of Anger and Action," uses the Soper photo of the mythical typhoid villain Dirty Baker as a frontispiece. Overall, though, his is a passionate, if somewhat muddled account of the epidemic that went further into the dark side than any article yet published.[17]

William T. Morris never spoke publicly about the epidemic, looking only to the future of his business. On March 17, 1906, while the water litigation was still under way, he incorporated a holding company for his utilities in part for the efficiencies this sort of arrangement provided. He called it Associated Gas & Electric Company, a name he had begun using for his utility business since 1903, after he purchased the Brush-Swan Electric Light Company of Ithaca for $100,000. The Brush Electric Company of Cleveland sold the soon-to-be-obsolete Brush-Swan technology for incandescent lighting to local power companies around the United States.

This was how it worked—the electric line to a customer's house charged storage batteries during the day, and those batteries powered incandescent lamps in the house for several hours at night. In a day before plug-in electric appliances, it made a certain amount of sense as a business model. Local companies that bought into the technology were not franchises but were allowed to incorporate "Brush-Swan" into their names as a form of marketing. This acquisition by Morris of his first real electric company—as opposed to the ludicrous Niagara Falls sewer-electric scheme—started his company down a long road that, surprisingly, ended in the Three Mile Island nuclear accident near Harrisburg, Pennsylvania, in 1979. We will get back to that later.[18]

There was another reason for incorporating Associated Gas & Electric. Morris had to have been aware of the rise of Charles Evans Hughes, a lawyer and dedicated utility reformer from New York City. Hughes was on a sleigh-ride to the Republican nomination for governor of New York. At the time he formally incorporated Associated Gas & Electric Company on March 17, 1906, Morris obviously did not know the details of Hughes's reform plan,

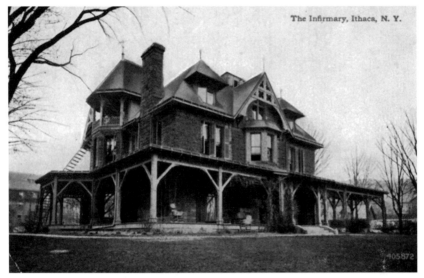

The Infirmary, Ithaca, N. Y.

Cornell Infirmary, the former Sage Mansion, was ground zero of the epidemic for students at the university. Overcrowded, offering substandard care, the typhoid death rate here was higher than at City Hospital. *The Leighton & Valentine Co.*

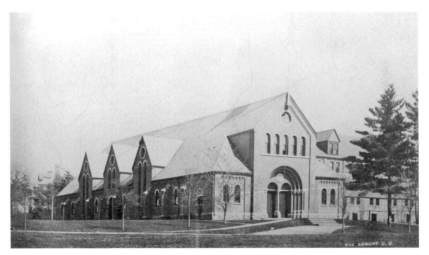

Cornell Armory was the scene of the doomed Junior Prom in 1903, held near the height of the epidemic. *Ira June Owens Scrapbook, Cornell University Rare and Manuscript Collections*

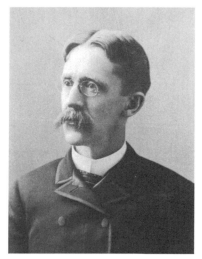

Brainard G. Smith was editor of the *Ithaca Daily Journal* during the epidemic. He was a professional colleague and rival of Duncan Campbell Lee. *Hamilton College Archives*

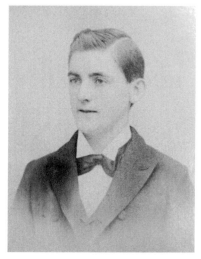

Frank E. Gannett was managing editor of the *Ithaca Daily News* under Duncan Campbell Lee when the typhoid epidemic broke out in Ithaca in 1903. He later built a newspaper empire and ran for the Republican nomination for President in 1940. *Gannett Collection, Cornell University Rare and Manuscript Collections*

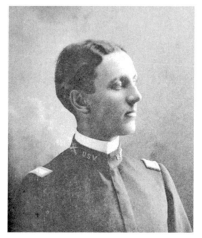

Ever the idealist, Duncan Campbell Lee took leave of the Cornell faculty in 1898 to join the Army to fight to free Cuba from Spanish rule. His unit, which never saw action, was hard hit by typhoid. When he returned home, Lee bought the *Ithaca Daily News* and hired Frank E. Gannett as managing editor. *Courtesy of Nancy Lee Gluck*

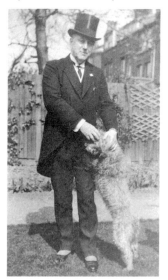

After his downfall in Ithaca, Duncan Campbell Lee went into exile in London, where he became a lawyer. *Courtesy of Nancy Lee Gluck*

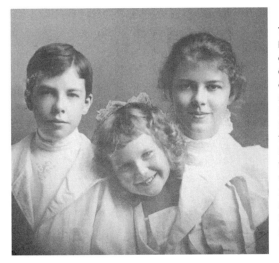

The three Griffis children were hard hit by the Ithaca typhoid epidemic. John Elliot Griffis, center, and Lillian Griffis, right, developed the disease but survived. Stanton Griffis, left, later chairman of Paramount Pictures and U.S. Ambassador to Argentina in the time of the Perons, escaped the fever but was a pallbearer for a friend who did not, Willis Dean, 17, an Ithaca High School classmate. *William Elliot Griffis Collection, Rutgers University Libraries*

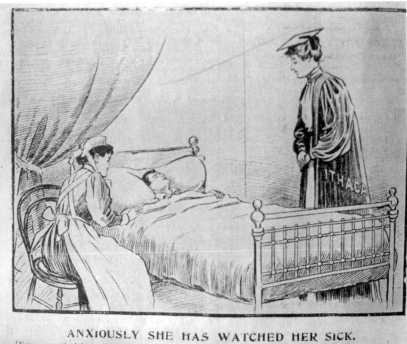

ANXIOUSLY SHE HAS WATCHED HER SICK.

[For a month Ithaca has been in sorrow over bed s of suffering. but hope has triumphed.]

This editorial cartoon captured the pathos of the 1903 typhoid epidemic. The cartoon was pasted into a student scrapbook and the newspaper which published it is unknown. *Kenneth Bertrand Turner Scrapbook, Cornell University Rare and Manuscript Collections*

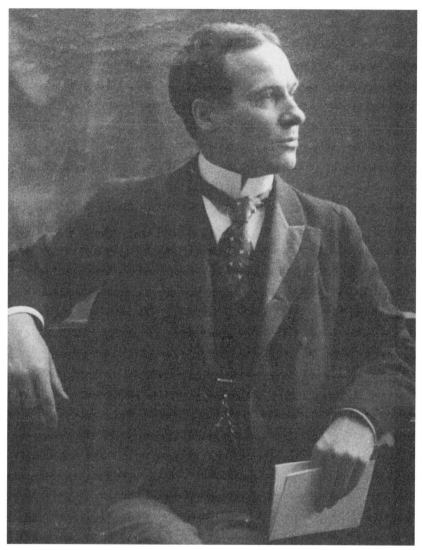

Jacob Gould Schurman was president of Cornell University during the typhoid epidemic.
Lillian Puris Heller Scrapbook, Cornell University Rare and Manuscript Collections

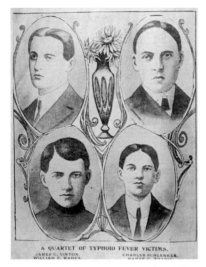

A QUARTET OF TYPHOID FEVER VICTIMS.
JAMES C. VINTON.   CHARLES SCHLENKER.
WILLIAM E. MAHER.

The Utica Journal on February 28, 1903, published these portrait illustrations of four of the Cornell men who died in the epidemic. *Kenneth Bertrand Turner Scrapbook, Cornell University Rare and Manuscript Collections*

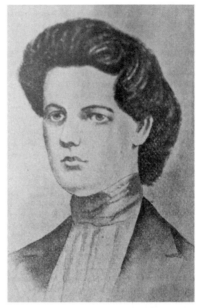

Charlotte Spencer was the second Cornell student and the first coed to die in the epidemic. *Kenneth Bertrand Turner Scrapbook, Cornell University Rare and Manuscript Collections. First published in Utica Journal, Feb. 28, 1903.*

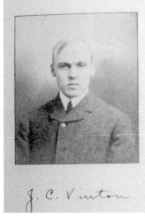

James Chapin Vinton, ΣΑΕ, came from Canal Dover, Ohio. He began his college career at the University of Colorado, and was received as a fellow Cornellian in our Sophomore year. The "Duke" had many warm friends, who deeply feel their loss in his sad death, so near the completion of his college course. He will be remembered by his classmates as a true friend and a "good fellow."

James C. Vinton's fellow students paid tribute to him in the Class Book after he died of typhoid during the epidemic. *Cornell University Rare and Manuscript Collections*

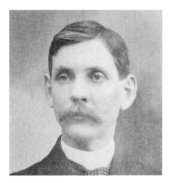

Professor Veranus A. Moore, who taught bacteriology at the Cornell Veterinary School, did important work to establish the cause of the typhoid epidemic. *Cornell University Rare and Manuscript Collections*

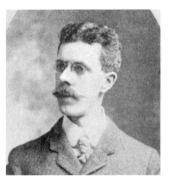

Professor Emile M. Chamot of Cornell had been concerned about the quality of Ithaca water for years. His methodical testing left no doubt that Ithaca's water was of poor quality even when it was not contaminated with typhoid germs. *Cornell University Rare and Manuscript Collections*

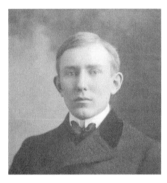

Shirley Clarke Hulse, a young assistant to Gardner S. Williams, failed to enforce camp sanitation during the Six Mile Creek Dam project. *Cornell University Rare and Manuscript Collections*

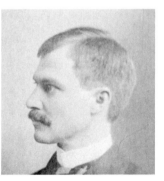

Gardner S. Williams, an engineering professor at Cornell, designed the star-crossed Six Mile Creek Dam for William T. Morris. *Cornell University Rare and Manuscript Collections*

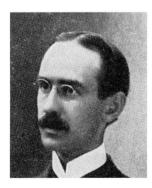

George A. Soper was dispatched to Ithaca by the New York State Health Commissioner to bring the typhoid epidemic under control. He carried out an intensive cleanup project in Ithaca aimed at stopping new secondary typhoid infections. *Rosenberg Library, Galveston, Texas*

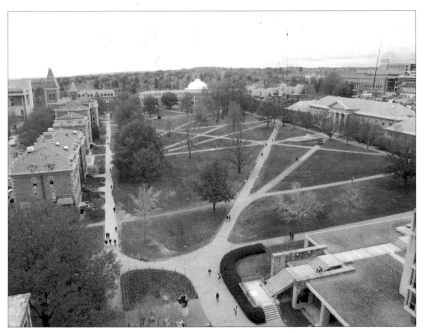

View from McGraw Tower of the Arts Quad of the Central Campus of modern day Cornell University. In 1903, this quad contained most of the school's classroom buildings and was at the heart of student life. *David DeKok*

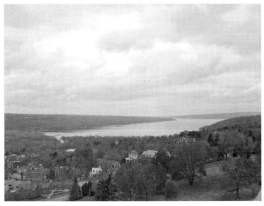

Cayuga Lake and part of Ithaca from McGraw Tower. *David DeKok*

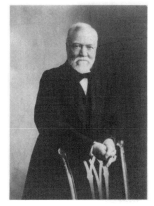

Cornell benefactor Andrew Carnegie. *Library of Congress*

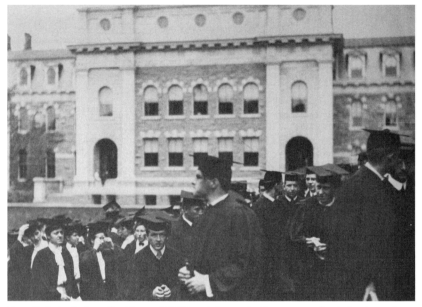

Cornell students from the Class of 1903 wait for graduation ceremonies to begin on June 18, 1903. Behind them is Sibley College, the Cornell engineering school. *Marie Paula Geiss Scrapbook, Cornell University Rare and Manuscript Collections*

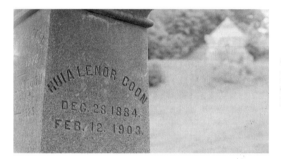

Grave of Ruia Coon, an Ithaca High School student who died of typhoid at age eighteen on Feb. 12, 1903. *David DeKok*

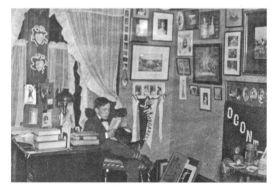

A typical Cornell University student room in Ithaca during the 1902–1903 school year. *Ira June Owens Scrapbook, Cornell University Rare and Manuscript Collections*

only that, if elected, he planned to pursue reform with a vengeance. Much of the talk in New York about utility reform centered on control of capital, namely requiring approval by a state utility regulatory commission of any plan by a monopoly utility to issue stocks and bonds or to purchase or sell other utility companies.

Associated Gas & Electric's charter gave it authority to do just about anything, but for a year it remained an empty vessel, not holding any of Morris's local utility companies such as Ithaca Gas Light. The headquarters were in Penn Yan, on the second floor of a downtown building, and Morris, Eben Treman, and Thomas W. Summers were the shareholders.[19]

Hughes won the election, defeating newspaper publisher William Randolph Hearst, in large part because of his vows to reform the utility industry, including the railroads. From January to May 1907, he campaigned hard for a law that would do just that, making speeches at forty dinners and debates.[20] The public was with him—oh, were they with him—but the utility industry fought him every step of the way. He encountered similarly tough sledding in the utility-dominated New York State Legislature, not broken until President Theodore Roosevelt met with legislative leaders and urged them to pass the bill. Resistance ended and the bill passed overwhelmingly on May 22, 1907.[21]

A week earlier, Associated Gas & Electric Company, at the direction of Morris, had issued $400,000 in common stock and $600,000 in preferred stock to buy out his stock holdings in the fifteen local utility companies he owned. All the new stock went to him, along with an additional $200,000 promissory note. It was unclear at the time whether the new New York Public Service Commission had the authority to regulate stock purchases by a utility holding company, as opposed to a local operating company. Morris, however, was taking no chances.[22]

On one level, things seemed to be going well for Morris in the spring of 1907. Despite the epidemic, he was not by any means a social pariah. Later in May, he received a letter from President Schurman of Cornell thanking him profusely for loaning his personal automobile to the university to transport visiting members of the Association of New York State Colleges and Universities. Despite having killed twenty-nine Cornell students in 1903, he was anything but persona non grata on campus.[23]

But on a deeper, more profound level, his business, like every other American business, was feeling the effects of a sharply declining economy that year. The stock market crashed on March 14, conditions worsened during the summer, and events culminated that fall in a severe banking crisis that became known as the Panic of 1907. Morris had started going farther afield for loans, including a visit in 1906 to a Philadelphia banking firm, probably Montgomery, Clothier & Tyler, whose partners he derided as "Quaker Jews" in a letter to Mynderse Van Cleef written from the posh Bellevue-Stratford Hotel in Philadelphia. Their sin was apparently imposing stiff terms for a $100,000 loan Morris needed. Another, bigger problem was that some of the companies he owned had been in sad shape when he acquired them and had not gotten any better with time. Remarkably, Ebenezer M. Treman revealed as much to Charles H. Blood when Blood inquired about the investment prospects of Associated Gas & Electric on behalf of another old friend.[24]

Morris might have hung on, but the newly minted New York Public Service Commission in 1909 took a dim view of a plan to float new bond issues for the underlying companies that made up Associated Gas & Electric. The commission objected to some of the proceeds going to Morris and not to the companies in whose name they were taken. It imposed stiff restrictions on how the proceeds could be used. So in the fall of 1909, Morris sold Associated Gas & Electric to Montgomery, Clothier & Tyler, a.k.a., the "Quaker Jews"; William S. Barstow, a former associate of Thomas A. Edison who ran a utility empire of his own; and a third investor, P. Chauncey Anderson. The price? Just $354,000, two-thirds less than the value of the underlying stocks Morris had sold to the company in 1907.[25]

~~~~~~~~~

Duncan Campbell Lee's life spiraled downward after he was cut loose from Cornell University. His newspaper continued to publish, of course, and the libel suits threatened by Tucker & Vinton and Morris never amounted to anything. An advertising boycott alluded to by Samuel Hopkins Adams is hard to quantify. No doubt some advertisers pulled their ads because of unhappiness with the newspaper's reporting of the epidemic, but not all or even most of them did. But Lee seemed to be cut off from his moorings, willing to throw the old journalism verities out the window. He began thinking of commercial printing as a new source of income—many newspapers did and still do this—but the client he envisioned was the State Democratic Committee. The annual printing contract for the Democratic Party was worth $200,000 a year, and Lee decided he would build a new, larger printing plant behind his current shop so he could get that contract. He and Frank E. Gannett parted ways in 1905 over this issue, if Gannett's biography is to be believed. Gannett thought such a move compromised the newspaper's objectivity, a strange complaint given that Lee never made any secret of his Democratic proclivities. Perhaps there was more to it than met the eye.[26]

Lee built the printing plant, and the newspaper's finances and his own went to hell. Whether the contract wasn't as lucrative as he believed, or his costs were higher than expected, is impossible to determine. But whatever the reason it happened, U.S. Comptroller of the Currency reports for the First National Bank of Ithaca, where his father-in-law, George R. Williams, was the president, and the records of court judgments filed against Lee and his wife, Elizabeth, tell an agonizing tale of financial collapse. On August 29, 1905, a federal bank examiner reported that a note of $14,610 owed by Lee and Ithaca Publishing Company was "doubtful" and one for $4,198 was a "loss," and "worthless," but was endorsed by George R. Williams. "Much of this past-due paper has been carried along," the examiner wrote. "Duncan C. Lee is a son-in-law of Pres. G.R. Williams; Mr. Williams is said to be good." Individuals and banks sued Lee or his wife for hundreds or thousands of dollars, huge amounts in that day. Even Gannett filed a lawsuit against him for nearly $400.[27]

Perhaps the most disturbing thing of all were the demands of country newspaper owners in New York for payments they claimed they were owed for "booming," or promoting the candidacy of the Democratic gubernatorial candidate, William Randolph Hearst. They began harassing Lee for payment early in 1907 in his capacity as chairman of the Democratic State Editorial Association. Lee told them Hearst owed the payments, which totaled $4,800. His degradation was nearly complete, and the finale came when he put Ithaca Publishing Company into bankruptcy in the spring of 1907.[28]

Neither Lee nor his wife, Elizabeth, saw any future for the family in Ithaca. One suspects that George R. Williams took care of their personal debts, and the business debts would disappear into the maw of bankruptcy court. Lee does not strike one as someone who would casually walk away from his debts, but he harbored a great deal of anger and guilt from the events of the past five years and wanted a fresh start. Sometime in 1908, Lee gathered up his family at the age of thirty-nine and sailed to Italy to begin a new life. He became secretary of the International Agricultural Institute in Rome. Edward Fitch, one of his Hamilton College classmates, ran into him on the Spanish Steps in 1909. Lee stayed in Rome for a little over a year, then moved the family to England, settling in Norwich. He had decided to become a British lawyer, which he did after an appropriate course of study.

"He was very, very happy living in England," said his daughter, Nancy Lee Gluck, who was interviewed in her nineties. "He was proud of what he accomplished. He liked the history and dignity that British law gave him."[29]

Her mother never wanted to live in Ithaca again or even visit there, Gluck recalled. She and the children did go back to see family every three years but stayed in the Williams family cottage on Cayuga Lake in Sheldrake, New York. Elizabeth Lee spoke often to her children about the terrible Ithaca water. Duncan Campbell Lee returned to America on business from time to time but never went back to Ithaca or even to Sheldrake. He lived in England until his death in 1943. His last wish was to have his body buried in Norwich, but his heart removed and interred in the Hamilton College Cemetery in Clinton, New York. The burial in the walled, tree-shaded cemetery at Hamilton was carried out by four of his college classmates on August 7, 1945. His brother, Rev. Dr. John Park Lee, officiated. "He was very religious on account of his father," Gluck said of her father. "He always tried to do the right thing."[30]

~~~~~~~~

Morris could not live without buying things, without spending. It is not always possible to figure out where he got the money, but Mynderse Van Cleef seems to have rarely turned off the spigot. Instead of easing into a sensible retirement after he sold Associated Gas & Electric, Morris seemed to want nothing but to add luxuries to his life.

Not that he waited until the sale was complete. In 1908, he purchased the Abraham Van Wagener mansion on Bluff Point, which jutted into Keuka Lake south of Penn Yan, where he retreated after his Ithaca dream died. The Greek Revival mansion sat on 181 acres and was surrounded on three sides by open fields and forests. The porch offered a view up and down the lake. Built in 1833, it was badly in need of restoration. He told the local newspaper he would bring in a prominent architect from Philadelphia and a landscape gardener from Boston to carry out his plans, and did.[31]

Nor was Morris finished buying places to live. On October 1, 1909, just four days after he sold Associated Gas & Electric, Morris purchased the Mary E. Wagener mansion on Main Street in Penn Yan as his primary residence. Seven weeks later, he purchased the Severn Wine Cellar property on Seneca Lake near Himrod, New York, for $10,575 at a foreclosure sale. The property came with one hundred acres of grape vines. In 1911, he spent $20,000 to renovate his Main Street mansion. The description of the planned renovations takes one's breath away. It was a Palace of Versailles for a single man and his servants. At the end of the summer of 1911, Morris purchased a forty-foot motor yacht with a half-inch-thick mahogany deck and hull. It was said to be the fastest boat on the Finger Lakes. He bought an office building in downtown Penn Yan for the Penn Yan Gas Light Company, which had not been part of the sale two years earlier, and the additional utility companies he was continuing to acquire for his new holding company, United States Gas & Electric. He was the president and his nephew, Morris Tracy, son of his sister Emma, was the manager. In 1912, William T. Morris commissioned an oil painting of himself in a lord of the manor pose. And on and on it went, even as Duncan Campbell Lee struggled to make a new life for himself and his family in England.

Morris's luck did not last. He tried to get into the shoe manufacturing business in 1912 and again in 1916, but both ventures failed. Morris went into decline during the war years, financially, physically, and eventually, mentally. The crisis seems to have come in 1918. Robert H. Treman wrote to Van Cleef in the spring of that year, telling a disturbing story about how "Billy Morris" had come to see him to try to collect some money. Morris then spoke of borrowing money to build up his farm, apparently the vineyard on Seneca Lake. "I should think the best thing for him would be to devote himself entirely to his farms and build himself up by outdoor living during the summer as he is almost a wreck. If his sister can secure us, I should be inclined to help him to a small necessary amount." But that did not happen. Emma's children, Morris and Lucy Tracy, objected to mortgaging their mother's house as security for the loan. Instead, Morris Tracy began to sell off some of his uncle's assets. Late in the year, he wrote to Van Cleef to tell him he had sold his uncle's forty-foot yacht, the *Lucy T.*, and the boathouse on Cayuga Lake that he had purchased from Van Cleef only a year earlier.[32]

He continued to spiral downward. At some point, Morris received a small sinecure, a position on the Willard State Hospital Board of Managers that he kept until his death. Properties were sold, and at the end he was living with relatives in Geneva, New York. The one thing that did not decline in him, however, was his devotion to Cornell University. When he died on November 4, 1928, the obituary in the *Ithaca Journal-News* (Gannett had acquired his old newspaper and merged it with the *Journal*) referred to him in the headline as "noted C.U. alumnus." The Associated Press story noted that he had never missed a commencement since his own graduation in 1873. None of the obituaries mentioned his role in the 1903 typhoid epidemic. No one seemed to remember.

~~~~~~~~

The legacy of William Torrey Morris was the company he created, Associated Gas & Electric. In 1922, the same people who had bought the company from Morris in 1909 sold it to John I. Mange and Howard Colwell Hopson. Mange was the president of the company but was largely a figurehead. Hopson was the brains and the id of Associated Gas & Electric. Born on a farm in Wisconsin, he was a whip-smart boy who excelled at the University of Wisconsin and at George Washington University. He was one of the first employees of the New York Public Service Commission, where he learned the tricks corporations used to deceive regulators and wondered if he could do better.

Hopson set out to build the utility empire that Morris could only have dreamed about. Using every means fair or foul, legal or illegal, including the bribing of public officials, Hopson spent the Roaring Twenties acquiring company after company. Associated Gas & Electric, which began life in 1906 with assets of $1,200,000, had upped that number to $641,820,000 by 1929, according to the Federal Trade Commission. By the time it all ended in 1940, Hopson and Mange owned companies in twenty-six states and two foreign countries.

Unfortunately for Hopson, he made an enemy of Franklin D. Roosevelt, tangling with Roosevelt repeatedly when he was governor of New York from

1929 to 1932. After he became president in 1933, Roosevelt took an almost personal interest in seeing Hopson brought to justice, even speaking about him at news conferences, and Hopson seemed to relish slapping back at the president. By this time, Hopson had descended into almost pure criminality, stealing from his shareholders, customers, even his employees. He was smart, and not until the Democratic Congress had passed the necessary laws was it possible for the Securities and Exchange Commission and the Justice Department to bring him down. That happened in 1940. Associated Gas & Electric was forced into bankruptcy and Hopson, insane or nearly so from the effects of tertiary syphilis, went to federal prison.

The bankruptcy lasted through World War II. Under SEC direction, the trustees gradually spun off most of the companies Hopson had acquired. In the end, all that was left was Metropolitan Edison Company and Pennsylvania Electric Company in Pennsylvania, and Jersey Central Power & Light Company in New Jersey, plus Manila Electric Company in the Philippines, which was not sold until the Kennedy administration. Under SEC rules designed to prevent another Hopson, owning more than one utility system was discouraged, and on the rare occasion when it was allowed, the utilities had to be contiguous, or border each other.

Emerging from bankruptcy in 1946 as General Public Utilities Corporation, the company soon turned its focus to an exciting new technology, atomic energy. Under the leadership of Edward W. Morehouse, GPU took the first step down a very rocky path that ended on March 28, 1979, when the Unit 2 reactor at the Three Mile Island nuclear plant of Metropolitan Edison Company had a core meltdown. More than one hundred thousand people fled the region around Harrisburg, Pennsylvania, racing to escape the invisible radiation drifting whichever way the wind blew.

Afterword

The Conquest of Typhoid

GEORGE A. SOPER, THE MAN WHO SAVED both Galveston, Texas, and Ithaca, New York, is fated never to be remembered for those achievements as much as he is for identifying and capturing the woman who came to be known as Typhoid Mary.

Mary Mallon was a typhoid carrier, little different from other typhoid carriers except that she refused to limit her opportunities to infect other people. Mary was a cook, quite a good one according to legend, and was employed in fine homes up and down the Eastern Seaboard, especially in the New York metropolitan area. Soper was hired in 1906 by George Thompson, who owned a summer rental house in Oyster Bay, Long Island, where six people in the household of eleven had become ill with typhoid. Worried that he would never be able to rent it again, Thompson asked Soper to investigate the causes of the outbreak.

In a 1939 letter to the *British Medical Journal* in London, Soper said that the techniques he used to identify and find Typhoid Mary were "an outcome of my work for the control of the epidemic of over 1,300 cases of typhoid at Ithaca, N.Y., in 1903, where I had seen typhoid spread from person to person and initiated energetic measures to prevent it." Once he learned that the hiring of Mary Mallon as the cook for the house coincided with the start of the epidemic, he began following her trail. "It was a difficult investigation, partly because I was not called for more than six months after the outbreak and the people had become separated and the house vacated. The cook (Miss

Mallon) could not be found for some months and then proved most refractory."[1] One definition of that last word is "obstinately resistant to authority or control." Mary was all that and more.

Other authors have explored the Typhoid Mary story in great depth, so we need not replicate their work here. Her importance is as an advertisement for the danger of typhoid carriers. While few people in America knew exactly what a typhoid carrier was before her detention (among them Soper, who thought that only the carrier's urine could spread the disease), through the magic of newspapers, the reality of typhoid carriers who spread their germs through both urine and feces became known.

The odd thing about Typhoid Mary is that she came to be widely blamed for the Ithaca epidemic even though she had absolutely nothing to do with it. This belief got started because there appeared to be a gap in her work history around the time of the Ithaca tragedy. But the only way Mary could have triggered the epidemic was if she had traveled to Ithaca and for some reason walked out into the bush to defecate on the banks of Six Mile Creek. The chances of that having happened seem decidedly remote. Even if for some reason she had decided to stop cooking in fine homes or institutions to sling hash in a rough immigrant work camp, the worst she could have done would be to infect some of the workers. Chances are the sick workers would have been sent away before they could take their own trip to the bank of the stream.

Yet this zombie story has made its way through the entire twentieth century and into the twenty-first, even finding its way into medical textbooks. Recitations of this myth can be found in the *Bismarck Tribune* of North Dakota on March 20, 1925, the *Fresno Bee* of Nov. 7, 1960, and the *Van Nuys News* of California on June 29, 1961. The newspapers can often blame syndicated columns and wire stories that they use without rechecking the information, but how about medical book publishers? The Mary Myth is found in Dr. Charles E. Simon's *Human Infection Carriers: Their Significance, Recognition and Management*, published in 1919; R. L. Huckstep's *Typhoid Fever and Other Salmonella Infections*, published in 1962; and *Microbiology for Surgical Technologists* by Paul Price and Kevin B. Frey, published in 2003. There are undoubtedly other examples. It is more comical than serious, perhaps only to be stamped out with better editing.

The greatest advances against typhoid early in the twentieth century came from better sanitation and cleaner water, especially after chlorine began to be used to kill germs in drinking water around 1909. The first usage, a dramatic success, was in Jersey City, New Jersey, and it spread rapidly after that. In the last years prior to chlorine, the average typhoid death rate in the United States was about 25 per 100,000, similar to the death rate from motor vehicle accidents now. By 1920, the death rate was down to about 8 per 100,000, and by 1948, to an almost imperceptible level.[2]

That was good, but still no cure for typhoid existed once you caught the disease. And outside of the developed world, typhoid remained endemic. In 1948, Paul Burkholder, a Yale University scientist, discovered a mold-like organism called an actinomycete in a soil sample that arrived from Venezuela. He was being funded by Parke, Davis & Company of Detroit, Michigan, to search for new antibiotics in soil samples from around the world. Actinomycete, later renamed chloramphenicol, proved effective against typhus, scrub typhus, and typhoid fever itself. Dr. Eugene Payne of Parke, Davis took a small amount with him on a trip to Bolivia and working with two Bolivian physicians, tried it on sixteen patients who were near death from typhus. All recovered.[3] At the end of 1948, Dr. Perrin Long, professor of preventive medicine at Johns Hopkins University, disclosed that chloramphenicol, now carrying the trade name of chloromycetin, had brought dramatic cures to ten typhoid patients at the University of Maryland Hospital.

Tests conducted by a team led by Theodore E. Woodward found that typical typhoid patients showed dramatic improvement beginning on the third or fourth day of treatment. Fever declined, the classic rose spots disappeared, and headaches became less painful. In one dramatic case, where perforation and bleeding had begun, chloromycetin eventually saved the man's life without doctors having to resort to surgery. The body healed the perforation.

The next step was to synthesize chloromycetin so it did not have to be made directly from the actinomycete organism. That was achieved by Dr. Mildred Rebstock, a twenty-eight-year-old chemist on the Parke, Davis staff. The final step was to produce the synthesized drug in industrial quantities of consistent quality, and Parke, Davis assigned that task to its production facility in Holland, Michigan.[4] The author's father, who was a young chemist working on the project, described it as complex, difficult work, but ultimately successful. "We essentially had to trick nature," Paul W. DeKok remembered. It was a heady time to be a chemist.

Chloromycetin became a big seller for Parke, Davis & Company but eventually fell out of favor because of potentially serious side effects, including deafness or even death. Other drugs, including ciprofloxacin, are more common treatments for typhoid now. There are no outbreaks in America anymore like the one in Ithaca in 1903. Typhoid is worrisome only for those Americans who travel to Third World countries, but even then they have the comfort of knowing that their chances for a quick recovery are high if they are so unlucky as to catch the disease.

ACKNOWLEDGMENTS

Sometimes a book takes much longer to finish than the author ever expects. In 1989, I set out to write a definitive account of General Public Utilities Corporation and the Three Mile Island nuclear accident of 1979. After some early unpleasantness initiated by the company, I discovered that GPU had a fascinating earlier history under the name of Associated Gas & Electric Company, led to ruin by a man named Howard C. Hopson. Instead of focusing only on the accident, I thought, why not write a book that would cover both the Hopson era and GPU's misadventures with nuclear energy? Then in 1993, while looking at New York Public Service Commission documents related to Associated Gas & Electric in Albany, New York, I found a brief mention of a typhoid epidemic in Ithaca, New York, and realized the company had two catastrophes in its long history. My book grew again. I eventually decided to divide my single GPU book into three; this is the initial volume in what I hope will be a trilogy.

I must first thank my wife, Lisa W. Brittingham, who was always supportive, and my lovely daughters, Elizabeth and Lydia DeKok. They grew from babies to teenagers while this book was in progress. Anyone writing a book spends hours huddled in a small room staring at a laptop or on the road doing research, and without a supportive family those tasks are far more difficult if they are even possible at all.

This book would not have been possible without the help of the staff at Cornell University Library's Division of Rare and Manuscript Collections. Even though the epidemic story does not reflect well upon the Cornell University of 1903, they helped me with enthusiasm and professionalism, especially Phil McCray, a skilled archivist who became a friend and hosted me at his home in Ithaca on numerous research trips. Other staff I should mention by name are Elaine Engst, director and university archivist, who helped in many ways but especially in guiding me through the process of unsealing the Cornell University Executive Committee files from the time of the epidemic, and Julia Parker and Laura Linke, who found and pulled many helpful documents during the years of my research. Special thanks also go to James J. Mingle, Cornell University counsel, who ultimately granted my request to unseal the Executive Committee papers.

I should also thank my cousin, Beth Zelony, and her husband, Rob, for loaning me their New York apartment on my research trips to the newspaper collections of the New York Public Library. Newspapers, especially the long defunct *Ithaca Daily News, New York Tribune,* and *New York Sun,* and the still publishing *Ithaca Journal,* played a critical role in my research. Their day-to-day coverage of the epidemic was invaluable to me. As a journalist, I could appreciate the hard work of these long dead and now anonymous reporters to write the first drafts of history. Some of the Ithaca reporters wrote their stories even while members of their own families lay ill with typhoid. I hope my second draft of history is a credit to their dedication.

It has become easier to access and make use of old newspaper articles with the advent of NewspaperArchive.com, which has gathered many of America's newspapers (though not yet all, and not yet those in Ithaca) into its database. When I found articles about the Ithaca epidemic in newspapers around the country, I knew it had been a national story. Researching my book was likewise made immensely easier by Google Books, the vacuum cleaner of our published past, the ultimate collector of digital copies of the "quaint and curious volumes of forgotten lore" that Poe once wrote about. Because Google Books allows keyword searching within its vast database, I was able to find any number of helpful books and articles that likely would have escaped my attention otherwise. I know many, including me, have qualms about how Google Books will ultimately affect writers and readers, especially if it chooses to begin charging for its services. For now, though, it is quite useful. But so are the older ways of research, and I am grateful to the staff of the Dauphin County Library in Harrisburg for finding many obscure titles for me via interlibrary loan. I'm sure some of my requests prompted some head scratching. The wide-ranging collections of the Pennsylvania State Library in Harrisburg were also invaluable. Thanks also to the Yates County Historical Society in Penn Yan, New York, for directing me to its collections of newspaper clippings relating to William T. Morris and for permission to photograph the 1912 oil painting of him that hangs in its museum. I also made good use of the collections of The History Center in Tompkins County, which gave me permission to use its photograph of Theodore Zinck. Photographs of George A. Soper, the savior of Galveston, Texas, and Ithaca, New York, who tracked down Typhoid Mary, are surprisingly rare, but Casey Greene at the Rosenberg Library in Galveston was able to provide me with one taken just two or three years before Soper arrived in Ithaca. Writing my book would have been much more difficult without the prior research done on Ithaca's founding families by Carol U. Sisler. Her excellent book, *Enterprising Families: Ithaca, New York*, was never far from my desk. Ulrike Folkens of the Robert Koch Institut in Berlin helped me find Dr. Koch's seminal writings on typhoid carriers.

Many people helped me find information about the Cornell University students who died in the epidemic, who often were the best and brightest in their hometowns. Maudine Bennum at the Harrison County Genealogical Society in Bethany, Missouri, and Gary Cox at the University of Missouri Archives in Columbia provided valuable information on the life and death of Oliver G. Shumard, the first Cornell student to die. Similarly, my thanks go to the Steuben County Historian's Office in Bath, New York, for help in finding a local news clip about the death of Charlotte Spencer; to Jean Ellis, reference librarian at the Passaic Public Library in Passaic, New Jersey, for clips on the death of George Wessman, Henry Schoenborn, and William J. Reinhart; to Fred Miller, president of the Tuscarawas County Historical Society in Ohio for clips on the death of James Vinton; to Susan L. Conklin, Genesee County historian, for a very helpful clip from the *Batavia Daily News* in Batavia, New York, on the death of Charles J. Schlenker; and to Robert J. Scheffel, local history librarian at the Rochester Public Library, for clips on the death of Otto Kohls.

Thanks also go to Jean Long, town historian of Alfred, New York, for material on the family of Charles Langworthy; to Lois A. Foxwell, archivist of Alfred University, for tracking down documents relating to the life of an alumnus, Dr. Daniel Lewis, who was the New York State health commissioner during the 1903 epidemic, as well as clips from the *Alfred Sun* about the death of Charles Langworthy; to Charlotte Garofalo of the Gouverneur Reading Room Association in Gouverneur, New York, for an obituary of George S. Hill; to Donna K. Baron and Ted Fuller of the Middlesex County Historical Society in Middletown, Connecticut, for clips on the death of

Lewis K. Hubbard, and to Barbara Goodwin at the Windsor Historical Society in Windsor, Connecticut, for information on Flavia Thrall, the clairvoyant healer who failed to save Hubbard from typhoid; to Wyoming County historian Doris A. Bannister in Warsaw, New York, for clips on the deaths of James Francis McEvoy and Henry Norris Rockwell; to the Sherburne Public Library in Sherburne, New York, for clips on the death of Fred J. Pray; and to the Oneida County Historical Society for clips on the death of Addison P. Lord.

I never cease to be amazed by New York's state system of 1,640 official local historians, which dates to 1919. Nearly every county has one, and so do many towns and villages. Historians are required to have a level of education appropriate to their work and are held to high standards of professionalism. I worry that this valuable service might become a juicy target in an era of government budget crises. Libraries themselves are no longer sacrosanct. In Pennsylvania, where I live, the current governor, Edward G. Rendell, a Democrat, has slashed funding for public libraries. Writing books like this one will become increasingly difficult if our society does not maintain the institutions that preserve our history.

David DeKok
Harrisburg, Pennsylvania
August 15, 2010

ENDNOTES

Abbreviations

ADW—Andrew Dickson White Papers, 01/02/02, Division of Rare and Manuscript Collections, Cornell University Library. White was the cofounder of and first president of Cornell University.

CUTP—Cornell University Typhoid Papers Collection, 35/4/42, Division of Rare and Manuscript Collections, Cornell University Library.

EC—Records of the Executive Committee of the Cornell University Board of Trustees, 2/5/5. The Executive Committee was made up of the members of the Board of Trustees who lived in or near Ithaca. It handled most of the business of the university.

JGS—Jacob Gould Schurman Papers, 3/4/6, Division of Rare and Manuscript Collections, Cornell University Library. Schurman was president of Cornell University from 1892 to 1920 and held office during the typhoid epidemic.

MVC—Mynderse Van Cleef Papers, #3088, Division of Rare and Manuscript Collections, Cornell University Library. Van Cleef was a lawyer and banker in Ithaca and a close friend of William T. Morris. He was a member of the university Board of Trustees and its Executive Committee.

Prelude: June 16, 1903

1. The average income in all American industries, excluding farm labor, in 1903 was $543. See, Scott Derks, ed., *Working Americans, 1880–1999, Vol. II, The Middle Class* (Lakeville, CT: Grey House, 2000), 53–54, 62.

2. President Jacob Gould Schurman of Cornell University to Andrew Dickson White, March 9, 1903; Samuel D. Halliday to Andrew D. White, March 2, 1903; Clara Newberry to Andrew Dickson White, February 27, 1903; Andrew White Newberry to Andrew Dickson White, February 22, 1903. All in ADW.

3. "Andrew D. White Talks to Seniors: Graduating Class Marches to Former President's House," *Ithaca Daily Journal,* June 16, 1903.

4. Tom Lutz, *American Nervousness 1903: An Anecdotal History* (Ithaca: Cornell University Press, 1991), 18.

5. "All Evidence Goes to Prove Theory Theodore Zinck Took His Own Life," *Ithaca Daily News,* June 17, 1903; "Theodore Zinck Drowns in Lake," *Ithaca Journal,* June 17, 1903. The *Daily News* was the morning paper and the *Journal* the evening paper. Most details about Zinck's drowning and the immediate aftermath come from these two articles. Zinck and his family used the original spelling of "Theodor," including on his tombstone, but the newspapers and Surrogate Court used the Americanized spelling of "Theodore."

6. Romeyn Berry, *Behind the Ivy: Fifty Years in One University With Visits to Sundry Others* (Ithaca: Cornell University Press, 1950), 164–65.

7. The March 9, 1903, date of Zinck's last will and testament is found in documents filed in the proceeding *In the Matter of the Estate of Theodore Zinck, deceased,* in Surrogate's Court of Tompkins County.

8. George A. Soper, "The Epidemic of Typhoid Fever at Ithaca, N.Y." *Journal of the New England Water Works Association* Vol. 18, No. 4 (January 1905): 431.

9. Charles-Edward Amory Winslow, "The War Against Disease," *Atlantic Monthly* (January 1903): 43–53.

10. William T. Sedgwick, "Typhoid Fever: A Disease of Defective Civilization," introductory essay to: George C. Whipple, *Typhoid Fever: Its Causation, Transmission and Prevention* (New York: John Wiley & Sons, 1908), xxxv.

11. "Treman's Box," *Ithaca Daily News,* June 16, 1903.

12. Charles H. Blood to John W. Dwight, May 18, 1903, Charles H. Blood Papers, Division of Rare and Manuscript Collections, Cornell University Library.

13. Complaint, *Tucker & Vinton, Inc., Plaintiff, against The Ithaca Publishing Company and Frank E. Gannett, Defendants,* Supreme Court, New York County, June 16, 1903, Collection #1900, Frank E. Gannett & Caroline Werner Gannett Papers, Division of Rare and Manuscript Collections, Cornell University Library.

Chapter 1: Ithaca and Its Kings

1. Carol U. Sisler, *Enterprising Families, Ithaca, New York: Their Houses and Businesses* (Ithaca: Enterprise Publishing, 1986), 11–29. Sisler's book tells well the story of the three Treman brothers and their offspring, as well as of other prominent Ithaca families.
2. T. W. Burns, "Reminiscences, Heroic and Historic, of Early Days of the Lehigh Valley System in Southern and Central New York," *Black Diamond Express*, Vol. IX, No. 1 (January 1905): 9.
3. Burns, 12.
4. "Over Half Century Ago, First Works Were Begun," *Ithaca Daily News*, December 31, 1904.
5. Ibid.
6. Andrew D. White, *Autobiography of Andrew Dickson White, Volume I* (New York: The Century Company, 1905), 342.
7. W.G.I., "Ithaca and the Gorge," *New York Times*, letter to the editor, July 11, 1872. The Fall Creek Gorge on the Cornell campus was fenced off for safety and liability reasons in 2009, making it impossible to repeat the climb today.
8. Ernest Earnest, *Academic Procession: An Informal History of the American College, 1636 to 1953* (Indianapolis: Bobbs-Merrill Company Inc., 1953), 144–45.
9. Cornell University president Jacob Gould Schurman to R. H. Jesse, president of the University of Missouri, JGS.
10. A. F. Weber, "Young and Wealthy: The Value of Cornell University Is $10,000,000," *Fort Wayne (Ind.) Weekly Sentinel*, syndicated article, June 19, 1895.
11. Morris Bishop, *A History of Cornell* (Ithaca: Cornell University Press, 1962), 224–32.
12. Eugene Hotchkiss, "Jacob Gould Schurman and the Cornell Tradition: A Study of Jacob Gould Schurman, Scholar and Educator, and His Administration of Cornell University, 1892–1920," (PhD diss., Cornell University, 1960), 51.
13. Freetown Historical Society, *Freetown Past & Present* (Freetown, PEI: Freetown Historical Society, 1985), 9.

14. Hotchkiss, "Schurman and the Cornell Tradition," 51–52.
15. Ibid., 58.
16. "No Great Minds Here: President Schurman of Cornell Says This Country Is Intellectually Weak," *New York Times,* June 21, 1901.
17. Berry, *Behind the Ivy,* 51.

Chapter 2: The Boys Club

1. Sisler, *Enterprising Families, Ithaca, New York,* 19.
2. Walter Wolcott, *Penn Yan, New York* (Penn Yan: Peerless Printing Co., 1915), 44; Lewis Cass Aldrich, ed., *History of Yates County, N.Y.* (Syracuse, N.Y.: D. Mason & Co., 1892) 190–91; entry on Daniel Morris, *Biographical Directory of the United States Congress,* http://bioguide .congress.gov/scripts/biodisplay.pl?index=M000974 (Sept. 21, 2009).
3. Cornell University Division of Rare and Manuscript Collections occasionally displays an official copy of the Thirteenth Amendment to the U.S. Constitution signed by the members of Congress who adopted it. The "D. Morris" signature of Daniel Morris is prominent among them.
4. William T. Morris alumni file, Collection 41/2/877, Public Affairs Records, Deceased alumni files, 1868–2008, Division of Rare and Manuscript Collections, Cornell University Library; "William T. Morris, Prominent Utility Owner and Former Penn Yan Resident, Died Monday," Penn Yan *Chronicle-Express,* November 8, 1928.
5. *Cornellian* yearbooks for 1870–73 for campus activities of William T. Morris, Division of Rare and Manuscript Collections, Cornell University Library.
6. Morris obituary, Penn Yan *Chronicle-Express,* November 8, 1928.
7. Records of Baldwin's Bank of Penn Yan vs. John H. Butler impleaded [sued] with William T. Morris, Yates County Historian's Office, Penn Yan, N.Y.
8. O. M. W. Sprague, *History of Crisis Under the National Banking System* (New York: Augustus M. Kelley, 1910 and 1968), 154, 167–68, 208–9; George E. Mowry, *The Era of Theodore Roosevelt: 1900–1912* (New York: Harper and Brothers, 1958), 2; Alexander Dana Noyes, *Forty Years of American Finance* (New York: G. P. Putnam's Sons, 1909) 266–67.

9. Mowry, 2; Noyes, 284; *Twelfth Census of the United States, Taken in the Year 1900*, Volume IV, Part 2, Statistics of Deaths (Washington: U.S. Census Office 1902), 175.

10. City of Ithaca, Plaintiff, v. Ithaca Water Works, et al, August 3, 1906, Vol. 21, p. 22. The voluminous transcript of the post-epidemic legal proceedings in which the citizens of Ithaca sought to seize Ithaca Water Works through eminent domain can be found in Box 4 of the Mynderse Van Cleef Papers (#3088) at the Cornell University Library's Division of Rare and Manuscript Collections. The collection also contains the Morris–Van Cleef correspondence. After this it will be referred to as the "water case transcript."

11. William T. Morris to Mynderse Van Cleef, January 14, 1901; P. W. Bailey to Van Cleef, February 22, 1901; Morris to Van Cleef, February 23, 1901; Bailey to Van Cleef, February 28, 1901. All in MVC.

12. Mark A. Schmidt, "Patriotism and Paradox: Quaker Military Service in the American Civil War." Written for History 480, West Chester University, West Chester, Pennsylvania, April 18, 2004. Read at: http://courses.wcupa.edu/jones/his480/reports/civilwar.html on September 19, 2009. Edited for the Web by Jim Jones.

13. "John Brown's Men Disinterred," *New York Times*, August 29, 1899.

14. *Catalogue for Five Years, Eagleswood Military Academy, Prospectus for 1866–67* (New York: John A. Grey and Green, Printers, 1866), Marcus and Rebecca Spring Collection, Stanford University Libraries.

15. Michael John Burlingham, *Behind Glass: A Biography of Dorothy Tiffany Burlingham* (New York: Other Press, 2002), 34–35, 37.

16. Allene M. Parker, "Eagleswood: An American Utopia in Transition, 1851–1890," (unpublished conference presentation), 11. Parker is on the arts and sciences faculty at Embry-Riddle Aeronautical University in Prescott, Arizona.

17. Frank Thornburg alumni file, Collection 41/2/877, Public Affairs Records, Deceased Alumni Files, 1868–2008, Division of Rare and Manuscript Collections, Cornell University Library; *Iowa State Gazetteer and Business Directory, 1884–85* (Des Moines: R. L. Polk & Co.), 284.

18. Graham Robb, *Strangers: Homosexual Love in the 19th Century* (New York: Norton, 2004), 30.

19. Sisler, *Enterprising Families, Ithaca, New York,* 100.

20. Detailed accounts of L. L. Treman's funeral can be found in the April 30, 1900, editions of the *Ithaca Daily News* and the *Ithaca Daily Journal.*

Chapter 3: Conflict of Interest

1. Noyes, *Forty Years of American Finance,* 294.

2. "For New Telephone Lines: Inter-Ocean Company to Be a Long Distance Branch of Connecting Company," *New York Times,* June 29, 1901. The company changed hands several times over the years and eventually became part of the International Telephone & Telegraph Company, or ITT, in 1951.

3. Naomi R. Lamoreaux, *The Great Merger Movement in American Business, 1895–1904* (Cambridge: Cambridge University Press, 1985), 1; Noyes, 286–87; *James Grant, Money of the Mind: Borrowing and Lending in America from the Civil War to Michael Milken* (New York: Farrar, Straus & Giroux, 1992), 18.

4. Water case transcript, August 3, 1906, Vol. 21, p. 38.

5. Water case transcript, August 3, 1906, Vol. 21, p. 23.

6. Water case transcript, August 3, 1906, Vol. 21, pp. 21, 25–26.

7. "Fraternity House Burned: Students Leaped from the Third Story Windows," *Ithaca Daily Journal,* January 29, 1900; "East Hill Aroused: The Question of Ampler Fire Protection Discussed," *Ithaca Daily Journal,* January 30, 1900; "Death of a Student: J. P. Lonergan's Injuries Prove Fatal," *Ithaca Daily Journal,* January 31, 1900.

8. "Fire Protection," *Ithaca Daily Journal,* February 8, 1900.

9. "Report of the Finance Committee of the Common Council of the City of Ithaca Upon Propositions of the Ithaca Water Works Co. to Sell Their Plant or Contract to Supply the City for a Long Term of Years" (Ithaca, N.Y., February 21, 1900), 4.

10. Ibid., 21.

11. John W. Bush to Mynderse Van Cleef, December 2, 1901, MVC.

12. William Irwin, *The New Niagara: Tourism, Technology, and the Landscape of Niagara Falls, 1776–1917* (University Park: The Pennsylvania State University Press), 99.

13. "Two Companies Consolidated: Will Be Known as the Niagara Falls Gas & Electric Light Company," *Niagara Falls Gazette*, January 3, 1900.

14. "To Tap the Trunk Sewer: Application for Permission to Do So Will Be Made to the Council Tonight by Gas and Electric Company," *Niagara Falls Gazette*, January 29, 1900; "Novel Plan for Municipal Plant: Sewage Used to Turn Turbines Which Will Generate Power," *Buffalo Sunday Times*, February 4, 1900.

15. Morris to Van Cleef, August 3, 1901, MVC.

16. "Pan-American Closes: Total of Eight Million People Saw Big Show in Buffalo," *Ithaca Daily News*, November 4, 1901.

17. "Ithaca Did Full Share for Pan-Am: Number Who Went to Buffalo Larger than Its Population," *Ithaca Daily News*, November 4, 1901.

18. *Pan-American Exposition, Buffalo, 1901*. Found in collection #2920, Division of Rare and Manuscripts Collection, Cornell University Library.

19. Isabel Dolbier Emerson scrapbook, Collection #37/5/2161, Division of Rare and Manuscript Collections, Cornell University Library.

20. Bush to Van Cleef, June 28, 1901, MVC; "Rites for Mrs. Bush: Prominent Buffalo Club Woman Passes Away at 86," *Buffalo News*, November 9, 1933.

21. McKinley's physicians billed Congress nearly $100,000 for their losing effort to save the president, which press reports said was almost twice the amount billed by physicians attending the mortally wounded President Garfield twenty years earlier. "M'Kinley's Doctor Bill Big," *Ithaca Daily News*, October 12, 1901.

22. "Opening of Cornell: President J. G. Schurman Talks to the Students About Anarchy," *New York Times*, September 28, 1901.

23. David Nasaw, *Andrew Carnegie* (New York: The Penguin Press, 2006), 360.

24 Ibid., 596–601.

25. "A Great Disaster: Forty-eight of Our Soldiers Fall in a Philippine Battle," *Ithaca Daily News*, September 30, 1901; "Schurman Speaks on the Philippines," *Ithaca Daily News*, January 11, 1902; "President Schurman Makes Reply to Opponents of Free Speech," *Ithaca Daily News*, January 27, 1902; "Our Humane War," *Ithaca Daily News*, April 9, 1902.

26. Bush to Van Cleef, October 7, 1901, MVC.

27. Morris to Van Cleef, October 2, 1901, MVC.

28. Solomon Stanwood Menken Scrapbook, 1890–1916, #37/5/2534, Division of Rare and Manuscript Collections, Cornell University Library.

29. Letter, Morris to Van Cleef, October 2, 1901, MVC.

30. The amount of Ithaca Light & Water Company bonds purchased by Cornell University came to light between February 18 and 21, 1903, in articles in the *Cornell Daily Sun*, *New York Sun*, and *New York Daily Tribune*. Although he had ample opportunity to be heard, President Jacob Gould Schurman did not deny the accuracy of the $100,000 figure. In fact, both he and the Board of Trustees acknowledged owning "a comparatively small part of the company's bonds" and saw nothing wrong with it.

31. "Statement of the Amount of Mortgages on the Property of the Ithaca Water Works Company," circa 1905, MVC.

32. "Cornell Heights Historic District," included on the City of Ithaca (N.Y.) municipal website, http://tinyurl.com/ye6tgtd (November 21, 2009).

33. "New Suburb Will Be Begun at Once: Syndicate Which Purchased Cornell Farm to Develop It," *Ithaca Daily News*, November 20, 1901.

34. John W. Bush to Mynderse Van Cleef, November 13, 1901, MVC.

35. Bush to Van Cleef, December 2, 1901, MVC.

Chapter 4: Newsmen

1. "Foreign Capitalists Negotiating Purchase of Ithaca's Waterworks," *Ithaca Daily News*, October 31, 1901. Today's reader might look askance at the wording of the headline, judging the *Daily News* to be a Marxist publication. But *foreign* meant "out of town," and mainstream newspapers commonly used *capitalists* to refer to wealthy individuals who bought and sold companies. It had not yet acquired a political meaning.

2. "Sale Concluded: Ithaca Gas and Water Companies Change Ownership," *Ithaca Daily Journal*, November 12, 1901.

3. James K. McGuire, *The Democratic Party of the State of New York: A History of the Origin, Growth, and Achievements of the Democratic Party of the State of New York, Including a History of Tammany Hall and Its Relation to State Politics* (New York: United States History Company, 1905), 391–95; "Duncan Campbell Lee," *The Shield* 9 (March 1893): 5–8; "Cornell University," *New York Times*, March 12, 1893.

4. "Brainard G. Smith, Herald's Owner and Publisher, Dies," *Ridgewood (N.J.) Herald*, December 12, 1930.

5. Duncan Campbell Lee to Jacob Gould Schurman, May 1, 1901, EC.

6. "Department of Elocution and Oratory, Course 23, Extemporaneous Speaking, 1897–98," 14/13/2305, Duncan Campbell Lee Collection, Division of Rare and Manuscript Collections, Cornell University Library.

7. "Cornell Professor Enlists: Prof. Lee, Head of the Department of Oratory, Now a Recruit," *New York Times*, July 22, 1898.

8. "Two Hundred and Third Regiment, Infantry," *New York in the Spanish-American War, 1898, Part of the Report of the Adjutant-General of the State for 1900, Volume III* (Albany: James B. Lyon, State Printer, 1900), 655–56.

9. *New York in the Spanish-American War, 1898, Part of the Report of the Adjutant-General of the State for 1900, Volume I* (Albany: James B. Lyon, State Printer, 1900) 214–50. The date and cause of death of any soldier in a New York unit is included in this list.

10. Victor C. Vaughan, *A Doctor's Memories* (Indianapolis: Bobbs-Merrill, 1926), 389.

11. *New York in the Spanish-American War, 1898, Vol. III*, 737.

12. McGuire, *The Democratic Party of the State of New York*, 393.

13. Schurman to Lee, September 28, 1898, Letterbook, Vol. 6, p. 776, JGS. Schurman and Lee discuss the latter's return to Ithaca, which Schurman says he confidently expects will not be later than October 15, 1898.

14. *The New York Tribune*, in a story about Duncan Campbell Lee on November 2, 1902, said his brief and lackluster military career became fodder for student verse, to wit: "Duke Lee is daily hoping some generous millionaire . . . Will listen to his pleadings and endow for

him a chair . . . Of military science, where Duncan may declaim . . . Of
his sanguinary battle against the hordes of Spain . . . Giving frequent
demonstrations how his famous battle went . . . With the murderous
mosquito that dared invade his tent." Lee may have encountered a few
northern mosquitoes in his brief Army service, but not the malarial
variety.

15. Nasaw, *Andrew Carnegie*, 544–45, 550.

16. Jacob Gould Schurman, *Philippine Affairs: A Retrospect and Outlook* (New
York: Charles Scribner's Sons, 1902), 1–2.

17. Samuel T. Williamson, *Frank Gannett: A Biography* (New York: Duell,
Sloan & Pearce, 1940), 32. This was Gannett's campaign biography
when he sought the Republican nomination for president in 1940,
losing to Wendell Willkie, a utility executive, who went on to lose to
President Franklin D. Roosevelt. One must tread carefully with this
book, which regrettably (along with a 1948 update) is almost the only
source of information about Gannett's early career. Scholars would
feel more comfortable with Williamson's book if there were alternative
sources to check some of its more self-serving claims on behalf of his
client, some of which are disprovable.

18. Ibid., 48–49.

19. Samuel T. Williamson, *Imprint of a Publisher: The Story of Frank Gannett
and His Independent Newspapers* (New York: Robert H. McBride & Co.,
1948), 70. This is essentially the same as Williamson's 1940 campaign
biography of Gannett and may have been published in anticipation
of Gannett making another run for the Republican nomination for
president that year. That didn't happen.

20. "The News Circulation," *Ithaca Daily News*, January 8, 1902; letter of
reference, Duncan Campbell Lee to newspaper in Terre Haute, Indiana,
May 15, 1903, Collection #1900, Frank E. Gannett and Caroline
Werner Gannett Papers, Division of Rare and Manuscript Collections,
Cornell University Library.

21. "Ice Trust and Tammany; State Convention Hastily Suppresses a
Resolution," *New York Tribune*, September 12, 1900.

22. Ibid.

23. David Hemenway, *Prices and Choices: Microeconomic Vignettes*, 3d ed. (Lanham, MD: University Press of America, 1993), Chapter 19, "The Ice Trust," 189-90.

24. Ibid., 191-93.

25. "Ice Trust and Tammany," *New York Tribune*, September 12, 1900.

26. Hemenway, *Prices and Choices*, 193-94.

Chapter 5: The Dam

1. "Water Analyzed: Chemist Chamot Makes an Unfavorable Report," *Ithaca Daily Journal*, February 12, 1902. This article mentions that Chamot followed the American Public Health Association testing protocols; American Public Health Association, *"Report of the Committee on Standard Methods of Water Analysis to the Laboratory Section of the American Public Health Association, 1897,"* published in *Journal of Infectious Disease*, Supplement #1, May 1905, 11.

2. *Lauby's Cornell Chemical Recollections, March 1972*, http://www.chem. cornell.edu/history/vignettes/LaubyChamot.htm; "Poison in Wall Papers: Remarkable Results of Analysis by Dr. Chamot of Cornell," *New York Times*, March 14, 1899; "Girl Accused of Murder," *New York Times*, October 19, 1902; "Chemist Declares Wells Dangerous: Instructor Chamot Says All in City Should Be Condemned," *Ithaca Daily News*, November 27, 1901.

3. "City Water Supply: Wells Strongly Condemned by Professor Chamot," *Ithaca Daily Journal*, November 27, 1901.

4. "Board of Health Plans Campaign: Center of City Must All Be Connected with Sewer Soon," *Ithaca Daily News*, October 9, 1901; "Increase Sewer Capacity: Commission Will Likely Arrange Tomorrow Night for Laying Another Pipe into Lake," *Ithaca Daily News*, January 29, 1902.

5. "City's Condition Much Improved: Health Officer Hitchcock Reviews Work of Past Year," *Ithaca Daily News*, December 12, 1901.

6. John W. Hill, a prominent evangelist for water filtration who in 1901 was designing filtration plants for the city of Philadelphia, Pennsylvania, denounced the dilution theory in his book *The Purification of Public Water Supplies* (New York: D. Van Nostrand Company, 1898), 16-17, 20-21.

7. *The Ithaca Daily News* provided a long account of the Ithaca Board of Health meeting in its November 27, 1901, issue. The *Ithaca Daily Journal* also covered the meeting and reported on it the following day. Both articles should be read to get the full flavor of what was said.

8. *Report of the Geological Survey of the State of Ohio*, Vol. VIII (Columbus, Ohio, January 1906), 181.

9. Water case transcript, Williams testimony, November 21, 1905, Vol. 5, 12–13.

10. Water case transcript, Vol. 5, 13–15, & Vol. 6, 162; Waterman Thomas Hewett, *Cornell University: A History, Volume 2* (New York: The University Publishing Society, 1905), 338–39.

11. Helmi Raaksa, *Finding Aid for Gardner Stewart Williams Papers, 1900–1945*, Michigan Historical Collections, Bentley Historical Library, University of Michigan, Ann Arbor.

12. Water case transcript, Vol. 5, 103.

13. Water case transcript, Vol. 5, 15.

14. Water case transcript, Vol. 5, 16, 48.

15. Amory Prescott Folwell, *Water Supply Engineering: The Designing, Construction, and Maintenance of Water-Supply Systems, Both City and Irrigation* (New York: John Wiley & Sons, 1900) 164–65; William T. Sedgwick, *Principles of Sanitary Science and the Public Health* (New York: The Macmillan Co., 1903), 246.

16. Water case transcript, Williams testimony, November 22, 1905, Vol. 6, 203–4, Vol. 8, 104.

17. *Purification of the Washington Water Supply: An Inquiry Held by Direction of the United States Senate Committee on the District of Columbia* (Washington: Government Printing Office, 1901), 131.

18. Folwell, *Water Supply Engineering*, 2–3; Allen Hazen, *The Filtration of Public Water Supplies* (New York: John Wiley & Sons, 1895), preface to first edition, iii–iv.

19. Hill, *The Purification of Public Water Supplies*, 131.

20. James H. Fuertes. *Water Filtration Works* (New York: John Wiley and Sons, 1901), 15.

21. *Washington Water Supply*, 22, 92; Folwell, *Water Supply Engineering*, 291; Whipple, *Typhoid Fever*, 240.

22. Hazen, *The Filtration of Public Water Supplies*, preface to first edition, iv.

23. Water case transcript, Williams testimony, November 21, 1905, Vol. 5, 20–21.

24. "Professor Williams's Report," *Ithaca Daily Journal*, January 28, 1902.

25. "Special Election: Taxpayers to Vote on Water Works Problem," *Ithaca Daily Journal*, February 6, 1902.

26. Water case transcript, Williams testimony, November 21, 1905, Vol. 5, 23; "Judge Finch's Views: Strongly Opposed to Municipal Ownership," *Ithaca Daily Journal*, February 12, 1902; "Person Can Vote Once on Question: City Attorney Makes Ruling Which Will Govern Election," *Ithaca Daily News*, February 23, 1903.

27. "Water Analyzed," *Ithaca Daily Journal*, February 12, 1902; American Public Health Association, 83. A book by Chamot and Harry W. Redfield, *The Analysis of Water for Household and Municipal Purposes* (Ithaca: Taylor & Carpenter, 1911) follows the AMHA protocols very closely; Hill, *The Purification of Public Water Supplies*, 24–25.

28. Water case transcript, Vol. 10, testimony of Thomas W. Summers, January 30, 1906, 50, 60–61.

29. Water case transcript, Williams testimony, Vol. 5, 22.

30. *A Study of the Conditions Governing the Water Supply of Large Cities*, a thesis presented to the College of Civil Engineering, Cornell University, by Herbert E. Fraleigh, for the degree of civil engineer, June 1902. Olin Library, Cornell University. Fraleigh's thesis is also a useful compendium of what was taught about water filtration to Cornell engineering students at the time, and proves that the department was entirely up to date. Even the meeting in New York City in January 1901 to discuss water filtration for Washington, D.C., is mentioned. Williams knew what had to be done in Ithaca.

31. Invitation to hear Lord Kelvin, with handwritten note from George S. Sheppard that he attended with William T. Morris, Laura Hosie Treman, and Mary Bott Treman, May 2, 1902, Oliver Sheppard Collection, Division of Rare and Manuscript Collections, Cornell University Library; "Greatest Interest in Famous Visitor," *Ithaca Daily News*, May 2, 1902; "Lord Kelvin: Royal Welcome Accorded Here Yesterday Afternoon," *Ithaca Daily Journal*, May 3, 1902; "Most

Picturesque in all the World: That Is Lord Kelvin's Opinion of Situation of University," *Ithaca Daily News*, May 3, 1902; "The Cornell Yell," *Cornell Daily Sun*, January 14, 1887.

32. Lord Kelvin's coronation honors are mentioned in *The Tribune Almanac and Political Register 1903* (New York: Tribune Associates), 44.

Chapter 6: Lives of the Students

1. Hendrik W. Van Loon, E. B. White, et al. *Our Cornell* (Ithaca: The Cayuga Press, 1939), 11–12.

2. *Descendants of John Carlisle, Generation No. 4,* http://familytreemaker. genealogy.com/users/b/o/m/Tom–Bombaci-jr/GENE6-0004.html, accessed January 14, 2010.

3. "In Loving Remembrance: Tribute to Oliver G. Shumard," *Bethany Democrat*, Bethany, Missouri, February 18, 1903.

4. "Death Ends Lengthy Career of Medical Missionary to India," *The Guardian*, Charlottetown, Prince Edward Island, January 22, 1957. In addition to information on Dr. Zella Marie Clark's life, the article provides details of the Clark siblings' living arrangements at Cornell.

5. *Time* magazine assessed the Pulitzer Scholar program in its January 1, 1940, issue and pronounced it an overwhelming success based on interviews with 268 of the 366 living graduates.

6. "International Recognition for Arthur Dove, County Artist," by Clyde M. Maffin, Ontario County historian, *Canandaigua Messenger*, Canandaigua, N.Y., December 5, 1967.

7. "Jarvis A. Wood Dead: Senior Member of Advertising Firm of N. W. Ayer & Son Was 71," *New York Times*, April 10, 1925; Edd Applegate, *Personalities and Products: A Historical Perspective on Advertising in America* (Westport, CT: Greenwood Press, 1998), 51; Ralph M. Hower, *The History of an Advertising Agency: N. W. Ayer & Son at Work, 1869–1949* (Cambridge, MA.: Harvard University Press), 98; Jarvis A. Wood to Jacob Gould Schurman, April 16, 1903, CUTP.

8. 1880 Federal Census, Troy, N.Y., http://www.connorsgenealogy.com /troy/Troy-H6.htm, accessed January 22, 2010; Margaret Harvey, warden of Sage College, to Jacob Gould Schurman, March 3, 1903, CUTP; Ithaca's claim to be the birthplace of the ice cream sundae is

explained at http://www.visitithaca.com/Media-Services/Birthplace-of-
the-Sundae.html, accessed on January 22, 2010.

9. "S. B. Newberry, Pioneer in Cement Industry, Passed Away Tuesday,"
Sandusky Register, Sandusky, Ohio, November 29, 1922; "She
Wants a Divorce and the Custody of Her Children," *Sandusky Daily
Star*, Sandusky, Ohio, June 25, 1901; "By His Own Hand: Son of
Ambassador White Ends His Suffering," *Sandusky Daily Star*, July 9,
1901; "Mrs. Clara White Newberry Gets an Absolute Divorce," *Sandusky
Daily Star*, August 15, 1901; "Ambassador White to Continue Work,"
Ithaca Daily News, October 7, 1901.

10. A good summary of the long Vonnegut family history in Indianapolis
can be found in *History and Genealogy of Lake Maxinkuckee-Vonnegut
Family*, which explores the lives of the families that owned cottages
around the Indiana lake. http://genwiz.genealogenie.net/lake_
maxinkuckee/vonnegut/vonnegut.htm, accessed January 23, 2010.
Anton Vonnegut's election as president of the Class of 1905 is
mentioned in "Junior Election," *Cornell Daily Sun*, October 13, 1903.

11. Bishop, *A History of Cornell*, 342; "Croker Boys Quit Cornell," *New
York Times*, October 13, 1901; "Silver Cups for Dogs," *New York Times*,
February 15, 1903; "Herbert Croker Dies on a Train in Kansas," *New
York Times*, May 13, 1905; "Richard Croker Jr. Will Seek Estate," *New
York Times*, May 8, 1922.

12. Bishop, *A History of Cornell*, 402; Van Loon, *Our Cornell*, 3.

13. Bishop, *A History of Cornell*, 342–43, 403.

14. Berry, *Behind the Ivy*, 50; Bishop, *A History of Cornell*, 341.

15. S. Harrison, et al, a.k.a. "Merchants of Ithaca," to President Jacob
Gould Schurman of Cornell, May 9, 1902; Major William P. Van Ness
to Schurman, May 10, 1902. Both letters in EC.

16. Burt G. Wilder to Emmons L. Williams, May 3, 1902, EC.

17. "Closing of Moving Pictures Tonight," *Ithaca Daily News*, December
21, 1901; Berry, *Behind the Ivy*, 62; Emily Dunning Barringer, *Bowery
to Bellevue: The Story of New York's First Woman Ambulance Surgeon*
(New York: W. W. Norton & Co., 1950), 56. Barringer describes her
undergraduate years at Cornell in Ithaca before transferring to the
Cornell School of Medicine's main campus in New York City.

18. John H. Selkreg, ed., *Landmarks of Tompkins County, New York, Including a History of Cornell University by Professor Waterman Thomas Hewett* (Syracuse, N.Y.: D. Mason & Co., 1894), 447; Bishop, *A History of Cornell*, 347; Barringer, *Bowery to Bellevue*, 51–52, 58.

19. Eleventh Annual Report of President Schurman, 1902–1903 (Ithaca, N.Y.: published by Cornell University, 1903), xxxix; George P. Bristol to Schurman, October 12, 1902, EC.

20. "President Takes Hand in Matter: Tells the Sophomores that Underclass Strife Must End," *Ithaca Daily News*, February 25, 1902.

21. "Freshmen Finally Have Their Feast: President Schurman Takes a Hand and Stops the Rioting," *Ithaca Daily News*, March 1, 1902.

22. "Bryan Holds Large Crowd by Magnificent Oratory," *Ithaca Daily News*, March 7, 1902; "Like Ithaca: W. J. Bryan Thinks City Pretty One," *Ithaca Daily News*, March 7, 1902; "*Journal* Methods," *Ithaca Daily News*, March 8, 1902.

23. Bishop, *A History of Cornell*, 346, 414.

24. "Cornell Oarsmen Sweep the River: Ithaca Crews Won All Three Races at Poughkeepsie," *New York Times*, June 21, 1902.

25. "Celebrating at Ithaca," *New York Times*, June 22, 1902.

26. "An Ideal City," *Ithaca Daily News*, March 1, 1902.

Chapter 7: The Valley of Death

1. "Agreement Between Ithaca Water Works and the City of Ithaca," August 25, 1902, MVC.

2. "Cornell May Get New Water Supply," *Ithaca Daily News*, October 11, 1902.

3. "Dam Contract Let: New York Firm Gets the Job for $34,225," *Ithaca Daily Journal*, September 11, 1902.

4. "Italians to Work on Hydraulic Dam: Local Laborers Not Willing to Accept Wages Offered," *Ithaca Daily News*, September 26, 1902.

5. "Yes or No? Shall Ithaca Acquire Water Works? What Many Taxpayers Say About It," February 22, 1902, MVC.

6. Jerre Mangione and Ben Morreale, *La Storia: Five Centuries of the Italian American Experience* (New York: Harper Perennial, Aaron Asher Books, 1993), xiii, 89, 131, 133, 139.

7. Articles about the Croton Dam strike can be found in newspapers all over the country in April 1900. Some the author consulted were: "Croton Dam Strike Extends: Entire Force of 700 Men Idle—The Superintendent Threatened," *New York Times*, April 4, 1900; "Troops Ordered to Big Cornell Dam," *New York Times*, April 16, 1900; "Carry Guns: Six Hundred Militiamen on the Way from New York City to Croton Dam," *Fort Wayne (Ind.) News*, April 16, 1900; "They May Use Dynamite," Davenport (Iowa) *Daily Republican*, April 17, 1900; "Victim Died: Young Sergeant Douglas Assassinated by Dagos," *The Evening Democrat*, Warren, Pennsylvania, April 17, 1900; "The Italian Strikers Are Making Trouble for the Cornell Dam Contractors," *The News*, Frederick, Md., April 19, 1900; "The Croton Dam Strike," letter to *New York Times*, April 24, 1900.

8. Frank Harvey Eno, "The Uses of Hydraulic Cement," *Geological Survey of Ohio*, Fourth Series, Bulletin No. 2, September 1904.

9. "Will Investigate Company's Plans: People Beginning to Worry over Building Enormous Dam," *Ithaca Daily News*, September 29, 1902; "Nervous Over Dam," *Ithaca Daily Journal*, October 2, 1902.

10. "Business Men Ask Aldermen to Act," *Ithaca Daily News*, October 14, 1902; "The People's Forum: The Reservoir Dam," *Ithaca Daily News*, October 15, 1902.

11. Ibid.; "How Volcanoes Work: Mt. Pelee Eruption (1902)," http://www.geology.sdsu.edu/how_volcanoes_work/Pelee.html, accessed March 1, 2010.

12. "Surveyors Begin on New Reservoir," *Ithaca Daily News*, March 14, 1902; "Have Begun Work on Big Reservoir," *Ithaca Daily News*, April 19, 1902.

13. "Working on Dam Days and Nights: Construction of Reservoir Will Be Hurried Very Fast," *Ithaca Daily News*, October 7, 1902.

14. "Will Start Work on a Second Dam: Tucker and Vinton Prepare to Build a Secondary Wall," *Ithaca Daily News*, October 21, 1902.

15. "Rushing the Work on the Great Dam," *Ithaca Daily News*, November 3, 1902; "Interest in the Dam," *Ithaca Daily Journal*, November 10, 1902.

16. Arthur Weston, *The Making of American Physical Education* (New York: Appleton-Century-Croft, 1962), 33.

17. Holmes Hollister to Veranus A. Moore, February 16, 1903, CUTP. Hitchcock's reaction reminds the author of the members of Centralia Borough Council in Pennsylvania in the 1960s. Confronted with the fact of an underground coal-mine fire moving toward their town, the Borough Council members said it was not their responsibility until the fire actually crossed the line from Conyngham Township into Centralia. By that time, it was too late to save Centralia. Today, nearly all of the town is gone. (See, David DeKok, *Fire Underground: The Ongoing Tragedy of the Centralia Mine Fire* [Guilford, CT: Globe Pequot Press, 2009].)

18. Veranus A. Moore and Emile M. Chamot to Jacob Gould Schurman, February 19, 1903, CUTP; statements of Elias J. Durand, Herbert H. Whetzel, and James M. VanHook, collected by Moore and Chamot, CUTP; water case transcript, Williams testimony, November 22, 1905, Vol. 6, 205–6, Collection #3088, MVC.

19. "Advertisements and Instructions to Bidders," p. 9, August 12, 1902, MVC. The specifications for the dam are included in this document, which in turn is incorporated into the contract between Ithaca Water Works and Tucker & Vinton.

20. "Cornell University's Needs," *New York Times*, October 26, 1902.

21. "Magnificent Plan for the Campus Adopted by Trustees of Cornell," *Ithaca Daily News*, October 27, 1902; Eve M. Kahn, "Pragmatic Visionaries," *Traditional Building*, February 2007.

22. Cornell University today lists Raymond Starbuck as the head football coach for 1902, but the *Cornell Alumni News* of October 15, 1902, identifies William J. Warner, team captain, as holding that position. Starbuck was one of the recent Cornell graduates who assisted Warner.

23. Lars Anderson, *Carlisle vs. Army: Jim Thorpe, Dwight Eisenhower, Pop Warner, and the Forgotten History of Football's Greatest Battle* (New York: Random House, 2008), 3, 19–21, 38; Waterman Thomas Hewett, *Cornell University: A History, Volume 3* (New York: The University Publishing Society, 1905), 308–10.

24. J. A. Wood to Jacob Gould Schurman, president of Cornell University, April 16, 1903. Wood cites passages from his son's diary in the letter. CUTP.

25. Andrew Newberry to Clara White Newberry, October 26, 1902, ADW.

26. "Work Progresses on Treman Houses," *Ithaca Daily News*, November 2, 1901.

27. Minutes of the Executive Committee, Cornell University Board of Trustees, November 18, 1902, EC.

28. Dr. Edwin O. Jordan, "The Typhoid Epidemic at Ithaca," March 14, 21, 28, and April 4, 1903, *Journal of the American Medical Association*, 913; "Snowfall Heavy for This Season," *Ithaca Daily News*, December 5, 1902; Andrew Newberry to Andrew Dickson White, December 7, 1902, ADW.

Chapter 8: Typhoid, and How the Epidemic Began

1. "Koch's Name for Institute," *New York Times*, April 28, 1912.

2. Hermann M. Biggs, M.D., "Robert Koch and His Work," *Review of Reviews*, September 1901, Volume 24, 324–27.

3. Ibid., 325.

4. "Die Bekämpfung des Typhus," from *Gesammelte Werke von Robert Koch*, Zweiter Band, Erster Teil (Leipzig: Verlag von Georg Thieme, 1912), 296–305, translated by the author. The German word for typhoid, confusingly enough for English speakers, is *typhus*, while the German word for the very different disease English speakers call typhus is *Flecktyphus*. The author has long wondered whether the death of Anne Frank, long attributed to typhus, was actually due to typhoid and misunderstood by the English troops who liberated the Bergen-Belsen camp in 1945.

5. Sedgwick, *Typhoid Fever*, 298–99, 300–303; Frederick P. Gay, *Typhoid Fever Considered As a Problem of Scientific Medicine* (New York: The MacMillan Co., 1918), 53; Sedgwick, 303–4; Gay, 53.

6. Edwin O. Jordan, "The Typhoid Epidemic at Ithaca—Preview," *Journal of the American Medical Association*, March 14, 1903, 267–68. The "per 100,000" statistic does not mean a city necessarily had that many people. Rather, it is a convenient way to compare apples-to-apples when judging the impact of typhoid or any disease on one city versus another.

7. "Osler Finds Nerves Chief War Problem: Typhoid Virtually Conquered through Lessons Learned in Other Great Conflicts," *New York Times*, July 9, 1916.

8. In a letter of May 26, 1902, to the minister of spiritual, educational, and medical affairs, Koch wrote that his original vision for cost-sharing by municipalities and regions had proven unworkable because of the amount of work that needed to be done to fight typhoid. He asked for "substantially higher funding" and an immediate advance of fifty thousand marks. This letter is also included in Koch's *Gesammelte Werke*.

9. Koch, *Gesammelte Werke*, 296.

10. Ibid., 299.

11. They were the villages of Waldweiler, Schillings, Heddert, and Mandern.

12. "Typhoid or Enteric Fever," *The Encyclopedia Britannica Dictionary of Arts, Sciences and General Literature, with American Revisions and Additions* (Chicago: The Werner Company, 1894), 678.

13. Koch, *Gesammelte Werke*, 920.

14. Gay, *Typhoid Fever Considered as a Problem of Scientific Medicine*, 6-7, 40.

15. For example, see Gay, 27, 45, 53. The Indian research is published in "Symposium: Typhoid Fever," *Journal of the Indian Academy of Clinical Medicine*, Vol. 2, Nos. 1 & 2, January-June 2001, 11-12. One tends to find typhoid research today in the countries where the disease is still a problem.

16. David D. Stewart, M.D., *Treatment of Typhoid Fever* (Detroit: George S. Davis, 1893), 4-5; William P. Mason, *Water Supply (Considered Principally from a Sanitary Standpoint)* (New York: John Wiley & Sons, 1901), 70; Edwin O. Jordan, M.D., *A Textbook of General Bacteriology* (Philadelphia: W. B. Saunders Company, First Edition, 1908) 274-75.

17. Water case transcript, testimony of Gardner S. Williams, November 22, 1905, Vol. 6, 225-26, MVC.

18. Caterina Rizzo, et al., "Typhoid Fever in Italy, 2000-2006," *Journal of Infection in Developing Countries*, Vol. 2, No. 6, December 2008, 466-68.

19. John Murray, *A Handbook for Travelers in Southern Italy* (London: John Murray, 1883), 94; J. Burney Yeo, M.D., "On Change of Air," *The Nineteenth Century: A Monthly Review*, Vol. 26, July-December 1889 (London: Kegan, Paul, Thench & Co.), 206.

20. George A. Soper, *Report on an Epidemic of Typhoid Fever at Ithaca, N.Y., 1903* (submitted to Dr. Daniel Lewis, commissioner, Department of

Health, State of New York, Albany, N.Y., June 30, 1904), 440; "Public Health: City's Death Rate for 1901 Has Been Low," *Ithaca Daily Journal*, December 21, 1901.

21. "Testimony of Olin Landreth," *Report of the Joint Committee of the Legislature to Investigate What Disposition Should Be Made as to the Sites at Yorktown, Westchester County.* Transmitted to the Legislature March 12, 1918 (Albany: J. B. Lyon Company, Printer), 288–89.

22. Rev. William E. Griffis, *Journal, May 18, 1901, Ithaca, to August 1, 1904* [accession 2074], William Elliot Griffis Collection, Alexander Library, Rutgers University, New Brunswick, N.J.

Chapter 9: Denial

1. "Students Return to Take Up Work," *Ithaca Daily News*, January 2, 1903.
2. "Salmonella Infections," *Merck Manual Home Edition, Second Edition*, 2004, http://www.merck.com/mmhe/sec17/ch190r.html, accessed May 2, 2010; Ronald L. Huckstep, *Typhoid Fever and Other Salmonella Infections* (Edinburgh, Scotland: E&S Livingstone Ltd., 1962), 35; Whipple, *Typhoid Fever*, 12.
3. Edwin O. Jordan, M.D., "The Typhoid Epidemic at Ithaca, Part 2," *Journal of the American Medical Association*, March 28, 1903, 848–49.
4. Landreth, 291; Sampurna Roy, M.D., "Typhoid Fever," *Histopathology-India.net*, 2009, http://www.histopathology-India.net/TyFev.htm, accessed May 3, 2010; Edwin O. Jordan, M.D., "The Typhoid Epidemic at Ithaca, Part III," *Journal of the American Medical Association*, April 4, 1903, 914.
5. George A. Soper, "The Epidemic of Typhoid Fever at Ithaca, N.Y.," presented September 15, 1904, to the New England Water Works Association, published in the *Journal of the New England Water Works Association*, Volume XVIII, No. 4, December 1904, 432, 438; Edwin O. Jordan, "The Typhoid Epidemic at Ithaca, Preview," *JAMA*, March 14, 1903, 715; Jordan, "Ithaca, Part III," *JAMA*, April 4, 1903, 915.
6. Whipple, *Typhoid Fever*, 103; Gay, *Typhoid Fever Considered as a Problem of Scientific Medicine*, 58–59; Huckstep, *Typhoid Fever and Other Salmonella Infections*, 44, 49; Whipple, 103.
7. "Rueteneyer (L.) on Ehrlich's Diazo Test in Typhoid Fever," *The Medical*

Analectic and Epitome: A Monthly Retrospective of Progress in All Divisions of Medico-Chirurgical Practice (New York: G. P. Putnam's Sons, 1890, Vol. VII), 534.

8. Hobart Amory Hare, M.D., *The Medical Complications, Accidents, and Sequelae of Typhoid or Enteric Fever* (Philadelphia: Lea Brothers & Co., 1899), 37. Dr. Julius Dreschfield's description of typhoid symptoms from *A System of Medicine,* edited by Clifford Allbutt, M.D., is quoted verbatim in Hare's book.

9. *The Standard Medical Directory of North America* (Chicago: G. P. Engehard & Co., 1902), 4.

10. Hewett, *Cornell University: A History, Volume 2,* 276.

11. Hill, *The Purification of Public Water Supplies,* 56–57.

12. Frederick E. Turneaure and Harry L. Russell, *Public Water Supplies: Requirements, Resources, and the Construction of Works* (New York: John Wiley & Sons, 1901), 124; Hill, *The Purification of Public Water Supplies,* 57.

13. Heinrich Curschman, M.D., *Typhoid Fever and Typhus Fever* (Philadelphia: W. B. Saunders Co., 1902), 425–26.

14. Lateef A. Olopoenia and Aprileona L. King, "Widal Agglutination Test—100 Years Later: Still Plagued by Controversy," *Post-Graduate Medical Journal* 2000, 76: 80–84; Luzerne Coville, M.D., "Ithaca Epidemic of 1903," *Transactions of the Medical Society of the State of New York* (1905), 209.

15. Huckstep, *Typhoid Fever and Other Salmonella Infections,* 70; Rueteneyer, 534.

16. "Grippe Prevails in This City," *Ithaca Daily Journal,* January 21, 1903; "Little Typhoid Found in Ithaca," *Ithaca Daily Journal,* January 22, 1903.

17. "Tie for Mayor in Ithaca: Democratic and Republican Candidates Each Receive 1,682 Votes," *New York Times,* November 14, 1902; *Tribune Almanac and Political Register 1903* (New York: Tribune Association), 120; "Ithaca Mayoralty Result: Close Inspection of Voting Machine Shows Democrat Received Majority," *New York Times,* November 25, 1902; "Legal Notes: Question as to the Number of Votes Indicated By a Voting Machine," *New York Times,* August 20, 1903; "Republican Mayor of Ithaca Resigns," *Elmira Advertiser,* January 31, 1903; "Mr. Miller Wins Mayoralty of Ithaca," *New York Times,* July 9, 1903.

18. "Final Exams On at Cornell," *Ithaca Daily Journal*, January 23, 1903; "University Promptly Removes All Danger," *Ithaca Daily News*, January 23, 1903.

19. Jordan, "Ithaca, Part III," *JAMA*, April 4, 1903, 915; Bishop, *A History of Cornell*, 333; Hewett, *Cornell University: A History, Volume 1*, 338. A description of the Cornell Infirmary is contained in *The Register* of Cornell University for 1902-03.

20. Dean and William H. Sage to the Executive Committee of Cornell University, November 30, 1897, EC.

21. "In Loving Remembrance: Tribute to Oliver G. Shumard," *Bethany Democrat*, Bethany, Mo., February 18, 1903; "Mark Twain Honored: Large Crowds at Railroad Stations Bid Him Godspeed," *Coshocton Daily Age*, Coshocton, Ohio, July 8, 1902. This was a wire story carried by a number of newspapers around the country; "Class of 1902," *The Missouri Alumnus*, September 1923.

22. William G. Shumard to Jacob Gould Schurman, April 15, 1903, CUTP.

23. "Many Fever Cases Reported in City: Number Suffer from Malady Which Differs from Typhoid," *Ithaca Daily News*, January 26, 1903; "Local Fever," *Ithaca Daily News*, January 26, 1903.

24. "Much Sickness: City Hospital Needs More Room—Many Cases at Infirmary," *Ithaca Daily Journal*, January 28, 1903.

25. Ben P. Poor to Jacob Gould Schurman, April 20, 1903, CUTP.

26. Judson F. Clark to Jacob Gould Schurman, March 2, 1903, and March 18, 1903, CUTP. Judson Clark was the brother of Zella Marie and Annie Sophia Clark and was an assistant professor of forestry at Cornell.

27. "Drinking Water Should Be Boiled: So Advise City Health Authorities," *Ithaca Daily Journal*, January 29, 1903; "Awaiting Report: Board of Health Not Certain About Cause of Prevailing Illness in City—Urge All to Boil Water," *Ithaca Daily News*, January 29, 1903. Williams is not quoted in the *Daily News* story.

28. "Third Assembly: Delightful Social Event Given at Masonic Hall," *Ithaca Daily Journal*, January 31, 1903. The author has warm thoughts for the newspaper clerk who typed in the names of the people at the gala so very long ago. These kinds of articles are drudgery for the writer but of great value in telling stories like this.

29. "Plea for Independence for the Filipino People: President J. G. Schurman's Fine Address in Cooper Union," *New York Times*, January 30, 1903.

30. "Philippine Problems: President Schurman and Gen. Greeley Address the Aldine Club," *New York Times*, December 12, 1902; "Public School Education: Dr. Schurman of Cornell before the Twentieth Century Club," *New York Times*, December 14, 1902; "Dr. Schurman to Speak in the West," *New York Tribune*, December 23, 1902; "Free Trade for Filipinos," *Iowa State Press*, January 14, 1903; "Favors Filipino Independence," *The Mansfield News*, Mansfield, Ohio, January 17, 1903, reporting on Schurman's speech at the University Club in Cleveland.

31. *Lowell Daily Sun*, Lowell, Mass., May 21, 1903.

32. "Third Assembly," *Ithaca Daily Journal*, January 31, 1903.

33. Samuel T. Williamson, *Frank Gannett*, 53.

34. Lee's presence in England during the 1901–1902 academic year is confirmed by a letter Schurman addressed to him at Oxford dated March 29, 1902, JGS. His presence in Ithaca during the 1902–1903 academic year is confirmed by a succession of news articles in which he is mentioned, including: "Fear Delivery's Wicked Tongue: Local Democrats Show Signs of Turning From Attack, *Syracuse Post-Standard*, Sept. 28, 1902; "Needs of Student Life: Professor D. C. Lee Gives Interesting Talk in Barnes Hall—Tells of Oxford University," *Ithaca Daily News*, Nov. 10, 1902; "Business Men's Banquet: Arrangements Completed or Pleasant Event Tonight," *Ithaca Daily Journal*, Feb. 10, 1903; and "Hill to the Front for the Presidency," *New York Times*, April 14, 1903. 35. Former U.S. President George W. Bush's great-great-grandfather, James Smith Bush, briefly taught Sunday school in the First Unitarian Church's original building, which burned in 1893, according to a church history.

35. "Epidemic Spreads throughout the City," *Ithaca Daily News*, January 31, 1903.

36. "Warning against Unboiled Water: Criminal Carelessness Alleged to Exist in City," *Ithaca Daily Journal*, February 24, 1903.

37. Burt G. Wilder to Andrew Dickson White, January 29, 1903, ADW.

38. "Claimed by Death," *Ithaca Daily News*, February 2, 1903.

39. "Danger in Junior Week," *Ithaca Daily Journal*, February 2, 1903; Sisler, *Enterprising Families, Ithaca, New York*, 22.

40. Minutes of the Ithaca City Board of Health, February 3, 1903, Ithaca City Archives; "Fifty New Fever Cases Reported by Physicians," *Ithaca Daily News*, February 3, 1903.

41. Editorial, "Fever Situation Becoming Dangerous," *Ithaca Daily News*, February 3, 1903; Editorial, "The *News*' Attitude on the Fever," *Ithaca Daily News*, February 5, 1903.

42. Bishop, *A History of Cornell*, 305; Berry, *Behind the Ivy*, 63.

43. "Necessary Precaution," *Ithaca Daily Journal*, February 3, 1903.

44. "In Loving Remembrance," *Bethany Democrat*, February 18, 1903.

45. "Ithaca's Typhoid Epidemic," *New York Sun*, February 6, 1903; Walter McCormick, acting mayor, and E. Hitchcock Jr., health officer, to *New York Sun*, February 6, 1903.

46. "Class of '04 Gives Brilliant Prom to Largest Number Ever at Junior," *Ithaca Daily News*, February 7, 1903; "Didn't Go Home Till Morning," *Ithaca Daily Journal*, February 7, 1903; Shumard letter to Schurman, April 15, 1903; "In Loving Remembrance," *Bethany Democrat*, February 18, 1903.

47. "Church Bells Silent: They Will Not Summon Worshipers to Service Tomorrow," *Ithaca Daily Journal*, February 7, 1903.

48. Ithaca Board of Health minutes, February 3 and 10, 1903, Ithaca City Archives.

49. Veranus A. Moore and Emile M. Chamot to President Jacob Gould Schurman, February 19, 1903, 4–5, Typhoid Papers, Collection #35/4/42, Department of Rare and Manuscript Collections, Cornell University.

50. Letter, Veranus A. Moore and Emile M. Chamot to President Jacob Gould Schurman, February19, 1903, 4-5, Typhoid Papers, Collection #35/4/42, Department of Rare and Manuscript Collections, Cornell University.

Chapter 10: Apocalypse

1. "Ithaca's Typhoid Epidemic," Philadelphia *Press*, February 7, 1903; "Fever Scourge Spreads; Ithaca in Great Panic," New York *Evening*

World, February 23, 1903; Susan E. Dufel, M.D., "CBRNE-Plague," Medscape, http://emedicine.medscape.com/article/829233-overview, accessed June 3, 2010. A typhoid epidemic, at least in the developed world, never approached the killing ferocity of bubonic plague. The "Black Death" in the pre-antibiotic era killed 40 to 60 percent of its victims, while typhoid killed 9 to 13 percent or less, depending on available treatment and luck.

2. William Budd, M.D., *Typhoid Fever: Its Nature, Mode of Spreading, and Prevention* (London: Longman's, Green & Co., 1873), 2.

3. Coville, "Ithaca Epidemic of 1903," 209; Huckstep, *Typhoid Fever and Other Salmonella Infections*, 187; Hare, *The Medical Complications, Accidents, and Sequelae of Typhoid*, 126; "Two More Deaths," *Ithaca Daily News*, February 3, 1903; "Charles E. Helm," *Ithaca Daily Journal*, February 3, 1903.

4. Hare, *The Medical Complications, Accidents, and Sequelae of Typhoid*, 78–79.

5. "James C. Vinton," *Ithaca Daily Journal*, February 14, 1903; "Student Dies," *Ithaca Daily News*, February 17, 1903.

6. Stewart, *Treatment of Typhoid Fever*, 13–17.

7. Hattie M. Greaves, "Nursing in Typhoid Fever," *The Trained Nurse and Hospital Review* (New York: Lakeside Publishing Co., July 1906, Vol. 37, No. 1), 287–89.

8. Stewart, *Treatment of Typhoid Fever*, 26; Gay, *Typhoid Fever Considered as a Problem of Scientific Medicine*, 217; "Ernest Brand, M.D.," *British Medical Journal*, Vol. 1, 1897 (London: British Medical Association), 692.

9. Stewart, *Treatment of Typhoid Fever*, 50; Luzerne Coville, M.D., "Typhoid Fever: With Especial Reference to Its Incubation Period and Reincubation Cycles," *New York State Journal of Medicine*, Vol. 6, 1906, 117; Charles E. Page, M.D., "The Successful Treatment of Typhoid Fever," *The Arena*, September 1892, 450–60.

10. *Hahnemannian Monthly*, Vol. 38, 1903 (Philadelphia: Homeopathic Medical Society of the State of Pennsylvania), 640.

11. "Two More Dead at Ithaca: Nearly 400 Cases of Typhoid Fever in That City," *Baltimore Morning Sun*, February 9, 1903; "More Than 20 New Fever Cases Being Treated by the Physicians," *Ithaca Daily News*, February 11, 1903; "Typhoid Spreading in Ithaca: Another Cornell

Student Dead—Nineteen New Cases in a Day," *New York Daily Tribune,* February 11, 1903; Luzerne Coville, M.D., "The Cornell Infirmary," unpublished manuscript, May 6, 1903, CUTP; "Fever Patients in City Number More Than 400," *Ithaca Daily News,* February 9, 1903.

12. "To Give Euchre Party for Hospital Benefit," *Ithaca Daily News,* February 6, 1903; "Fever Patients in City Number More Than 400," *Ithaca Daily News,* February 9, 1903; Griffis Journal, February 11, 1903; "Open-Handed Charity: Rich and Poor Responded Nobly to the Need of the Hour," *Ithaca Daily Journal,* March 17, 1903.

13. James C. Bayles, M.D., "Outlook for Ithaca Growing Brighter," *New York Times,* March 14, 1903; "Cornell Medical Faculty and Trustees at Odds," *New York Times,* March 20, 1903; Dr. Abram Kerr to Schurman, February 18, 1903, CUTP. The prohibition on medical school involvement may have had something to do with the disputes between homeopathic and allopathic physicians. Dr. Luzerne Coville noted in his lengthy protest screed of May 6, 1903, "The Cornell Infirmary," previously cited, that the infirmary normally hired only homeopathic nurses. The medical school was allopathic.

14. Samuel Hopkins Adams, "Typhoid: An Unnecessary Evil," *McClure's Magazine,* June 1905, 151; Coville, "The Cornell Infirmary," Ibid.

15. "More Than 20 New Fever Cases Being Treated by the Physicians," *Ithaca Daily News,* February 11, 1903.

16. In the Matter of the Estate of Edwin Besemer Deceased, Filed March 6, 1903, Tompkins County Surrogate Court, Ithaca, N.Y.; "Arthur Besemer, M.D.," *History of Rochester and Monroe County, Volume II* (New York: The Pioneer Publishing Co., 1908), 1165.

17. "Funeral of Willis Dean," *Ithaca Daily News,* February 20, 1903; "Stanton Griffis Marries," *Palm Beach Post,* September 15, 1973.

18. "Children Safe in Local Schools: Superintendent Explains the Precautions Which Are Observed," *Ithaca Daily Journal,* February 26, 1903; "Warning Against Unboiled Water: Criminal Carelessness Alleged to Exist in City," *Ithaca Daily Journal,* February 24, 1903.

19. "Victim of Typhoid," *Ithaca Daily News,* February 20, 1903; "Cesar Larrinaga," *Ithaca Daily Journal,* March 7, 1903; "Dr. Lewis, State Expert, Does Some More Talking," *Ithaca Daily News,* February 28, 1903. "The

air is filled with farewells to the dying" comes from Henry Wadsworth Longfellow's poem, *Resignation*. See, Thomas R. Lounsbury, ed. *Yale Book of American Verse* (New Haven, CT: Yale University Press, 1912), Bartleby.com, 1999. www.bartleby.com/102/, accessed June 11, 2010.

20. Mentions of Louise Zinck's illness can be found in the *Ithaca Daily News* editions of Feb. 18, 20, 21, 23 and 24. A brief account of her visit to a rooftop party in Syracuse, N.Y., is found in the Syracuse *Sunday Herald* of July 23, 1899.

Chapter 11: The Fixer

1. "Board of Health Adopts Measures to Check the Prevailing Epidemic," *Ithaca Daily News*, February 4, 1903; "Water Analysis," *Ithaca Daily Journal*, February 2, 1903.

2. "Inspectors Officially Report on Awful Conditions along Buttermilk Creek Watershed," *Ithaca Daily News*, February 17, 1903; "Health Report: Findings of City Inspector about Ithaca Water Are Sickening," *Cornell Daily Sun*, February 17, 1903.

3. "The Condition of Ithaca's Water Supply," Editorial, *Ithaca Daily News*, February 17, 1903; "Prominent Business Men Speak Out against the Big Dam and Bad Water," *Ithaca Daily News*, February 18, 1903.

4. "Water Company States Position," *Ithaca Daily Journal*, February 12, 1903. It is probably hard for any twenty-first-century reader not to think of O. J. Simpson and his search for the "real killer" after reading that quotation from Summers.

5. "Committee Begins Exploring Creeks; Canvass of City Progressing," *Ithaca Daily News*, February 13, 1903; "The People's Forum," letter to *Ithaca Daily News*, February 19, 1903; "Work of Local Health Officers," *Ithaca Daily Journal*, February 16, 1903; "Mild Occipito-Spinal Faradization a Sure Cure of Diabetes Mellitus," *The Medical Council*, Vol. 6 (Philadelphia: The Medical Council, 1901), 170.

6. See, Joel A. Tarr, "Urban Pollution: Many Long Years Ago," *American Heritage*, October 1971, for the environmental impact of horses on American cities in the early twentieth century.

7. "Filth in the Streets Not Epidemic's Cause," *Ithaca Daily News*, February 10, 1903; "Find Dead Horse Near Creek's Bed: Putrid Carcass Drained

into Source of City Water Supply," *Ithaca Daily News*, February 10, 1903; "Water Very Bad," *Ithaca Daily News*, February 18, 1903.

8. "May Be Cause of Scourge," *Ithaca Daily Journal*, February 23, 1903; "Report False: Health Authorities Had Informed Journal Story Was Untrue, Yet It Was Published," *Ithaca Daily News*, February 24, 1903; "Was Not Typhoid," *Ithaca Daily Journal*, February 24, 1903.

9. Water rental billing, May to November 1903, Ithaca Water Works to Edwin Besemer, Edwin Besemer estate file, Tompkins County Surrogate Court, Ithaca, N.Y.

10. "Swears Official of Water Company Claimed City Supply Was Not Impure," *Ithaca Daily News*, February 27, 1903.

11. Richard Summers and Louisa Waterman were on the patient list printed by the *Ithaca Daily News* on February 18, 1903. Allen Treman is mentioned in a story in the *Daily News* on March 2, 1903. Charles E. Treman's departure to Europe is mentioned in a regrets note he submitted in advance of the February 21, 1903, meeting of the Cornell Board of Trustees, Executive Committee Files, #2/5/5, Department of Rare and Manuscript Collections, Cornell University Library; "R. T. Summers, 28, Dies Following Brief Illness," *Ithaca Daily Journal*, October 5, 1923.

12. "Minor Accident: T. W. Summers Felled by a Mail Bag," *Ithaca Daily Journal*, January 30, 1903; "A Gas Explosion Occurred in Hornellsville Last Evening," *Elmira Advertiser*, February 3, 1903; "Explosion at Hornellsville: Accident at Plant of Hornell Gas Light Company," *Elmira Daily Gazette & Free Press*, February 3, 1903.

13. Veranus A. Moore and Emile M. Chamot to Jacob Gould Schurman, February 19, 1903, CUTP.

14. "Cornell to Probe Causes of Fever: President Schurman Promises That Something Will Be Done," *Ithaca Daily News*, February 11, 1903; "Pres. Schurman on City's Health: Says Emphatically There Is No Cause for Alarm," *Ithaca Daily Journal*, February 11, 1903.

15. Minutes of the Cornell University Executive Committee, February 16, 1903, EC; Gardner S. Williams to Jacob Gould Schurman, February 13, 1903, CUTP; "Businessmen Indignant over Water Co.'s Scheme," *Ithaca Daily News*, February 17, 1903; "Campus," *Ithaca Daily Journal*, February 17, 1903, 3, 7.

16. "Cornell Students Want Pure Water," *Ithaca Daily News*, February 17, 1903; "C. J. Schlenker Died at Cornell Today," *Batavia Daily News*, Batavia, N.Y., February 17, 1903.

17. "Student Petition to the President and Board of Trustees," February 17, 1903, Records of the Executive Committee, #2/5/5, Department of Rare and Manuscript Collections, Cornell University Library; "Minutes of the Special Meeting of the Executive Committee," February 17, 1903, Records of the Executive Committee.

18. "University Men Want Safeguard," *Ithaca Daily News*, February 18, 1903.

19. "Common Council Gives Ithaca Chance to Own Water Works," *Ithaca Daily News*, February 19, 1903; "Pure Water for Ithaca By Next September," *Ithaca Daily Journal*, February 19, 1903; "Filtering Plant for Cornell: City Council Accepts the Proposition Made by the University," *New York Tribune*, February 19, 1903.

20. Editorial, "Let There Be No Halfway Business," *Ithaca Daily News*, February 19, 1903.

21. Jacob Gould Schurman to Arthur W. Hickman, February 11, 1903, JGS; Jacob Gould Schurman to Andrew D. White, March 9, 1903, ADW.

22. "What Matters the Ten-Cent Sale?" *Ithaca Daily News*, February 14, 1903; "Sad, Sad Story," *Ithaca Daily News*, February 16, 1903. The increase in the circulation of the *Ithaca Daily News* is derived from two documents. "The News Circulation," an editorial published on January 8, 1902, says that the average daily circulation during the previous month was 2,929. A letter of recommendation written for Frank E. Gannett Jr. by publisher Duncan Campbell Lee on May 15, 1903, states the current circulation to be 4,200, or a 43 percent increase over January 1902.

23. There was clearly at least one other important student stringer, based on a vituperative letter to the *Ithaca Daily Journal* on February 24, 1903, written by Sidney Graves Koon, a student. Koon claimed the stringer boasted that he "owned the *Associated Press*" and "all of the New York papers except one." Koon mentions that this stringer had already received his bachelor's degree and was working on another degree, which eliminated Lynn George Wright as a candidate. Wright received his bachelor's degree in 1903.

24. "The Death of Lynn G. Wright, Managing Editor of *Printer's Ink*," *Printer's Ink*, article published in 1919. Copy of obituary found in Lynn George Wright's alumni file at Division of Manuscripts and Archives, Cornell University Library; Constance Frick, *The Dramatic Criticism of George Jean Nathan* (Port Washington, N.Y.: Kennikat Press, 1972. Reissue of original Cornell University Press edition), 6–7.

25. Frank E. Gannett Jr. to Jacob Gould Schurman, February 15, 1903, CUTP; affidavit of A. T. Seaman, Watson W. Lewis, L. G. Wright, and Charles A. Stevens, reporters for the *Ithaca Daily News*, February 14, 1903, CUTP.

26. Jean Folkerts and Dwight L. Teeter Jr., *Voices of a Nation: A History of Media in the United States* (New York: MacMillan, 1989), 248; "Class of 1872, Brainard Gardner Smith," Hamilton College Archives, Clinton, New York.

27. Alumnus, "Communication," letter to *Cornell Daily Sun*, February 18, 1903.

28. "Many Students Hear President," *Ithaca Daily Journal*, February 19, 1903; "Cornell Will Run Boarding House for Men During Present Epidemic," *Ithaca Daily News*, February 19, 1903.

29. "Goes With Bryan: Manton M. Wyvell an Enthusiastic Cornell Student," *The Sunday Herald*, Syracuse, N.Y., October 28, 1900; "The Mass Meeting," *Cornell Daily Sun*, February 21, 1903.

30. "A Dastardly Outrage," *Ithaca Daily Journal*, February 20, 1903.

31. Schurman comments on the *New York Tribune* in a letter to Andrew D. White of March 9, 1903. ADW.

32. "Schurman's Statement: Reports Unfair, He Says," *New York Tribune*, February 21, 1903; "A Better Outlook at Cornell," *New York Tribune*, February 21, 1903.

33. "Pure Water at Cornell," *Ithaca Daily Journal*, February 21, 1903.

34. Coville, "Report on Cornell Infirmary," May 6, 1903.

35. "Dr. Coville Leaves the University Because of Management of the Infirmary—Another Student Dead," *New York Times*, March 20, 1903.

36. "Cornell Alumni Meet in Buffalo," *Ithaca Daily Journal*, February 23, 1903. Courtney said that when the student stringer had been "lying at death's door," clearly before the typhoid epidemic, he was taken to the

student infirmary and nursed back to health by the university. This
points to Lynn George Wright, who dropped out of Cornell for the
1899–1900 academic year.

37. Folkerts and Teeter, *Voices of a Nation*, 278; Henry R. Ickelheimer to
Jacob Gould Schurman, February 25, 1903, CUTP.

38. Jacob Gould Schurman to Henry R. Ickelheimer, February 23, 1903, JGS.

39. Ickelheimer letter to Schurman of February 25, 1903.

40. "Typhoid at Ithaca," *New York Times*, February 26, 1903; Schurman to
Ickelheimer, February 28, 1903, JGS.

41. "J. C. Bayles Dies from Pneumonia," *New York Times*, May 9, 1913;
"Obituary: James C. Bayles," *The Iron Age*, May 15, 1913, Vol. 91, 1213;
Ickelheimer to Schurman, March 5, 1903, Typhoid Papers, Cornell
University Library.

42. Telegram, Adolph S. Ochs to Jacob Gould Schurman, March 4, 1903,
CUTP.

Chapter 12: Going Home

1. "Cornell's Refugees: They Can Stay at Columbia as University Guests,
Dr. Butler Says," *New York Sun*, March 6, 1903; "Epidemic Spreads:
Three Deaths and Eight New Cases in Ithaca Yesterday—Patients Sent
Out of Town," *Rochester Herald*, February 17, 1903; Columbia University
in the City of New York, *Annual Reports of the President and Treasurer to
the Trustees, with Accompanying Documents, for the Year Ending June 30, 1903*
(New York: Printed for the University, 1903).

2. Two Letters, Jarvis A. Wood to Jacob Gould Schurman, April 16, 1903,
CUTP; "Student Wood Dies at Camden," *Ithaca Daily Journal*, April 8,
1903.

3. "Five Cornell Men Ill with Fever at Auburn," *Ithaca Daily News*, February
23, 1903; Fred A. Sieder to Jacob Gould Schurman, March 1, 1903,
CUTP; "Graduate Student Dies: Paul A. Wanke Succumbs to Typhoid
at His Home in Auburn," *Ithaca Daily News*, February 28, 1903; "Paul
Wandke Funeral Notice," *Auburn Bulletin*, February 28, 1903. Cornell
University spelled the name as Wanke, but his parents spelled it
"Wandke." They were German immigrants, and their son appears to
have Americanized the family name.

4.   "Agricultural Student Dies," *New York Times*, February 22, 1903; "Death of Young Man: Charles S. Langworthy Succumbs to Typhoid Fever, Contracted at Ithaca," Alfred *Sun*, Alfred, N.Y., February 25, 1903; Alfred Historical Society and Baker's Bridge Association. "Langworthy, William Henry, of East Valley." *History of Alfred, New York* (Curtis Media Corp., 1990), 220.

5.   "Healer Fails to Heal the Fever: Father of Cornell Student Refuses to Call a Physician," *Ithaca Daily News*, February 28, 1903; untitled and undated article about Flavia Thrall published in the *Windsor Journal*, Windsor, Connecticut, and found in the files of the Windsor Historical Society; "World Famous Healer, Mrs. Thrall, Is Dead: Windsor Woman Consulted by People from Many Lands," *Hartford Courant*, January 24, 1910; "Overcome by Sad News," *Ithaca Daily Journal*, February 27, 1903.

6.   Samuel D. Halliday to Andrew D. White, March 2, 1903, ADW; "Students Leaving: Exodus from Town on Account of Epidemic Continues—Said That 1,000 Have Gone Home," *Ithaca Daily News*, February 17, 1903.

7.   A good example of student sentiment on the danger of missing classes is found in a letter to the editor of the *Cornell Daily Sun* published on February 11, 1903. It is signed simply "1903."

8.   "Cornell to Probe Causes of Fever," *Ithaca Daily News*, February 11, 1903.

9.   "Terse Tales," *Ithaca Daily Journal*, February 26, 1903; "Milestones in AT&T History," http://www.corp.att.com/history/milestones, accessed June 30, 2010.

10. "Dixon Public Library: Library History," http://www.dixonpubliclibrary .org/history.html, accessed July 2, 2010; "The Ronald Reagan Trail: Dixon Public Library," http://www.ronaldreagantrail.net, accessed July 2, 2010; Orris B. Dodge to Jacob Gould Schurman, February 18, 1903, CUTP.

11. G. B. Rose to Jacob Gould Schurman, February 24, 1903, CUTP; "Rose Law Firm: Our History," http://www.roselawfirm.com/about /history_01.asp, accessed July 2, 2010; "George B. Rose Dies Today," *Hope Star*, Hope, Ark., July 20, 1942.

12. Hattie E. Cochrane to Jacob Gould Schurman, March 12, 1903, CUTP. Telegram, Schurman to Cochrane, March 14, 1903, CUTP.

13. George G. Cotton to Jacob Gould Schurman, March 11, 1903, CUTP; Andrew W. Newberry to Andrew D. White, February 22, 1903, ADW. Newberry mentions the Slaterville water used at Psi Upsilon to his grandfather in the letter.

14. Mary D. Huestis to Jacob Gould Schurman, February 22, 1903, CUTP; Charles S. Francis to Schurman, March 2, 1903, CUTP; letter with attached statements, Margaret Harvey, warden of Sage College, to Schurman, March 3, 1903, CUTP.

15. Margaret Harvey to Jacob Gould Schurman, March 3, 1903, CUTP.

16. *Isabel Dolbier Emerson Scrapbook*, Collection #37/5/2161, Division of Rare and Manuscript Collections, Cornell University Library.

17. Delta Gamma, Chi Chapter, *The Anchora* (Baltimore: Psi Chapter, Women's College of Baltimore, editors, 1902-03), 138-39; Clarence Brett Piper, "Alpha Psi—Cornell University" (published by the Alpha Psi Fraternity, Vol. 20), 220.

18. "Cornell Loses," *Ithaca Daily News*, February 28, 1903; "Cornell Hurt by the Fever," *New York Evening World*, February 18, 1903; "Student Victims of Typhoid Now Number 16," *New York Sun*, March 1, 1903; Hugh Jennings, "Baseball," *The 1904 Cornellian, The Yearbook of Cornell University, Being the Complete Record of the Collegiate Year 1902–1903* (Ithaca: Cornell University, 1903), 366; "Ten Cornell Students Dead: Many Hasten to Leave Ithaca and Classes Are Depleted," *Baltimore Morning Sun*, February 22, 1903.

19. Jordan, *A Textbook of General Bacteriology*, 277.

20. Duane L. Atkyns to Jacob Gould Schurman, May 4, 1903, CUTP; Rev. Alan G. Wilson to Jacob Gould Schurman, June 4, 1903, CUTP.

21. Alice P. Nourse to Jacob Gould Schurman, April 28, 1903, CUTP.

22. O. M. Searles, secretary of the Downers Grove Board of Education, to Jacob Gould Schurman, CUTP; Alice Tisdale Hobart, *Gusty's Child* (New York: Longmans, Green & Co., 1959), 41–42; Jerry N. Hess, oral history interview with Dr. Edwin G. Nourse, March 7, 1972 (Independence, Mo.: Harry S. Truman Library), http://www.trumanlibrary.org/oralhist /nourseg.htm, accessed July 3, 2010; "Biographical Note," *Guide to the Alice Tisdale Hobart Papers, 1916–1967*, University of Oregon Libraries,

Special Collections & University Archives, http://nwda-db.wsulibs.wsu
.edu/findaid/ark:/80444/xv89611, accessed July 3, 2010.

23. "Son Better; Father Dead," *Ithaca Daily News*, April 29, 1903; "Alfred
Eugene Mudge," *New York Times*, April 29, 1903; "A. E. Mudge Dead;
Lawyer 40 Years," *New York Times*, August 24, 1945.

24. Jacob Gould Schurman to Stewart L. Woodford, March 6, 1903, JGS.

25. Rev. William L. O'Hara to Jacob Gould Schurman, February 21, 1903,
CUTP.

Chapter 13: The Man Who Saved Ithaca

1. "'Typhoid Mary' Has Reappeared: Human Culture Tube, Herself
Immune, Spreads the Disease Wherever She Goes," *New York Times*,
April 4, 1915; George A. Soper, "Typhoid Mary," *The Military Surgeon*,
Vol. XLV, July 1919, No. 1, p. 14.

2. "As to Sanitation: Observations of Dr. George A. Soper of Matters
Pertaining to Health in Texas," *Galveston Daily News*, Galveston, Texas,
May 9, 1901.

3. "The City Is to Be Cleaned," *Galveston Daily News*, October 3, 1900; "As
to Sanitation," Ibid.

4. "Dr. G. A. Soper Dies; Fought Epidemics," *New York Times*, June 18, 1948.

5. Frederick C. Curtis, M.D., "Typhoid Fever at Ithaca," *Twenty-fourth
Annual Report of the New York State Department of Health*, 1903.

6. "Daniel Lewis, M.D., Ph.D.," *The Alfred University*, Vol. IV, No. 4, May
1892 (Alfred Centre, N.Y.: The Trustees of Alfred University), Alfred
University Archives, Herrick Memorial Library; "The State Board of
Health: Dr. Daniel Lewis of New York Was Re-elected President," *New
York Times*, May 12, 1899; "State Health Commissioner: Dr. Daniel
Lewis of the Former State Board of Health Appointed," *New York Times*,
March 1, 1901.

7. Samuel Hopkins Adams, "Typhoid: An Unnecessary Evil," *McClure's
Magazine*, June 1905, 145–56; "Infirmary Visited: Dr. Lewis Satisfied—
Condition of Fever Patients," *Cornell Daily Sun*, February 27, 1903.

8. Adams, op cit.

9. "Health Board States Wherein Danger Lies," *Ithaca Daily News*, February
27, 1903.

10. "To Make Up Lost Time," *New York Tribune*, February 26, 1903.

11. "Attitude Changed on Return of Men: President Schurman Won't Say It Is Safe for Students Here," *Ithaca Daily News*, February 28, 1903.

12. "Some Students Are Returning," *Ithaca Daily Journal*, March 3, 1903.

13. "Dr. Lewis, State Expert, Does Some More Talking: Says Our Health Board Has Been a Little Slow," *Ithaca Daily News*, February 28, 1903.

14. Dr. Daniel Lewis to Jacob Gould Schurman, March 3, 1903, CUTP.

15. Jacob Gould Schurman to Dr. Daniel Lewis, March 5, 1903, JGS; "Ithaca's Typhoid Epidemic," *New York Sun*, February 27, 1903; "Lessons of the Ithaca Epidemic," *Medical Record: A Weekly Journal of Medicine and Surgery*, Vol. 64, 1903, 639–40.

16. "Fever Worse in Ithaca: Seven New Cases and Another Death Alarm Authorities," *Passaic Daily News*, Passaic, N.J., February 27, 1903; "Dr. George H. Soper Here to Investigate Epidemic," *Ithaca Daily News*, March 4, 1903.

17. Chart, "Disinfectants Prepared by the Board of Health," *Ithaca Daily Journal*, March 9, 1903.

18. "Will Spend Money to Stop Epidemic: Common Council Takes Warning and Acts Promptly," *Ithaca Daily News*, March 5, 1903; "Money to Fight Fever Epidemic," *Ithaca Daily Journal*, March 5, 1903; "Health Officers Working for City," *Ithaca Daily Journal*, March 7, 1903; "Disinfectants Prepared by the Board of Health," *Ithaca Daily Journal*, March 9, 1903; Soper, "The Epidemic of Typhoid Fever at Ithaca," 442.

19. "Health Officers," Ibid. "Two More Deaths at Ithaca," *New York Times*, March 8, 1903; "Getting Control of Typhoid," *New York Tribune*, March 8, 1903.

20. "To Disinfect the City Water Mains," *Ithaca Daily Journal*, March 9, 1903. Water case transcript, Oct. 19, 1905, Vol. 4, p. 51.

21. Shirley Clarke Hulse, "Reminiscences of a Field Engineer," *Civil Engineering*, Vol. 14, No. 5, May 1944.

22. Cornell University Board of Trustees minutes, March 19 and April 19, 1903, Division of Manuscripts and Archives, Cornell University Library.

23. "To Disinfect the City Water Mains," *Ithaca Daily Journal*, March 9, 1903.

24. "Large Meeting of Physicians," *Ithaca Daily Journal*, March 9, 1903.

25. "Ithaca's Typhoid Fever Epidemic," *New York Times*, March 11, 1903.
26. Ibid.
27. "Citizens Protest against Article: Physicians Point to Errors in Statement of Mr. Bayles," *Ithaca Daily News*, March 12, 1903.
28. "Great Injustice Done to the City," *Ithaca Daily News*, March 10, 1903.
29. Soper, "The Epidemic of Typhoid Fever at Ithaca," 44530.
30. Urotropin entry, Online Encyclopedia, http://encyclopedia.jrank.org /TUM_VAN/UROTROPIN_hexamethylenetetramin.html, accessed July 14, 2010. The Online Encyclopedia incorporates articles from the 1911 *Encyclopedia Britannica*.
31. The letters to Walter Stevenson Finlay Jr. are contained in his scrapbook, Collection 37/5/1888, Division of Rare and Manuscript Collections, Cornell University Library. One of Finlay's relatives, George D. Finlay Sr., was a director of the P. Lorillard Tobacco Company. Another relative, Winifred Finlay Fosdick, George's daughter, shot her children and herself to death in 1932. She was said to suffer from progressive paranoia. Her brother-in-law was Rev. Harry Emerson Fosdick, longtime pastor of Riverside Church in New York City.
32. Soper, "The Epidemic of Typhoid Fever at Ithaca," 445.
33. "Typhoid Situation: Dr. Soper Says Ithaca Will Be Safe in Summer—Epidemic Declining," *Cornell Daily Sun*, March 30, 1903; Office of the President to Unnamed Cornell University Student, March 27, 1903, Typhoid Papers, Collection #35/4/42, Division of Manuscript and Archives, Cornell University Library.
34. "Cremate Garbage to Destroy Germs," *Ithaca Daily News*, March 11, 1903; "Comments by Shirley Clarke Hulse," *Transactions of the American Society of Civil Engineers*, 1905, Vol. 54, 327.
35. Soper, "The Epidemic of Typhoid Fever at Ithaca," 444; Cornell Board of Trustees minutes, April 19, 1903, Division of Rare and Manuscript Collections, Cornell University Library; "Extension of Sewer Systems: An Improvement to Stop Drainage into Six Mile Creek," *Ithaca Daily Journal*, March 16, 1903.
36. "Nearly Thousand Had the Typhoid: Dr. Soper Compiles Figures in Regard to Recent Epidemic," *Ithaca Daily News*, May 7, 1903; "Was Truly a Great Epidemic," *Ithaca Daily News*, May 8, 1903.

37. "Musical Comedy Star of *The Billionaire* Infected While Playing in Ithaca," New York *Evening World*, April 30, 1903.

38. "Epidemic Scare Is Fast Abating: More Than Half of Absentee Students Have Returned," *Ithaca Daily Journal*, March 25, 1903.

39. Cornell Infirmary patient roster for April 1, 1903, CUTP; Cornell Board of Trustees Executive Committee records, April 2, 1903, Collection #2/5/5, Division of Rare and Manuscript Collections, Cornell University Library; Earl Blough leave request, April 15, 1903, EC.

40. Walter S. Lenk to Jacob Gould Schurman, March 25, 1903, Cornell University Board of Trustees, EC.

41. John C. Gifford, *On Preserving Tropical Florida*, Compiled and with a Biographical Sketch by Elizabeth O. Rothra (Coral Gables, Fla.: University of Miami Press, 1972) 3, 23–24.

42. Cornell University Board of Trustees minutes, April 19, 1903, Division of Rare and Manuscript Collections, Cornell University Library; mortality rates from typhoid in the 1902–1903 time frame in large American cities come from charts in "The Role of Public Health Improvements in Health Advances: The 20th Century United States," by David Cutler and Grant Miller, http://www.economics.harvard.edu/faculty/cutler/files/cutler_miller_cities.pdf, accessed July 15, 2010.

43. "Dr. Alice Potter a Victim of Fever," *Ithaca Daily News*, May 2, 1903; Deborah Bruch Bucki writes about Dr. Matthew D. Mann's controversial treatment of President McKinley in her article, "A History of the Century House: 100 Lincoln Parkway in Buffalo, New York," http://www.buffaloah.com/a/linc/100/hist/index.html, accessed July 15, 2010; Dr. Alice Potter's will is on file in Tompkins County Surrogate Court, Ithaca, N.Y.; "Pass Resolutions," *Ithaca Daily News*, May 6, 1903.

44. "Infirmary Reports During Fever Epidemic," CUTP.

45. *The 1904 Cornellian, The Year Book of Cornell University, Being the Complete Record of the Collegiate Year 1902–1903* (Ithaca: Cornell University, 1903), 162.

Chapter 14: The Man Who Saved Cornell University

1. Warren S. Barlow medical claim, CUTP; Howard C. Smith to Edith M. Fox, regional historian, Cornell University Library, March 19, 1952, Howard C. Smith Reminiscence, Collection #42/2/m.317, Division of Rare and Manuscript Collections, Cornell University Library.

2. In 1903 it was still possible to teach with only a high school education, so Odell's course of being a high school teacher for ten years and then going off to college was not as odd as it may seem in the twenty-first century. Mrs. D. D. Hammond to Jacob Gould Schurman, February 26 and March 4, 1903, CUTP; James P. Howe, University of Chicago Law School, to Jacob Gould Schurman, March 22, 1903, CUTP217217.

3. Editorial, *Cornell Daily Sun*, March 27, 1903; "Large Subscription," *Cornell Daily Sun*, March 28, 1903.

4. Dean Thomas F. Crane to President Schurman, March 18, 1903, CUTP.

5. "Will Build Palace of Peace: Carnegie Negotiating for an Estate at The Hague," *New York Sun*, February 21, 1903; "Carnegie Aids an Old Friend," *New York Sun*, February 16, 1903.

6. George G. Cotton to Andrew Carnegie, with handwritten Carnegie note to Jacob Gould Schurman, March 23, 1903, JGS; "History of the Solvay Public Library," http://www.solvaylibrary.org/Solvay%20 Process/splhistory.htm, accessed July 22, 2010.

7. Joseph Frazier Wall, *Andrew Carnegie* (New York: Oxford University Press, 1970), 419.

8. Jacob Gould Schurman to Andrew Carnegie, April 1, 1903, JGS; minutes of the Executive Committee of the Cornell University Board of Trustees, April 6, 1903, EC; Caroline G. A. Slater to Jacob Gould Schurman, April 7, 1903, CUTP; form letter about Carnegie offer from Jacob Gould Schurman, April 7, 1903, CUTP; "Opens His Wallet: Carnegie Asks That Money be Returned to Other Donors," *Times-Democrat*, Lima, Ohio, April 15, 1903; R. A. Franks, president, Home Trust Company, Hoboken, N.J., to Jacob Gould Schurman, April 25, 1903, EC.

9. Jacob Gould Schurman, *Eleventh Annual Report of President Schurman*, 1902–1903 (Ithaca: Cornell University, 1903), 5.

10. Homer S. Sackett to Jacob Gould Schurman, May 1, 1903, Typhoid Papers, Cornell University Library.

11. Hannah Spencer to Jacob Gould Schurman, April 22, 1903, CUTP.

12. Jarvis A. Wood to Jacob Gould Schurman, April 16, 1903, CUTP.

13. Editorial, *Oakland Tribune*, Oakland, California, April 16, 1903.

14. "Pay the Doctor Bills," *Ithaca Daily News*, May 20, 1903.

15. Minutes of the Executive Committee of Cornell University, February 14, 1905, EC. New York was actually the first state to adopt a compulsory workers' compensation law in 1910, but it was overturned as unconstitutional by the courts. The state then adopted a constitutional amendment and passed a new compulsory law in 1913. See, http://eh.net/encyclopedia/article/fishback.workers .compensation, accessed August 4, 2010. The purpose of workers' compensation laws was to eliminate fault from the system. In return for the worker giving up his right to bring a lawsuit, the employer agreed to pay his medical expenses and about two-thirds of his wages or survivor benefits if he died.

Chapter 15: Retribution

1. "Person Can Vote Once on Question: City Attorney Makes Ruling Which Will Govern Election," *Ithaca Daily News*, February 23, 1903.

2. "Water Company's Plans," *Ithaca Daily Journal*, February 26, 1903.

3. "Large Vote Cast for Water Works," *Ithaca Daily News*, March 2, 1903; "People Vote on Water Ownership: Sexes Meet on Equal Terms at the Polls," *Ithaca Daily Journal*, March 2, 1903; "Overwhelming Victory," *Ithaca Daily News*, March 3, 1903; the number of taxpayers in Ithaca is found in "Petition Worded Satisfactorily," *Ithaca Daily News*, March 27, 1903.

4. Jacob Gould Schurman to David Roe Jr., February 12, 1903, JGS; Jacob Gould Schurman to Latin Prof. H. C. Elmer, February 28, 1903, JGS; Jacob Gould Schurman to Henry R. Ickelheimer, March 6, 1903, JGS; Jacob Gould Schurman to Rev. C. H. Parkhurst, March 2, 1903, JGS; Jacob Gould Schurman, to Mr. Palmer, February 28, 1903, JGS.

5. R. S. Tarr, "Artesian Well Sections at Ithaca, N.Y.," *The Journal of Geology*, Vol. 12, No. 2 (February-March 1904), 69–82; Robert H. Thurston to Jacob Gould Schurman, March 5, 1903, CUTP.

6. Editorial, "Pure Water in City Mains in Two Week's Time," *Ithaca Daily News*, March 3, 1903; "Seeking Pure Water Supply: Committee of 100

Proceeding with Much Energy," *Ithaca Daily Journal*, March 3, 1903; Editorial, "Now for Pure Water," *Ithaca Daily Journal*, March 3, 1903.

7. Jared Treman Newman to Jacob Gould Schurman, March 4, 1903, CUTP; "Pure Water for Ithaca," *New York Times*, March 12, 1903; "Water Plant for Ithaca," *New York Times*, March 24, 1903.

8. Jared Treman Newman to Jacob Gould Schurman, March 25, 1903, CUTP.

9. The typhoid case of Stewart's wife is mentioned in "New York Legislature: Five Republicans Bolt the Leadership of Senator Raines," *New York Times*, February 25, 1903; "A Health Department Bill," *Elmira Advertiser*, February 6, 1903; editorial, "For the Public Health," *New York Tribune*, March 10, 1903.

10. Water case transcript, Williams testimony, January 2, 1906, Vol. 8, p. 9.

11. William T. Morris to the Finance Committee of the Board of Trustees of Cornell University, April 15, 1903, EC.

12. Minutes of the Cornell University Board of Trustees, April 19, 1903, Division of Rare and Manuscript Collections, Cornell University Library.

13. "Pushing Work Hard in the Six Mile Gorge," *Ithaca Daily News*, April 27, 1903.

14. Cornelius Vermeule to the Committee of 100, March 21, 1903, CUTP.

15. Mayor George W. Miller to William T. Morris, April 28, 1903, MVC; Water Works Company States Selling Price," *Ithaca Daily News*, May 6, 1903; "Water Company Meets New Board," *Ithaca Daily Journal*, May 6, 1903; Ithaca Water Board minutes, May 5, 1903, Ithaca City Archives.

16. "Alderman Howell Opposes the Dam," *Ithaca Daily Journal*, May 21, 1903; "Common Council Says Stop the Dam," *Ithaca Daily Journal*, May 27, 1903.

17. Editorial, "An Insult to Public Intelligence," *Ithaca Daily News*, April 29, 1903.

18. Editorial, "Will the Water Company Be Fair," *Ithaca Daily News*, May 2, 1903.

19. Editorial, "Nothing Less Than an Outrage," *Ithaca Daily News,* May 28, 1903.

20. Henry Woodward Sackett, *The Law of Libel: What Every Tribune Employee Is Expected to Know about It; How to Guard against Libel Suits; and How*

to Be Prepared to Defend Them When Brought (New York: The Tribune Association, 1885), 6.

21. Complaint, Tucker & Vinton, Inc., Plaintiffs, against the Ithaca Publishing Company and Frank E. Gannett, Defendants, Supreme Court of the State of New York, New York County, June 16, 1903, Frank E. Gannett & Caroline Werner Gannett Papers, Division of Rare and Manuscript Collections, Cornell University Library; editorial, "We Shall Know the Facts," *Ithaca Daily News,* June 20, 1903.

22. Henry W. Sackett to Mynderse Van Cleef, July 24, 1903, MVC.

23. "Beautiful Society House Damaged by the Flames: Chi Phi Members Lose Large Amount of Goods," *Ithaca Daily News,* May 18, 1903; "Fire Damages Chi Phi House: Loss Estimated at Fifteen Thousand Dollars," *Ithaca Daily Journal,* May 18, 1903.

24. "Will Rebuild Chi Phi House," *Ithaca Daily Journal,* May 19, 1903.

25. Charles H. Blood to John W. Dwight, May 18, 1903, Charles H. Blood Papers, Division of Rare and Manuscript Collections, Cornell University Library; "Cornell's Second Varsity Crew Wins, Pennsylvania Second, Harvard Third," *Ithaca Daily News,* June 1, 1903.

26. Minutes of the Cornell University Executive Committee, May 12, 1903, EC; Minutes of the Cornell University Board of Trustees, June 17, 1903, Division of Rare and Manuscript Collections, Cornell University Library.

27. Samuel Hopkins Adams, "Typhoid: An Unnecessary Evil," *McClure's Magazine,* June 1905, 152.

28. Hotchkiss, "Jacob Gould Schurman and the Cornell Tradition," 208–11.

Epilogue: Getting Away with Murder

1. "Many Students at Cornell," *New York Times,* September 26, 1903.

2. "Schurman Tells of Cornell Gain," Syracuse *Herald,* Syracuse, N.Y., October 7, 1907.

3. "Campus Supplied with Pure Water: Carnegie Filtration Plant Now in Operation," *Ithaca Daily Journal,* May 29, 1903.

4. "Pure Water for Ithaca," *New York Times,* August 24, 1903; "Penalty for Drinking Filtered Water: Ithaca Householders May Have to Break

Law to Avail Themselves of New Plant," *New York Tribune*, August 30, 1903. The headline referred to a municipal ordinance enacted during the epidemic that levied a $50 fine on anyone who drank city water without boiling it first; Emile M. Chamot to William T. Morris, October 10, 1903, CUTP.

5. Dorothy Harris, *History of Ithaca's Water & Sewer Systems* (Ithaca: City of Ithaca, 1956), 4, 6; Tarr, "Artesian Well Sections at Ithaca, N.Y.," 69, 69n.

6. William T. Morris to Mynderse Van Cleef, June 29, 1904, MVC; Ithaca Water Works to Ithaca Water Board, July 12, 1904, MVC.

7. Nathan Mathews Jr. to William T. Morris, October 21, 1905, MVC. Mathews wrote to Morris because the expert witnesses in the case, including Allen Hazen and Gardner S. Williams, were upset by a flip remark Morris made to the effect that they should seek their witness fees from the city of Ithaca, or in other words, work on a contingency basis and only be paid in the event of a victory. Morris gave in and agreed to pay them from his company accounts.

8. "Examiner's Report of the Tompkins County National Bank, April 16–17, 1907," and letter, Robert H. Treman to William B. Ridgley, Comptroller of the Currency, May 8, 1907, Record Group 101, U.S. Comptroller of the Currency, National Archives, College Park, Md.

9. Final ruling, water case, December 27, 1906, Jared Treman Newman Papers, Division of Rare and Manuscript Collections, Cornell University Library; Nathan Mathews Jr. to Mynderse Van Cleef, January 5, 1907, MVC; Mathews to Van Cleef, January 30, 1907, MVC.

10. Jacob Gould Schurman to Samuel D. Halliday, January 26, 1907, JGS.

11. Minutes of the Cornell University Executive Committee, January 22, 1907, 192, Division of Rare and Manuscript Collections, Cornell University Library; final settlement, water case, February 23, 1907, MVC; Sisler, *Enterprising Families, Ithaca, New York*, 23; minutes of the Ithaca Water Board, September 9, 1907, Ithaca City Archives.

12. Charles H. Blood to William T. Morris, April 29, 1903, Charles H. Blood Papers, Division of Rare and Manuscript Collections, Cornell University Library; Jared Treman Newman to Cornell University Executive Committee, December 13, 1904, EC.

13. Editorial, *Journal of the American Medical Association*, March 28, 1903, 852.

14. See Chapter 8.

15. Soper, "The Epidemic of Typhoid Fever at Ithaca," 437, 442; Robert H. Thurston to President Schurman and the Executive Committee, September 20, 1902, EC. Thurston's letter refers to "the unusual frequency and magnitude of the summer rains" in the summer of 1902.

16. Adams, "Typhoid: An Unnecessary Evil," *McClure's Magazine*, June 1905, 150–52; Samuel Hopkins Adams to Jacob Gould Schurman, April 1, 1905, EC; Emmons L. Williams to Samuel Hopkins Adams, April 5, 1905.

17. Hewett, *Cornell University: A History*; Berry, *Behind the Ivy*; Bishop, *A History of Cornell*; David L. Schiller, "The Social History of the 1903 Ithaca Typhoid Fever Epidemic: A Study of Anger and Action," submitted for History 435, Cornell University, Spring Term 1973.

18. "Light Company Changes Hands," *Ithaca Daily Journal*, June 9, 1903. Brush Electric Company of Cleveland eventually became a part of General Electric Company.

19. Charles Nodder, *Report of the Examination of the Accounts and Records of Associated Gas & Electric Co. as of Dec. 31, 1929*, Vol. 1, p. 29 (Washington, D.C.: Federal Trade Commission); Associated Gas & Electric Certificate of Incorporation, March 17, 1906, Archives of the New York Public Service Commission, Albany, N.Y.

20. At one of them, in a debate before the Chamber of Commerce in Elmira, N.Y., on May 3, 1907, Hughes, a future chief justice of the U.S. Supreme Court, uttered his famous remark that the U.S. Constitution "is what the judges say it is." See, *Addresses and Papers of Charles Evans Hughes, Governor of New York, 1906–08* (New York: G. P. Putnam's Sons, 1908), 139.

21. Merlo J. Pusey, *Charles Evans Hughes, Vol. 1* (New York: Columbia University Press, 1963), 202, 226; Robert F. Wesser, *Charles Evans Hughes: Politics and Reform in New York, 1905–1910* (Ithaca: Cornell University Press, 1967), 167, 169.

22. FTC Report, Vol. 4, 29–31; Barbara H. Brock, author of *The Development of Public Utility Accounting in New York* (East Lansing:

Graduate School of Business Administration, Michigan State University, 1981), p. 91, says that New York's 1907 Public Service Law regulated only local utility operating companies, not holding companies like Associated Gas & Electric. Donald C. Baldwin, author of *Capital Control in New York* (Menasha, Wis.: The Collegiate Press, 1920), p. 9, says the 1907 law "essentially" banned gas and electric holding companies.

23. Jacob Gould Schurman to William T. Morris, May 31, 1907, JGS.
24. William T. Morris to Mynderse Van Cleef, May 2, 1906, MVC.
25. FTC, Vol. 4, p. 31.
26. Samuel T. Williamson, *Imprint of a Publisher*, 79.
27. W. Emerson Barger, "Examiner's Report of the First National Bank of Ithaca," August 29, 1905, R.G. 101, U.S. Comptroller of the Currency, National Archives, College Park, Md.; Frank E. Gannett vs. Ithaca Publishing Company, January 22, 1907, Onondaga County Supreme Court, Syracuse, N.Y.
28. The story about Duncan Campbell Lee and the country newspaper owners was printed in the *New York Tribune* of January 12, 1907.
29. Interview with Nancy Lee Gluck, Nokesville, Va., April 19, 1996. Mrs. Gluck, who died at age ninety-nine in 2003, married into the family that discovered the long-missing half of the original manuscript of Mark Twain's *Huckleberry Finn* in a trunk in the attic of their Los Angeles home around 1991. www.nytimes.com/1992/08/02/books /arts-artifacts-more-huck-finn-adventures-to-buffalo-via-hollywood .html.
30. Ibid.; "Last Request of Hill Alumnus Carried Out by Classmates of '91," *Utica Daily Press*, August 8, 1945, Hamilton College Archives.
31. David C. Tomlinson, a later owner of the Van Wagener Mansion, provided information on the history of the house in an e-mail to the author, May 18, 2004.
32. Robert H. Treman to Mynderse Van Cleef, May 1, 1918, MVC; William T. Morris to Mynderse Van Cleef, May 6, 1918, MVC; Morris Tracy to Mynderse Van Cleef, December 19, 1918, MVC.

Afterword: The Conquest of Typhoid

1. George A. Soper, "The Discovery of Typhoid Mary," *British Medical Journal*, January 7, 1939.

2. Keith Christman, "The History of Chlorine," http://www .waterandhealth.org/drinkingwater/history.html, accessed August 11, 2010.

3. Frank Carey, "New Soil-Derived Drug Proves to Be the Only Enemy of Rickettsia," *Associated Press*, June 27, 1948; Frank Carey, "Doctor Takes Big Chance as He Shows New Wonder Drug's Effect on Typhus," Associated Press, July 19, 1948.

4. William E. Lawrence, "Wonder Drug, Foe of Plagues, Is Made Artificially in Quantity," *New York Times*, March 27, 1949.

BIBLIOGRAPHY

Abt, Henry. *Ithaca*. Ithaca, NY: Ross W. Kellogg, 1926.

Adams, Samuel Hopkins. "Typhoid: An Unnecessary Evil." *McClure's Magazine*, 1905: 145–56.

Aldrich, Lewis Cass, ed. *History of Yates County, N.Y.* Syracuse, NY: D. Mason & Co., 1892.

Applegate, Edd. *Personalities and Products: A Historical Perspective on Advertising in America*. Westport, CT: Greenwood Press, 1998.

Baker, Moses N., ed. *The Manual of American Water Works*. New York: Engineering News Publishing Co., 1897.

Baldwin, Donald C. *Capital Control in New York*. Menasha, WI: The Collegiate Press, 1920.

Baron, Abraham L. *Man Against Germs*. New York: E. P. Dutton & Co., 1957.

Barringer, Emily Dunning. *Bowery to Bellevue: The Story of New York's First Woman Ambulance Surgeon*. New York: W. W. Norton, 1950.

Bayles, James C. "The Prevention of Typhoid Fever." *World's Work*. 6 (1903): 3647–50.

Berry, Romeyn. *Behind the Ivy: Fifty Years in One University with Visits to Sundry Others*. Ithaca, NY: Cornell University Press, 1950.

Bishop, Morris. *A History of Cornell*. Ithaca, NY: Cornell University Press, 1962.

Brock, Barbara H. *The Development of Public Utility Accounting in New York*. East Lansing: Graduate School of Business Administration, Michigan State University, 1981.

Brock, Thomas D. *Robert Koch: A Life in Medicine and Bacteriology*. Madison, WI: Science Tech, 1988.

Budd, William. *Typhoid Fever: Its Nature, Mode of Spreading, and Prevention*. London: Longmans, Green & Co., 1873.

Burns, T. W. "Reminiscences, Heroic and Historic, of Early Days of the Lehigh Valley System in Southern and Central New York." *Black Diamond Express* 9[1] (1905): 7–18.

Burton, William K. *The Water Supply of Towns and the Construction of Water-works*. London: Crosby, Lockwood & Son, 1898.

Chamot, Emile M., and Harry W. Redfield. *Part I: The Analysis of Water for Household and Municipal Purposes*. Ithaca, NY: Taylor & Carpenter, 1911.

The City of Ithaca, N.Y., plaintiff, vs. Ithaca Water Works Co., Ithaca Light & Water Co., Henry L. Hinckley as Trustee for first mortgage bond holders of Ithaca Water Works Col, Ithaca Trust Co. as trustee for subsequent mortgage bond holders of Ithaca Water Works Co. and Ithaca Light & Water Co., Myron Van Orman, Lucy R. Hollister, defendants., Tompkins County Court, Ithaca, N.Y., 1903.

Chudacoff, Howard P. *The Age of the Bachelor*. Princeton, NJ: Princeton University Press, 1999.

Cirillo, Vincent J. *Bullets and Bacilli: The Spanish-American War and Military Medicine*. New Brunswick, NJ: Rutgers University Press, 2004.

Clarkson, Grosvenor B. *Industrial America in the World War: The Strategy Behind the Lines, 1917–1918*. Boston & New York: Houghton Mifflin Co., 1923.

Coville, Luzerne. *Ithaca Epidemic of 1903*. Symposium on Typhoid Fever, Medical Society of the State of New York, 1905.

——. "Typhoid Fever: With Especial Reference to Its Incubation Period and Reincubation Cycles." *New York State Journal of Medicine* 6 (1906).

Curschmann, Heinrich. *Typhoid Fever and Typhus Fever*. Philadelphia: W. B. Saunders & Co., 1902.

Danelski, David J., and Joseph S. Tulchin, eds. *The Autobiographical Notes of Charles Evans Hughes*. Cambridge, MA: Harvard University Press, 1973.

Earnest, Ernest. *Academic Procession: An Informal History of the American College, 1636 to 1953*. Indianapolis: Bobbs-Merrill Co., Inc., 1953.

Emerson, Isabel Dolbier. Scrapbook. *Isabel Dolbier Emerson*. Ithaca, NY: Cornell University Rare and Manuscript Collections, 1903.

Finch, Joyce. H., ed. *As I Remember: Recollections of Allan H. Treman*. Ithaca, NY: Department of Manuscripts and Archives, Cornell University Libraries, 1979.

Folkerts, Jean, and Dwight L. Teeter Jr. *Voices of a Nation: A History of Media in the United States*. New York: MacMillan, 1989.

Folwell, Amory Prescott. *Water Supply Engineering: The Designing, Construction, and Maintenance of Water-Supply Systems, Both City and Irrigation*. New York: John Wiley & Sons, 1900.

Freetown, Past and Present. Freetown, Prince Edward Island: Freetown Historical Society, 1985.

Fuertes, James H. *Water Filtration Works*. New York: John Wiley & Sons, 1901.

Gabert, T. A., Alexandra C. Lipsky, and Elaine D. Engst, eds. *Guide to Frank E. Gannett and Caroline Werner Gannett Papers*. Ithaca, NY: Division of Rare and Manuscript Collections, Cornell University Library, 1987.

Garbat, Abraham. L. *Typhoid Carriers and Typhoid Immunity*. New York: The Rockefeller Institute for Medical Research, 1922.

Gay, Frederick P. *Typhoid Fever Considered as a Problem of Scientific Medicine*. New York: The MacMillan Company, 1918.

Gerhard, William P. *Sanitation and Sanitary Engineering*. New York: Published by the author, 1909.

Gifford, John C. *On Preserving Tropical Florida*. Coral Gables, FL: University of Miami Press, 1972.

Gillespie, Charles Coulston, ed. *Dictionary of Scientific Biography*. New York: Charles Scribner's Sons, 1971.

Grant, James. *Money of the Mind: Borrowing and Lending in America from the Civil War to Michael Milken*. New York: Farrar, Straus & Giroux, 1992.

Graves, Ross. *William Schurman, Loyalist, of Bedeque, Prince Edward Island, and His Descendants*. Summerside, PEI: Harold B. Schurman, 1973.

Gurock, Jeffrey S., ed. *Central European Jews in America, 1840–1880*. American Jewish History, a thirteen-volume history sponsored by the American Jewish Historical Society. New York: Routledge, 1998.

Hare, Hobart Amory. *The Medical Complications, Accidents, and Sequelae of Typhoid or Enteric Fever*. Philadelphia: Lea Brothers & Co, 1899.

Hazen, Allen. *The Filtration of Public Water Supplies*. New York: John Wiley & Sons, 1895.

Hill, John W. *The Purification of Public Water Supplies*. New York: D. Van Nostrand Company, 1898.

Hobart, Alice Tisdale. *Gusty's Child*. New York: Longmans, Green & Co., 1959.

Hotchkiss, Eugene I. "Jacob Gould Schurman and the Cornell Tradition: A Study of Jacob Gould Schurman, Scholar and Educator, and His Administration of Cornell University, 1892–1920." *Graduate School*. Ithaca, NY: Cornell University, 1960.

Howard, Leland O. *Fighting the Insects: The Story of an Entomologist*. New York: Arno Press (reprint of original Macmillan edition), 1980.

Hower, Ralph M. *The History of an Advertising Agency: N. W. Ayer & Son at Work, 1869–1949*. Cambridge, MA: Harvard University Press, 1949.

Huckstep, Ronald L. *Typhoid Fever and Other Salmonella Infections*. Edinburgh, Scotland: E & S. Livingstone Ltd., 1962.

Hughes, Charles Evans. *Addresses and Papers of Charles Evans Hughes, Governor of New York, 1906–08*. New York: G. P. Putnam's Sons, 1908.

Hulse, Shirley Clarke. "Comments on Making Garbage Burn." *Transactions of the American Society of Civil Engineers* 54 (1905): 327.

———. "Reminiscences of a Field Engineer." *Civil Engineering* 14^5 (1944): 191–94.

Hungerford, Edward H. The American City and Its Utilities. Rochester, NY: Public and Municipal Education Committee, Rochester Board of Education, 1926.

Jacobs, Lawrence. *Early Boyhood Days in Ithaca*. Ithaca, NY: Dewitt Historical Society of Tompkins County, 1971.

Jordan, Edwin O. "The Typhoid Epidemic at Ithaca, Preview." *Journal of the American Medical Association*. (1903).

———. "The Typhoid Epidemic at Ithaca, Part I." *Journal of the American Medical Association* (1903): 781–83.

———. "The Typhoid Epidemic at Ithaca, Part II." *Journal of the American Medical Association*. (1903).

———. "The Typhoid Epidemic at Ithaca, Part III." *Journal of the American Medical Association*. (1903).

———. *A Textbook of General Bacteriology*. Philadelphia: W. B. Saunders Company, 1908.

Keen, William W. *The Surgical Complications and Sequels of Typhoid Fever*. Philadelphia: W. B. Saunders, 1898.

Kerr, Richard D. *Ithaca Street Railway*. Forty Fort, PA: Harold E. Cox, 1972.

Kindleberger, Charles P. *Manias, Panics & Crashes: A History of Financial Crises, Revised Edition.* New York: Basic Books, 1989.

Kober, George M. "The Progress and Achievements of Hygiene." *Science* 6(152) (1897): 789–99.

Koch, Robert. "Uber die Bazillentragerfrage" (On the Bacillus Carrier Question). *Robert Koch: Gesammelte Werke II, 2, S. 917.* (1902)

Kotkin, Stephen. *Magnetic Mountain: Stalinism as a Civilization.* Berkeley: University of California Press, 1995.

Kraut, Alan M. *Silent Travelers: Germs, Genes, and the "Immigrant Menace."* New York: Basic Books, 1994.

Kurtz, D. Morris. *Ithaca and Its Resources: Being an Historical and Descriptive Sketch of the "Forest City" and Its Magnificent Scenery.* Ithaca, NY: Journal Association Book and Job Printer, 1883.

Lamoreaux, Naomi R. *The Great Merger Movement in American Business, 1895– 1904.* Cambridge: Cambridge University Press, 1985.

Last, John M. "Winslow, Charles-Edward Amory," eNotes.com. 2006: website.

Lumsden, Leslie L., and Arthur M. Stimson. "Examination of Excreta for Typhoid Bacilli." *Public Health Reports* XXVII[21] (1912): 3–6.

Lutz, Tom. *American Nervousness 1903: An Anecdotal History.* Ithaca, NY: Cornell University Press, 1991.

Mangione, Jerre, and Ben Morreale. *La Storia: Five Centuries of the Italian American Experience.* New York: Harper Perennial–Aaron Asher Books, 1993.

Marsh, M. C., recording secy. "The Biological Society of Washington, 429th Meeting." *Science* 25(648) (1907): 862–65.

Mason, O. T. "Oysters as a Means of Transmitting Typhoid Fever." *Science* 1[2] (1895): 49–50.

Mason, William P. *Water Supply (Considered Principally from a Sanitary Standpoint).* New York: John Wiley & Sons, 1902.

McGuire, James K. *The Democratic Party of the State of New York: A History of the Origin, Growth, and Achievements of the Democratic Party of the State of New York, Including a History of Tammany Hall in Relation to State Politics.* New York: United States History Company, 1905.

McLaughlin, Allen J. *The Effect of Safe Water Supplies on the Typhoid Fever Rate.* Association of Life Insurance Presidents, New York: U.S. Public Health Service, 1912.

McTavish, Jan R. "Antipyretic Treatment and Typhoid Fever, 1860–1900." *Journal of the History of Medicine and Allied Sciences Online* 42 (1987): 486–506.

Merriman, Mansfield. *Elements of Sanitary Engineering.* New York: John Wiley & Sons, 1906.

Moody, Robert E. *America's First Rushville.* Rushville, N.Y, 1991.

Mosher, William E., and Finla G. Crawford. *Public Utility Regulation.* New York: Harper & Brothers, 1933.

Nasaw, David. *Andrew Carnegie.* New York: The Penguin Press, 2006.

New York (State), AGSO. *New York in the Spanish-American War, 1898.* Albany, NY: J. B. Lyon, 1900.

Nodder, Charles. Report of the Examination of the Accounts and Records of Associated Gas & Electric Company as of Dec. 31, 1929, Vol. 1. Washington, D.C.: Federal Trade Commission, 1929.

Novy, Frederick G. "Disease Carriers." *Science* 36(914) (1912): 1–10.

Noyes, Alexander Dana. *Forty Years of American Finance.* New York: G. P. Putnam's Sons, 1909.

———. *The War Period of American Finance: 1908–1925.* New York: G. P. Putnam's Sons, 1926.

Page, Charles E. "The Successful Treatment of Typhoid Fever." *The Arena* (1892): 450–60.

Phillips, Kevin. *William McKinley.* New York: Times Books, Henry Holt & Company, 2003.

Piper, Clarence Brett. "Alpha Psi—Cornell University." *The Purple and Gold* 20 (1903): 220–21.

"Plea for Independence of the Filipino People: President J.G. Schurman's Fine Address in Cooper Union." *Ithaca Daily News.* Ithaca, N.Y., 1903.

Poole, Murray Edward. *A Story Historical of Cornell University, with Biographies of Distinguished Cornellians.* Ithaca, NY: The Cayuga Press, 1916.

The Purple and Gold. Ithaca, N.Y., Chi Psi Fraternity, Alpha Chapter, Cornell University, 1903.

Pusey, Merlo J. *Charles Evans Hughes, Volume 1.* New York: Columbia University Press, 1963.

Reed, Walter, Victor C. Vaughan, and Edward O. Shakespeare. *Report on the Origin and Spread of Typhoid Fever in the U.S. Military during the Spanish War of 1898.* Washington, DC: U.S. Government Printing Office, 1904.

"Report of the Committee on Standard Methods of Water Analysis to the Laboratory Section of the American Public Health Association, 1897." *Journal of Infectious Disease, Supplement #1* (May 1905).

"Report of the Geological Survey of the State of Ohio." *Report of the Geological Survey of the State of Ohio* VIII, 1906. Rotundo, E. Anthony. *American Manhood: Transformations in Masculinity from the Revolution to the Modern Era.* New York: Basic Books, 1993.

Schiller, David L. "The Social History of the 1903 Ithaca Typhoid Fever Epidemic: A Study of Anger and Action." *History.* Ithaca, NY: Cornell University, 1973.

Schurman, Jacob Gould. Letter of Reference for Frank E. Gannett. Frank E. Gannett Papers, Cornell University. Ithaca, NY, 1902.

——. *Philippine Affairs: A Retrospect and Outlook.* New York: Charles Scribner's Sons, 1902.

——. *Eleventh Annual Report of President Schurman, 1902–1903.* Ithaca, NY: Cornell University, 1903.

——. *Cornell University: Twelfth Annual Report, 1903–1904.* Ithaca, NY: Cornell University, 1904.

Schuyler, James D. *Reservoirs for Irrigation, Water-Power and Domestic Water Supply.* New York: John Wiley & Sons, 1908.

Sedgwick, William T. *Principles of Sanitary Science and the Public Health.* New York: Macmillan, 1903.

——. "Typhoid Fever: A Disease of Defective Civilization." *Typhoid Fever: Its Causation, Transmission, and Prevention, by George C. Whipple.* New York: John Wiley & Sons, 1908.

Selkreg, John H., ed. *Landmarks of Tompkins County, N.Y., Including a History of Cornell University by Prof. W.T. Hewett.* Syracuse, NY: D. Mason & Co., 1894.

Sheldon, George H. *Advertising Elements & Principles.* New York: Harcourt, Brace & Co., 1925.

Simon, Charles E. *Human Infection Carriers: Their Significance, Recognition and Management*. Philadelphia: Lee & Febiger, 1919.

Soper, George A. "Filtration and Typhoid: Report of Dr. George A. Soper upon the Causes of the Epidemic of Typhoid Fever at Butler, Pennsylvania." *The Engineering Magazine* 26(February 1904): 754–55.

——. "The Epidemic of Typhoid Fever at Ithaca, N.Y." *Journal of the New England Water Works Association* XVIII[4] (1904).

——. "The Work of a Chronic Typhoid Germ Distributor." *Journal of the American Medical Association* XLVIII[24] (1907): 2019–22.

——. "Typhoid Mary." *The Military Surgeon* XLV[1] (1919).

——. "The Curious Case of Typhoid Mary." *Bulletin of the New York Academy of Medicine* 15 (1939): 698–712.

The Standard Medical Directory of North America, 1903-04. Chicago: G.P. Engelhard & Co.

Stewart, David D. *Treatment of Typhoid Fever*. Detroit: George S. Davis, 1893.

Swaine, Robert T. *Volume I, The Cravath Firm and Its Predecessors, 1819–1947*. New York: Ad Press, 1948.

Teachout, Terry. *The Skeptic: A Life of H. L. Mencken*. New York: Harper Collins, 2002.

Treman, Ebenezer Mack, and Murray E. Poole. *The History of the Treman, Trumaine, Truman Family in America*. Ithaca, NY, 1901.

The Tribune Almanac and Political Register 1903. New York, The Tribune Association.

Turneaure, Frederick E., and Harry L. Russell, *Public Water Supplies: Requirements, Resources, and the Construction of Works*. New York: John Wiley & Sons, 1901.

U.S. Census. Census Reports, Vol. IV, Twelfth Census of the United States Taken in the Year 1900, Vital Statistics, Part II, Statistics of Deaths. W. R. Merriam. Washington: U.S. Census Office, 1902.

Vaughan, Victor C. *A Doctor's Memories*. Indianapolis: Bobbs-Merrill, 1926.

Wall, Joseph Frazier. *Andrew Carnegie*. New York: Oxford University Press, 1970.

Wegmann, Edward. *The Design and Construction of Dams*. New York: John Wiley & Sons, 1908.

Wesser, Robert F. *Charles Evans Hughes: Politics and Reform in New York, 1905–1910.* Ithaca, NY: Cornell University Press, 1967.

Weston, Arthur. *The Making of American Physical Education.* New York: Appleton-Century-Crofts, 1962.

Whipple, George C. *Typhoid Fever: Its Causation, Transmission and Prevention, with an introductory essay by William T. Sedgwick.* New York: John Wiley & Sons, 1908.

White, Andrew Dickson. *The Autobiography of Andrew Dickson White.* New York: The Century Company, 1905.

Williams, G. S. "Discussion of Multiple Arch Dams." *Transactions of the American Society of Civil Engineers* 81 (1917): 899–900.

Williamson, Samuel T. *Frank Gannett: A Biography.* New York: Duell, Sloan and Pearce, 1940.

——. *Imprint of a Publisher: The Story of Frank Gannett and His Independent Newspapers.* New York: Robert H. McBride & Co., 1948.

Winslow, Charles-Edward Amory. "The War Against Disease." *Atlantic Monthly.* 91 (1903): 43–53.

Wolcott, Walter. *Penn Yan, New York.* Penn Yan, NY: Peerless Printing Co., 1915.

Wolman, Abel, and Arthur E. Gorman. "The Significance of Waterborne Typhoid Fever Outbreaks, 1920–1930." *Journal of the American Water Works Association* 23^2 (1930): 160–201.

——. "Waterborne Typhoid Fever Still a Menace." *American Journal of Public Health and The Nation's Health* XXI^2 (1931): 115–29.

INDEX

A

Abraham Van Wagener mansion, 208–9

actinomycete, *see* chloromycetin

Adams, Abigail, 83

Adams, Samuel Hopkins, 157, 194, 203, 206

agar, 95

Alfred, New York, 143, 179

Alfred University, 179

Allen, William P., 67

allopathy, 94–95

Alma Mater, Cornell song, 79

Alpha Delta Phi fraternity, 64

Alpha Psi fraternity, 149

ALUMNUS letter, 135

American Ice Company, 43–44

American Public Health Association, water testing protocols, 46

Amherst College, 76

Anchora, 149

Anderson, P. Chauncey, 206

artesian water, 56, 119, 131, 147, 184, 185, 189, 197, 199; problems with Ithaca artesian wells, 198

Associated Gas & Electric Company, 205–6; bankruptcy, 211; birth of, xviii, 204; Howard Hopson years, 210–11; William T. Morris sells, 206, 208–9

Associated Press, 36, 133

Association of New York State Colleges & Universities, 205

Atlantic Monthly, xv

Atwater, Leslie, last Cornell typhoid victim, 169

B

Bailey, Edward, 174

Baker, Helen M., 116

Baldwin's Bank of Penn Yan, 14

Ballantine, J. Herbert, 18

Bancroft, Wilder D., xvi

Barber, Jennie, typhoid victim, 118

Barlow, Warren S., 147, 173, 177

Barringer, Emily, 65–66

Barstow, William S., 206

Barton, Clara, American Red Cross, 157

Bayles, James C., 140–41, 169; *New York Times* articles, 164–65

Beaux-Arts, 78, *see also* Carrère & Hastings

Beebe Lake, 8, 65

Behind the Ivy (Berry), 204

Benjamin, Charles M., co-publisher of *Ithaca Daily Journal,* 35, 42–43, 102, 135

Bergholtz, Herman, 32

Berry, Romeyn, author, xiii, 8, 203

Besemer, Dr. Arthur, 117–18, *see also* homeopathy

Besemer, Edwin, typhoid victim, 117–18

Besemer, Ethel, 117–18

Besemer, Dr. H. Burr, says "Ithaca Fever" not typhoid, 165–66

Bethany, Missouri, 99, *see also* Shumard, Oliver

Biggs, Dr. Chauncey P., 140

Biggs, Dr. Hermann M., 82, 140, 141

Bishop, Morris, author, 8, 64, 204

Blazing Saddles, 203

Blood, Charles H., co-developer of Cornell Heights, xv, 19, 80, 103, 109, 136, 163, 186, 199–200, 206; Cornell Heights, 19, 32; Memorial Day regatta, 193; Umphville men's club, 19

Blood, Louise (Mrs. Charles H. Blood), 19

Blough, Earl, 169

Bluff Point on Keuka Lake, 208

Boynton, Frank David, superintendent of schools, 118–19

Brand, Dr. Ernest, developed ice bath treatment protocol, 114–15

Bristol, George P., 66

British Medical Journal, 212

Brookings Institution, 152

Brookside Cemetery, Newfield, New York, 118

Brown University, 154

Brush Electric Company of Cleveland, 204

Brush-Swan Electric Light Company of Ithaca, 204

Brush-Swan technology, 204

Bryan, William Jennings, Democratic candidate for U.S. president, 15, 40, 67, 136

bubonic plague, 111

Budd, Dr. William, typhoid researcher, 112

Buddenbrooks (Mann), 83

Buddenbrooks, Hanno, literary typhoid victim, 83

Burdick, Daniel W., 105; appeals for Ithaca City Hospital donations, 116

Burkholder, Paul, soil researcher, 214

Burlingham, Michael J., author, 17, *see also* Eagleswood Military Academy

Burr, George Lincoln, 170

Bush, John W., Treman in-law, 2, 24, 27, 32; doubts utility sales will go through, 30; dubious about value of water company stock, 33

Bush, Kate Treman, 2, 23–24, 33

Butler, Nicholas Murray, president of Columbia University, 142

Buttermilk Creek, 9, 31, 46, 48, 50, 92, 161; filthy condition in watershed, 122, 203

Buttermilk Falls, 199
Buttermilk Falls State Park, 199

C

Calkins, Marcus E., president
of Cayuga Lake Cement
Company, 185
Camus, Albert, author, 97
Canandaigua, New York, 56
Carlisle, Floyd L., student leader, 59,
129, 130
Carlisle (Pa.) Indian School, 78–79
Carnegie, Andrew, 4, 21, 73;
anti-imperialist, 28, 39;
experience with typhoid, 177;
letters from Cornell parents,
178–79; opposes annexation
of Philippine Islands, 40;
pays for Cornell filtration
plant, 163, 177; pays Cornell
student medical bills, 175–81;
philanthropy and peace
activism, 28, 176–77
Carrère and Hastings, 78
Cascadilla Creek, 49–50, 188
Cascadilla School, 37
Caveney, Katherine, child typhoid
victim, 119
Cayuga Lake, ix, 10, 32, 74, 78,
131, 161, 168, 185, 195; barge
traffic, 3; description, 2; ice
boating, 65; inlet, xi, 197;
pollution, 9, 47, 49, 163
Cayuga Lake Cement Company,
185, *see also* Calkins, Marcus E.

Chamot, Emile M., Cornell
professor, 45, 48, 50, 54, 110,
119, 122, 163, 197; explains
danger of private wells, 47;
maps and tests Ithaca private
wells, 46; passion for safe
drinking water, 45–46; report
to Schurman, 127; witnesses
excrement along Six Mile
Creek, 77
Chapman, Claire, 112
Chapman, Helen, 112
Chapman, Margery, 112
Chestnut Hill Academy,
Philadelphia, 148
Chi Phi fraternity, 11, 15–17, 20,
29, 67, 71, 112, 193; Chi Phi
House Association, 15, 18; fire
in fraternity house, 193; revival
at Cornell, 18
Chi Psi fraternity, 64
chloromycetin, anti-typhoid drug,
214–15, *see also* Parke, Davis &
Co.
cholera, 89; New York city
outbreak, 83
Christ Church Cemetery,
Sherburne, New York, 151
ciprofloxcin, modern typhoid
drug, 215
Civil Engineering magazine, 163
Clark, Annie Sophie, 60, 101, 108
Clark, Clemmie, 99
Clark, John Artemas, 60
Clark, Judson, 60

Clark, Zella Marie, 60, 99, 101, 108, 117

Clemens, Samuel L. (Mark Twain), 99

Clinton, Miles L., 18, *see also* Treman, Ebenezer M.

Cochrane, Hattie E., mother of ill student, 146

Columbia University, 156, 200; College of Physicians & Surgeons, 95; welcomes Cornell students fleeing epidemic, 142

Commission of Appraisal, 199

Committee of 100, 183, 185, 189, 197

Conover, R.T., inspector for Board of Health, 122, 124

Conradi, Hermann, assistant to Dr. Robert Koch, 86

Conway, Patrick, leader of Ithaca Band, 18, 109

Coon, Kate, mother of Ruia, 113

Coon, Ruia, Ithaca High School typhoid victim, 113, 118

Cornell, Alonzo B., son of Ezra, 188

Cornell, Ezra, co-founder of Cornell University, 3–5, 8, 15, 25, 58–60

Cornell, Franklin C., son of Ezra, 5, 25, 31, 116, 129

Cornell Daily Sun, 36, 41, 107, 133, 135, 174, 196

Cornell Heights development, 19, 32, 103, 116, 185, 199, 200; water supply, 32, 199–200

Cornell Infirmary, 98, 101, 114–16, 137–40; complaints about quality of care during epidemic, 100, 116–17, 138, 140, 147, 149, 152, 169, 174–75; higher typhoid death rate than Ithaca City Hospital, 116; last typhoid patient discharged, 171; terms of Sage endowment, 116

Cornell Livery, 65

Cornell University, ix, x, xiv, 25, 31, 33, 49, 57, 59, 63, 70, 102, 186, 190, 196, 200; abortive attempt to teach journalism, 37; Armory, 27, 57–58; campus master plan, 78; close ties to Ithaca, 64; College of Medicine, 78, 95, 167; control by local trustees, 6; Cornell Yell, 58, 68; crew team, 68; criticism of Ithaca Water Works investment, 135; criticized as "Godless," 4; disparity between rich and poor students, 64; enrollment statistics, 78; flowers to student funerals, 109; football team, 78–9; founding, 3; fraternities, 11, 15–16, 17, 20, 29, 64, 67, 71, 112, 146–47, 149, 193; Junior Prom, 66, 106–7, 112; Law School, 25; loan to William T. Morris to acquire Ithaca Water Works, 30–32, 126,

135–36, 138, 175, 200; McGraw
Tower, ix, 63; Percy Field, 79;
philosophy of founders, 4;
plans for growth, 78; Sage
Chapel, ix, 7, 42; Senior
Dance, xv; Sibley College, 159;
sororities, 148–49; Student
Agencies, 63; student demands
during epidemic, 126, 129,
136; student stringers for
newspapers, 36, 133; students
flee epidemic, 126, 128–29,
142, 144–45, 150, 169; students
return, 157–59; town–gown
conflict, 65; waterfalls, 5; where
students lived, 63–64
Cornell University Board of
Trustees, 135, 160, 163, 186,
187–8, 199–201; more loans to
Morris, 188; settles scores with
Duncan Campbell Lee, 194–95
Cornell University Executive
Committee (of the Board of
Trustees), 31, 32, 37, 126,
129–30, 135, 178, 180, 200;
exacts boil-water pledges
from student boardinghouse
operators, 128; protects
Treman and VanCleef
mansions from encroachment,
80; rejects student demands
during epidemic, 130
Cornell University: A History (Hewett),
201, 203
Cornell Veterinary College fire, 23

Cornellian yearbook, 61, 150, 171;
"The ABC of Cornell," 178
Cosmopolitan magazine, 16
Cotton, Donald Reed, 146–47, 176
Cotton, George C., father of
Donald, 146–47, 176–77, see
also Carnegie, Andrew
Couch, William, discovered dead
horse, 124
Courtney, Charles, Cornell crew
coach, 68–69, 138, 150
Coville, Dr. Luzerne, Ithaca
physician, 95–96, 101, 114,
116–17, 138
Crane, Thomas F., Cornell dean, 9,
174–75
Crawford, Mary Merritt, 148
Croker, Herbert, 62–63
Croker, Richard, Jr., 62–63
Croker, Richard, Sr., Tammany
leader, 43–44, 62–63
Cross-Ways, 99, see also Langtry,
Lilly
Curschman, Dr. Heinrich, 96
Curtis, Dr. Frederick C., 157
Czolgosz, Leon, assassin of
President McKinley, 27

D

Dean, Willis, Ithaca High School
typhoid victim, 118
DeKok, Paul W., Parke, Davis
chemist, 215
Delaware, Lackawanna & Western
Railroad, 59, 75

Delta Chi fraternity house fire, 23
Delta Gamma sorority, 149
Democratic State Editorial
	Association, 207
Depew, Chauncey, U.S. senator, 60
Diazo urine test for typhoid, 96, 167
Dirty Baker, 202–4, *see also* Soper,
	George A.
disinfection of Ithaca, 161–64,
	167–68; mucking out and
	disinfection of outhouses,
	163, 168
Dodge, John O., 145
Dodge, Orris B., father of John, 145
Dome dam, 53, *see also* Williams,
	Gardner Stewart
Dormitories for Cornell male
	students, 196; Sheldon
	Court, 197
Dove, Arthur Garfield, American
	painter, 60–61
Dreschfield, Dr. Julius, 93–94
Driscoll Brothers & Company, 71, 90
Dryden, New York, 188
Dudley, Frank A., business partner
	of Morris, 25
Durand, Elias J., excrement
	witness, 77

E

Eagleswood Military Academy,
	16–17, 22, *see also* Treman,
	Ebenezer M.
East Hill, 9, 32, 49, 63–64, 66, 100,
	196; epicenter of typhoid

epidemic, 92–93; three
	mansions, 12, 80
East Hill School, 119
E coli bacteria, 47–48, 85–86
Edison, Thomas, 206
"Edison moving picture," 65
Edward VII (King of England),
	58, 99
Ehrlich, Paul, 96
Emerson, Isabel Dolbier, 27, 109,
	149, 172
Enfield Creek, 50
Enfield Falls, 199
Enterprising Families, Ithaca, New York
	(Sisler), 12
epidemic blame shifting, 160,
	164–65, 201–3
"Epidemic Spreads Through the
	City," 104, *see also Ithaca Daily
	News*

F

Fall Creek, 32, 46, 50, 53, 70, 92,
	127–28, 161–62, 188, 201
"Fall Creek Fallacy," 137–38,
	162–63, 201–3
Farmer, W.H.P., 154
Federal Trade Commission,
	U.S., 210
Fernow, Edward, 148
filth, 124; definition of, 87
filtration plant, Cornell, 163,
	175, 197
filtration plant, Ithaca, 130, 157,
	182, 187, 189, 190, 197, 198

financial toll of epidemic, 173–74,
180; Bernard Reilly case, 180;
student mass meeting, 174
Finch, Francis Miles, banker and
lawyer, 25, 31, 54, 183
Finlay, Walter Stevenson, Jr., 167
First National Bank of Ithaca, 42,
136, 207
First Presbyterian Church, 113
First Unitarian Church, 105, see also
Heizer, Rev. Cyrus W.
Fisk, Harvey E., 29
Fisk & Robinson, Wall Street bond
house, 26, 29–30
Fiske, Daniel Willard, 6–7
Fiske, Jennie McGraw, 6, 64
Fitschen, Rev. John Frederick,
113, see also First Presbyterian
Church
Follis, Nellie, 169
Folwell, Amory Prescott,
author, 50
Foote, Dr. Charles J., 84
Forty Years of American Finance
(Noyes), 21
Foster & Thomson law firm, 13, 25
Fraleigh, Herbert E., 57
Francis, Charles S.
Francis, Harry C., Jr., Cornell
typhoid victim, 113
Francis, Nellie, other woman, 62
Freeville, New York, 188
Fulkerson, Edna, typhoid
victim, 113

G

Gala at Masonic Hall, 102–4
Galveston Central Relief
Committee, 156–57
Galveston, Texas; hurricane of 1900,
155–56; George A. Soper role in
clean-up, 156–67, 212
Gannett, Frank E., managing editor,
Ithaca Daily News, xvi, 34, 67,
69, 102–4, 132–33, 191–92,
207, 210; accepts job offer
from Lee, 41–42; accompanies
Schurman to Philippines,
40–41; campaign biography
claim about Lee, 103–4; denies
plot to close university, 134;
early life, 40–41; fails to get
GOP presidential nomination
in 1940, 104; splits with Lee
over politics, 207
General Public Utilities
Corporation, (GPU), xviii, 74,
76, 211
George family, 112, 169
George Washington University, 210
Gifford, John C., Cornell
professor, 170
Gilbert, Harold A., 175
Gluck, Nancy Lee, daughter of
Duncan Campbell Lee, 208
Goldman, Emma, anarchist, 27
Grace Robinson Hospital, 101
The Great Train Robbery, xi
Greaves, Hattie M., typhoid
nurse, 114

Green, Edward V., 143–44

Greenwood, Ernest H., head of Junior Prom committee, 112

Griffis, John Elliot, 105

Griffis, Lillian, Vassar student, 106

Griffis, Sarah, 119

Griffis, Stanton, 105–6, 118

Griffis, Rev. William Elliot, 91, 105, 116, 119, *see also* First Congregational Church

Griggs, Dr. Elma C., 115, *see also* homeopathy

Gunderman, William R., mayor of Ithaca, 70, 97

Gusty's Child (Hobart), 153, *see also* Nourse, Alice

H

Hahnemann, Dr. Samuel, father of homeopathy, 94

Hall, Quincy A., 144, *see also* Hubbard, Lewis K.

Halliday, Samuel D., president of Cornell board of trustees, x, 103, 129, 144, 186, 199

Hamilton College, 36–37

Hammond, Mrs. D. D., typhoid nurse, 174

Hanna, Mark, strategist for President McKinley, 83

Harvard University, 193

Harvey, Margaret, warden of Sage College, 66, 147–49

Hawes, Dr. John B., physician employed by Ithaca Water Works, 123

Hazen, Allen, water filtration expert, 52, 56, 188

Head, Walter L., xi

Hearst, William Randolph, 205, 207

Heizer, Rev. Cyrus W., Unitarian minister, 105

Helm, Charles E., typhoid victim, 113

Hewett, Waterman Thomas, author and Cornell professor, 143, 201, 203

hexamine, *see* urotropin

Hill, George, Cornell typhoid victim, 60

Hill, John W., author, 51

Hirsch, Elsie, 58

A History of Cornell (Bishop), 204

Hitchcock, Dr. Edward, Jr., Ithaca health officer, 76–77, 96–97, 100, 108, 121, 161; ignores excrement report from Hollister, 77; issues boil-water advisory, 101; ridicules notion of typhoid epidemic, 97

Hitchcock, Edward, Sr., physical education expert, 76–77

Hobart, Alice Tisdale, 153, *see also* Nourse, Alice

Hochwald, 86–87, *see also* Koch, Dr. Robert

Holland, Michigan, 214

Hollister, Holmes, 76–77, 96, 101, 127

homeopathy, 94–95, 115, 117–18

Hopkins, James B., 97

Hopson, Howard Colwell, xviii, 210–11; sent to prison, 211

Hornellsville Gas Light Company, 126

Horton, Randolph, Ithaca city attorney, 185–86, 190

Hospital of the Good Shepherd, Syracuse, N.Y., 146

hospitals, 116; complaints about quality of care during epidemic, 100, 116–17, 138, 140, 147, 149, 152, 169, 174–75; Cornell Infirmary, 98, 101, 108, 114–16, 137–40; Grace Robinson Hospital, 101; higher death rate than Ithaca City Hospital, 116; Hospital of the Good Shepherd, Syracuse, 146; Ithaca City Hospital, 90, 100, 105, 113, 115–16, 160; last typhoid patient discharged, 171; overcrowding, 115, 152; terms of Sage endowment, 116

Hotel Brunswick, xii, 92, 119, *see also* Zinck, Theodor

Howell, Charles C., father of Esther, 113, 185, 189, *see also* Ithaca Common Council

Howell, Esther, youngest typhoid victim, 113, 185, 189

Hubbard, Lewis K., Cornell typhoid victim, 144

Huestis, Edna, Cornell student, 147–49

Huestis, George, father of Edna, 147

Huestis, Mary D., mother of Edna, 147

Hughes, Charles Evans, governor of New York, 204–5

Hulse, Shirley Clarke, in charge of Six Mile Creek dam project sanitation, 77, 89, 121–22, 163, 202; mucks out Fall Creek outhouses, 163

I

Ice Trust, 43, *see also* Lee, Duncan Campbell

Ickelheimer, Henry R., Schurman's emissary to Adolph Ochs, 138–41, 166, 184

Illston Artesian Water Company, 185

Illston well, 188–89; *see also* artesian water

immigrant workers, 71–72; Italians, 71–72, 75, 81, 89, 91, 156, 163, 165, 188, 201; New Croton Dam incident, 72

incinerator, 167–68

Institute for the Investigation of Infectious Diseases, 82

International Agricultural Institute, Rome, 208

intestinal perforation by
typhoid, 113
Ithaca Band, 18, 20, 109, *see also*
Conway, Patrick
Ithaca Board of Health, 46–48, 54,
119, 124–25, 158, 160–62, 167,
169, 185; adopts ordinance
banning drinking of city water,
125; blindsided by State Health
Commissioner, 158; huddles
on epidemic response, 107,
110; links epidemic to city
water, 121
Ithaca Board of Public Works, 76
Ithaca Board of Sewer
Commissioners, 47
Ithaca Businessmen's Association,
53, 105, 184
Ithaca City Cemetery, 20
Ithaca City Hospital, 90, 100, 105,
113, 115–16, 160; lower death
rate than Cornell infirmary
during epidemic, 116
Ithaca Common Council, 54, 74,
90, 185; debates public water,
53; focuses on dam threat, 100,
190; funds Soper's disinfection
campaign, 162; schedules new
referendum on public water,
182–83
Ithaca Conservatory of Music
(Ithaca College), 11, 19, 57, 105
Ithaca Cycle Club, 113, *see also*
Coon, Ruia

Ithaca Daily Journal, 2, 34–35, 37,
41–42, 53–55, 67–68, 72, 75,
97, 100–2, 105, 108, 112, 119,
122–24, 128, 134–36, 159,
166, 185, 187, 190; describes
appearance of Zinck's body, xvii;
description of lake blasting to
recover Theodor Zinck's body,
xvii; establishment newspaper
in Ithaca, 35; stresses personal
responsibility to avoid getting
typhoid, 105, 134
Ithaca Daily News, xv, 32, 34, 36–37,
42, 46–47, 49, 56, 60, 67,
70–71, 74, 97, 101–2, 108, 112,
120, 122–24, 132, 161, 166,
171, 180, 183, 185, 189–90,
192, 194; business unease
over epidemic coverage,
107; condemns attitude of,
"profits over people," 133;
editorial, "An Ideal City," 69;
editorial, "Nothing Less Than
an Outrage," 191; first major
epidemic story, 100; prints
patient lists, 105, 107; reaffirms
typhoid epidemic is real, 104
Ithaca Democrat, 36
"Ithaca Fever," 97, 100, 165
Ithaca Gas Light Company, 2, 20,
22, 24, 30, 78, 205; acquisition
by Morris, 21, 22, 26, 29;
economic boom in United
States, 21; trend toward
business combinations, 22

Ithaca High School, 94, 120; student congress, 118–19

Ithaca Hotel, 80, 163

Ithaca Light & Water Company, 29–30, 32, 187, 199

Ithaca, New York, 89; description, 2, 3; fire problems, 3, 9, 23, 193; Flats, 64, 100; hills of, 3; newspapers, 32; physician-to-population ratio, 94, 111; population of, 2, 94; railroads to, 5; tie in mayoral race, 97; typhoid before 1903, 90, 164

Ithaca Post Office, 144–45

Ithaca Publishing Company, 192, 207

Ithaca Savings Bank, 98

Ithaca Trust Company, 2, 15, 25–26, 30, 54, 116, 183

Ithaca typhoid epidemic, 88–89, 92, 96–97, 139; church bells silenced, 109–10; Class of 1903 song, 172; collateral deaths, 150–51; cut across social classes, 105; disinformation campaign by Ithaca Water Works, 161–64, 167–68; effect of weather on, 90–91, 110; epidemic statistics, 169–70; financial toll of, 173–74, 180; first Cornell student dies, 109; first Ithaca citizen dies, 106; first patient admitted to hospital, 93; impact on Cornell sports, 149–50; no lawsuits, 181; prayers for Divine intervention, 153–54; press coverage of, xiv; secondary infections from, 110, 150; social events during and after, xv, xvi; triggered by storm, 91, 93; use of Widal Reaction for diagnosis, 96; was statistically one of worst, x, 111

Ithaca Water Board, 186–90, 197, 199–200; litigation with William T. Morris, 198–99, 204; Morris wins litigation, 199; settlement with Morris, 199; takes over Ithaca Water works, 197

Ithaca Water Works, x, 2, 20, 22–23, 30, 32, 46, 49, 52–55, 70, 74–76, 78, 81, 88–89, 100–101, 121–22, 124–25, 131, 140, 166, 182, 184–86, 189–92, 197, 200, 202; agrees to build filtration plant, 130, 157; capital stock problem, 29; disinfects mains, 164; exonerated by Bayles, 165; outlines expansion plans, 56; promises to supply clean water, 70; refuses to cooperate in epidemic response, 100; sends bills to typhoid victims, 190–91; Treman offer in 1900 to sell to city, 23–24; tries to prove it wasn't responsible for typhoid, 123

J

Jennings, Hugh, Cornell baseball
    coach, 150
Jersey Central Power & Light
    Company, 211
Johns Hopkins University, 214
Johnson, Gabby, 203
Johnstown Flood of 1889, 73, 75
Jordan, Dr. Edwin O., bacteriologist,
    84, 93, 150, 200
*Journal of the American Medical
    Association*, 93, 150, 200
*Journal of the New England Water
    Works Association*, 201
Junior Prom, 66, 106–7, 109, 112,
    148; popular with Ithaca
    elite, 107
Junior Week, 106–8, 148; newspaper
    health warnings for, 108

K

Kaiser Wilhelm Institute, 83, 155
Kappa Alpha fraternity house
    fire, 23
Kappa Kappa Gamma sorority, 148,
    see also Huestis, Edna
Kerr, Dr. Abram, 116, 167
Keuka Lake, 12, 208
Knapp, Robert, Cornell typhoid
    victim, 150
Koch, Dr. Robert, German
    bacteriologist, 82–83, 86–87,
    95, 155, 166, 202; how
    typhoid spreads, 85; method
    for stopping epidemics, 85;

typhoid carriers, role of, 87;
    typhoid research, 83–86
Kohls, Otto, Cornell typhoid victim,
    112, 129

L

Lake View Cemetery, xiii, xviii
Lancet, 87
Landreth, Olin H., absorption of
    excrement into soil, 90, 202
Langdon, Jervis, nephew of
    Clemens, Samuel, xvi
Langtry, Lilly, 99
Langworthy, Charles, Cornell
    typhoid victim, 143–44
Larrinaga, Cesar, Ithaca High
    School typhoid victim, 119
*La Storia: Five Centuries of the Italian
    American Experience* (Mangione
    & Morreale), 72
Law, Dr. James, 124
Lee, Duncan Campbell "Duke,"
    publisher of *Ithaca Daily
    News*, ix, 34, 45, 60, 102–3,
    130, 132, 136, 184, 188, 191,
    198, 203; becomes a British
    lawyer, 208; crusading editor,
    36; Democratic Party ties,
    36; denied promotion to full
    professor, resigns, xvi, xvii,
    194, 203; denounces Ice Trust,
    43–44; description of, 42; early
    life, 36–37; exile in Europe,
    208; experience with typhoid,
    38–39; financial collapse, 207;

heart buried in Hamilton College Cemetery, 208; hired as oratory professor at Cornell, 37; life spirals downward, 206-7, 209; revives Cornell debate program, 37; sabbatical myth, 104; Spanish–American War service, 38-39; support for better water in Ithaca, 44, 122

Lee, Elizabeth Williams (Mrs. Duncan Campbell Lee), 42, 207

Lee, Rev. J. Beveridge, brother of Duncan, 36

Lee, Rev. James B., father of Duncan, 36

Lee, Rev. John Park, 36, 208

Lehman Brothers, 139

Lehman, Pauline, 139, see also Ickelheimer, Henry R.

Lehigh Valley Railroad, 5, 59

Lehigh Valley Station, 92, 108

Lenk, Walter S., 169-70

Leonard brothers, body recovery business, 2; recover Theodor Zinck's body, xvii

Lewis, Dr. Daniel, New York Commissioner of Health background, 157; "Perfectly safe" statement, 157-58; sends George A. Soper to clean up Ithaca, 159-60

libel actions, xvi, 191–93

Lincoln, President Abraham, 103

Lincoln, Willy, 83

Long, Dr. Perrin, 214

long-distance telephone calls, 145

Lord, Addison P., Cornell typhoid victim, 60

Lord, Burt, 129

Lord Kelvin, see Thompson, Sir William

Low, Seth, mayor of New York, 44

Lucy T., yacht owned by Morris, 210

Lyceum Theatre, 18, 67, 99, 116

Lyford, Percy L., 149

M

Mack, Ebenezer, 2, 35

malaria, 89

Mallon, Mary, 156, 212, see also Typhoid Mary

Malone, Molly, fictional typhoid victim, 83

Maloney, Dan, a.k.a., Dynamite Dan, xvii

Mange, John Isaac, 210

Mangione, Jerry, 72

Manila Electric Co., 211

Mann, Dr. Matthew, 27, 171

Mann, Thomas, author, 83

Mantel, Frank A., 143

manufactured gas, 14, 21

Martinique disaster of 1902, 74

Mary E. Wagener mansion, 209

The Masque of the Red Death (Poe), 109

Massachusetts Agricultural College, 77

Matthews, Nathan, Jr., lawyer for Morris, 198–99

McClure's Magazine, 157, 194, 203

McCormick, Walter, 108

McEvoy, James Francis, 60

McKinley, President William, 21,
39–40, 67, 72, 83, 133, 136,
171; appoints Schurman to
head Philippine Commission,
40; assassination of, 27

Memorial Day regatta, xvi, 193

Menken, S. Stanwood, 29–30

Merchants Association and
Chamber of Commerce of New
York, 156

Metropolitan Edison Company, 211

miasma theory, 48, 87, 100, 123–24

microscopy, 45, 85, 95, 96

Miller, George W., mayor of Ithaca,
97, 186, 189

Montgomery, Clothier & Tyler,
206; Morris derides as "Quaker
Jews," 206

Moore, Dr. Veranus A., Cornell
professor, 46, 107, 110, 123;
letter from Holmes Hollister,
76; report to Schurman, 127

Morehouse, Edward W., father of
GPU nuclear program, 211

Morgan, J. P., 21, 29, 176

Morreale, Ben, author, 72

Morrill Act, 25

Morris, Daniel, U.S. congressman,
father of William T. Morris, 13

Morris, Dr. Robert T., 113

Morris, William Torrey, owner of
Ithaca Water Works, x, xv, xvi,
10–11, 17, 20, 25, 32–34, 46,
49, 54–55, 57, 70, 73–74, 78,
80, 88, 102, 109, 112, 124, 126,
128, 130, 134–35, 160, 181–83,
189, 190, 192, 200, 204–7;
acquires small-town utilities,
12–15, 17–19; approves
90-foot dam, 52; begins
negotiations with Treman to
purchase Ithaca Gas Light
Co. and Ithaca Water Works,
21–24; closes law practice,
15; demands high price for
Ithaca Water Works, 198–99;
early life, 12; financing of
deal, 25, 26, 29, 30; friendship
with Ebenezer M. Treman,
11–12, 15–16; incorporates
Associated Gas & Electric Co.,
204; later years and decline,
208–9; legacy, 210; legal
training, 13; litigation costs,
198; Memorial Day regatta,
193; moves to Ithaca, 55;
Niagara Falls boondoggle,
25; rejects building filtration
plant before dam, 56–57;
resumes social life after
epidemic, xvi; sexuality, 16;
student at Cornell, 13

Morrison, Olive, 148

Morse, Charles W., 43

Mount Saint Mary's College, 153

Mudge, Alfred E., Jr., 153

Mudge, Alfred E., Sr., collateral
typhoid victim, 153, 169

Mudge, Rose, Guthrie & Alexander, law firm, 153
Murphy, Frank J. H. "Senator," xiv
Murray, John, 89

N

Nathan, George Jean, xiii, 133
Newberry, Andrew White, 61–62, 79–81; 147
Newberry, Clara White, x, 62
Newberry, Spencer B., 61–62
Newfield, New York, 118
Newman, Jared Treman, co-developer of Cornell Heights, 19, 31–32, 42, 80, 103, 116, 185–86, 199–200
New York City Board of Health, 157
New York *Evening World,* 111, 169
New York *Herald,* 66, 133
New York and Pennsylvania Telephone & Telegraph Co., 145
New York Public Service Commission, 205–6, 210
New York State Department of Health, 157
New York State Legislature, 185
New York Sun, 37, 135–37, 160; first outside article on Ithaca epidemic, 108
New York Times, 69, 138–40, 164, 166, 169; James Bayles articles, 164–65
New York Tribune, 42, 137, 192
Niagara Falls, New York, 24

Niagara Falls Gas & Electric Light Co., 25, 204
Nichols, Charles Worthington, Jr., 61, 142
Nicholls, Samuel, friend of Andrew Carnegie, 176
North American Review, 40
Northwestern University, 152
Nourse, Alice (sister) 152
Nourse, Alice P. (stepmother), 152
Nourse, Edwin G. (son), 151–52
Nourse, Edwin H. (father), collateral typhoid victim, 152, 169
Noyes, Alexander Dana, 21

O

Oakland Tribune, 179
Ochs, Adolph S., publisher of *New York Times,* 138–41, 166
Odell, Benjamin, governor of New York, 187
Odell, Letitia R., 173–74
O'Hara, Rev. William L., 153–54, *see also* Mount Saint Mary's College

P

Pan-American Exposition, 26–27, 171
Panic of 1907, 206
Park, Dr. Roswell, 27
Parke, Davis & Company, 214–15
Payne, Dr. Eugene, 214
Pennsylvania Electric Company, 211
Penn Yan Gas Light Company, 209

Penn Yan, New York, 10, 12, 15, 205, 208, 209

Phi Delta Theta fraternity, 112

Philadelphia Press, 111

Philbin, Beekman, Menken & Griscom, 29

Philippine-American War, 28, 39, 40; Schurman lectures against, 102-3

Philippine Commission, 41

Philomatheon debating society, 118

Pickert, Nellie, 151

The Plague (Camus), 97

Platt & Colt Pharmacy, Ithaca, 148

Plymouth, Pennsylvania, typhoid epidemic at, 88, 110

Poe, Edgar Allan, 109

Poor, Ben, 101

Potter, Dr. Alice M., 94, 134; dies of typhoid complications, 170-71

Potter, Dr. Bina, 94

Potter, Dr. Charles, 94

Potter, Dr. Jaennette, 94

Poughkeepsie Regatta, 68-69, 138

Pray, Emma, 151

Pray, Fred J., Cornell typhoid victim, 151

Pray, James A., collateral typhoid victim, 151, 169

Pray, Nettie, 151

Priest, George E., co-publisher of *Ithaca Daily Journal*, 20, 35, 42, 102, 135

Prime, Commander Edward L, 174-76

Prime, Edward L., Jr. , Cornell typhoid victim, 174

Prince Albert (husband of Queen Victoria), 83

Prince Edward Island, 7, 60, 99, 196

Principles of Sanitary Science and the Public Health (Sedgwick), 50

Progressive Party of Ithaca, 97

Psi Upsilon fraternity, 146-47

public water, 53, 122, 130; first water referendum, 53-55; Morris campaign tactics, 54-55; petitions in favor, 53; promised land, 184

Pulitzer, Joseph, newspaper publisher, 60

Pulitzer Scholarship, 60

The Purification of Public Water Supplies (Hill), 51

R

Rebstock, Dr. Mildred, synthesized chloromycetin, 214

Rensselaer Polytechnic Institute, 156

Renwick Pier, eyed as incinerator site, 168

Richard Wallace boardinghouse, 112

Robb, Graham, author, 18

Robert H. Treman State Park, 199

Robinson, Dean G., typhoid victim, 113, 118

Rockefeller Hall of Physics, 78

Roosevelt, Franklin D., governor of New York, 210

Roosevelt, President Franklin D. xviii, 104, 129, 211

Roosevelt, Theodore, governor of New York, 72

Roosevelt, President Theodore, 205

Rose, Clarence E. (son), 146

Rose, George B. (father), 146

Rose Law Firm, 146

Rossiter, Maida, 148

S

Sackett, Henry W., libel lawyer, xvi, xvii, 192

Sackett, Homer S., 178

Sage, Henry W., 6, 7, 66; endows Cornell Infirmary, 98

Sage College, 19, 63, 66, 92, 147–49; basketball games, 66; gymnasium converted to emergency housing during epidemic, 136

St. John's Episcopal Church, 18, 20

sanitation habits of construction workers, 50, 76, 89; no liability threat from bad water, 51; several witness excrement along Six Mile Creek, 76–77, 89

Schiller, David L., writer, 204

Schlenker, Charles J., Cornell typhoid victim, 129

Schoenborn, Henry A., Cornell typhoid victim, 113–14, 129

Schurman, Barbara F. (Mrs. Jacob Gould Schurman), 102

Schurman, Jacob Gould, president of Cornell University, x, xiv, xvi, 7–9, 37, 57, 64–65, 67, 98, 102, 106, 126, 129–30, 132–33, 135–36, 138–41, 143–44, 160, 166–67, 170, 174, 176–77, 182, 184, 186, 194, 199, 201, 203; away on lecture tour when epidemic starts, 102; commissions faculty report on causes of epidemic, 127; deals with student demands, 128; draws up talking points in university's defense, 137–38; emotions regarding epidemic, 153; exploits "perfectly safe" statement, 157; family history, 7; leads Philippine Commission at President McKinley's request, 40–41; letters from concerned parents, 145–46, 152; letters of support, 147–48, 153–54, 157; mentors Frank E. Gannett, 40–41; praises Andrew Carnegie, 27; sends thank-you letter to Morris, 205; support for Darwin and evolution, 8; views on academic freedom, 194; voices opposition to Philippine-American War, 8; war against press, 128, 132, 137–40; writes epitaph for dead students, 157

Second Philippine Commission, 41

Securities and Exchange
    Commission, U.S., 211

Sedgwick, William T., xv, 50

Severn Wine Cellar, 209

Sheehy, Margaret, confrontation
    with Summers, 125

Sheppard, George S., lawyer for
    Morris, 55, 57

Shumard, Oliver G., first Cornell
    student to die in epidemic, 59,
    98–99, 108–9; funeral, 109

Shumard, William (father), 108–9

Sieder, Fred W., 143

Simpson, Edna, 149, see also Huestis,
    Edna

Sincebaugh, Alvin, police officer, xii

Sisler, Carol U., author, 12

Six Mile Creek, 9, 31, 46–48, 50, 53,
    75–77, 89–92, 100, 110, 121,
    124, 127–28, 134, 161, 168,
    184, 198–99

Six Mile Creek dam project, 70–71,
    75, 81, 156, 187, 189–90;
    comparison to nuclear debate,
    74; fear of dam, 72–74, 100;
    poor sanitation at, 76–77, 89,
    101, 121, 127, 202

Slaterville Water, 147, see also
    artesian water

Slingerland, Mark V., 170

smallpox scare, 97

Smith, Brainard G., editor of Ithaca
    Daily Journal, 37, 102, 107,
    135–37

Smith, Emma H., 106

Smith, Goldwin, 78

Smith, Howard C., cross-country
    runner, 173

Snowdon, William H., 112

"The Social History of the 1903
    Ithaca Typhoid Epidemic: A
    Study of Anger and Action
    (Schiller)," 204

Solvay, New York, 146, 177

Solvay Process Company, 146, 177

Soper, George A., sanitarian, 93,
    155–57, 159–61, 163–64,
    166–69, 201–3, 204, 212; writes,
    "The Epidemic of Typhoid
    Fever at Ithaca, New York," 201;
    used Ithaca experience to find
    Typhoid Mary, 212

Sophomore Cotillion, 148

South Fork Hunting & Fishing
    Club, 73

Spencer, Charlotte E., Cornell
    typhoid victim, 113

Spencer, Hannah, 179; husband
    blames her for Charlotte's
    death, 179

Spriggs, Edward, 97

Spring, Rebecca, 16–17, see also
    Eagleswood Military Academy

Stalin, Josef, 49

Standard Medical Directory of North
    America, 94

Stanford University, xv, cancels
    Senior Dance in sensitivity to
    campus typhoid deaths

Stewart, Dr. David, 114

Stewart, Edwin, New York state senator, 30, 187

Stimson Hall, ix, 78, 115, 167

Strangers: Homosexual Love in the 19th Century (Robb), 18

Summers, Richard, 125–26

Summers, Thomas W., key manager for Morris, 35, 55, 122, 124, 126, 182 189, 205; confrontation with Margaret Sheehy, 125

Syracuse Herald, 41

A System of Medicine, 93

T

Taft, William Howard

Tammany Hall, 43–44

Theta Delta Chi fraternity, 112

Thilly, Frank, mentor to Oliver G. Shumard, 99, 109

Thompson, George, 212

Thompson, Sir William (Lord Kelvin), 57–58

Thornburg, Frank, business partner of Ebenezer M. Treman, 17–18

Thrall, Flavia, clairvoyant healer, 144

Three Mile Island nuclear accident, xviii, 211

Three Mile Island nuclear plant, 74, 211

Thurston, Robert H., 185

Tiffany, Charles (father), 17, *see also* Eagleswood Military Academy

Tiffany, Louis Comfort, 17, *see also* Eagleswood Military Academy

Tompkins County National Bank, 2, 11, 198

Tompkins County Supreme Court, 97, 199

Tompkins County Surrogate Court, 117, 171

Toothless Ben, 202, *see also* Soper, George A.

Tracy, Emma Morris, sister of William T. Morris, 209

Tracy, Lucy, niece of William T. Morris, 209

Tracy, Morris, nephew of William T. Morris, 209–10

Treman, Allen, 125

Treman, Arthur, 125

Treman, Belle Norwood, second wife of Ebenezer M. Treman, 9

Treman brothers, 3; childhood, 1; move to Ithaca, 1

Treman, Charles E., xv, 10–11, 15, 19, 22, 26, 29–30, 32, 57, 103, 109, 125, 136, 188; builds mansion on East Hill, 12, 80; Memorial Day regatta, 193; returns from Europe, 188

Treman, Ebenezer Mack, son of Lafayette L. Treman, 2, 9, 11, 15, 17, 20, 27, 30, 31, 34–35, 112, 125, 189, 200, 205-6; begins negotiations with Morris over sale of Ithaca Gas Light Company, 21–23;

choirmaster of St. John's Episcopal Church, 18; death of first wife, 18; demands Morris also buy Ithaca Water Works, 22–23; Eagleswood Military Academy, 16–17; interest in the arts, 16; Lyceum Theatre, 18; Memorial Day regatta, 193; sexuality, 16, 18; Thornburg, Frank, 17–18

Treman, Elias, brother of Lafayette L. Treman, 1, 2, 10, 22, 125

Treman, Eliza A., wife of Lafayette L. Treman, 11, 20, 22

Treman, Elizabeth Lovejoy, widow of Elias Treman, 22, 25, 193

Treman, Eugenie MacMahan, 9; death in childbirth, 18; marriage to Ebenezer M.' Treman, 18

Treman, King & Company, 1, 22, 62

Treman, Lafayette L., patriarch of Treman family, 1, 7, 9–11, 26, 35, 125–26; business career, 2; death of, 10; funeral of, 20; mansion, 9, 11; relationship with son 16

Treman, Laura Hosie (Mrs. Robert H. Treman), 57, 103, 107, 109, 193

Treman, Leonard, brother of Lafayette L. Treman, 1, 2, 22

Treman, Louisa, 9, 11, 22

Treman, Mary Bott (Mrs. Charles E. Treman), 57, 103, 109, 193

Treman, Robert H., xv, 10, 11, 15, 22, 26, 30–32, 57, 103, 109, 128–29, 136, 198, 209; builds mansion on East Hill, 12, 80; donates lands to state for parks, 199; Memorial Day regatta, 193; obtains litigation properties from Morris, 199; son ill with typhoid, 125

Troy Times, 147

Truman, President Harry S., 152

tuberculosis, 96; death rate, 82

Tucker & Vinton construction firm, xvi, 71, 75, 77, 89, 121, 191, 192, 203, 206; hires immigrant labor to build Six Mile Creek dam, 71

typhoid, absorption into soil, 90; Boer War, 84; Brand ice baths, 114–15, 147; carriers, 39, 75, 86, 89–90, 165–66, 201, 212–13; cure, 214–15; death rates of, 83–84, 93; diagnosis of, 85–86; disease of teens and young adults, 93; effect of chlorine on typhoid, 214; famous victims, 48, 62, 83, 87; Franco–Prussian War, 84; how typhoid kills, 113; incubation period, 93; national security issue, 84–85; oyster threat, 84; Spanish–American War, 38–39, 84, 103; stomach acid, effect of, 82; survival time of bacilli outside human host,

88; symptoms, 93–95; toll
on families, 112; treatment,
114–15, 147; typhoid in Italy,
89–90; Wesleyan University
outbreak of 1894, 84
Typhoid Mary, 156, 212–13;
wrongly blamed for Ithaca
epidemic, 213
Typhusbazillentrager, 86

U

Umphville men's club, 19, 163
Union College, 90
United States Gas & Electric, 209
University of Buffalo Medical
School, 94, 171
University of Maryland
Hospital, 214
University of Missouri, 99
University of Pennsylvania, 142,
193, 200
University of Wisconsin, 210
urotropin, kills germs in urine, 167
Utica Herald–Dispatch, 37
Utter, Joseph, 121

V

Van Anda, Carr, 139
Van Cleef, Elizabeth Treman (Mrs.
Mynderse Van Cleef), 10, 32
Van Cleef, Mynderse, xvii, 10, 15–16,
22, 25, 27 30, 31, 33, 54, 47
136, 189, 192, 206, 208–10;
early life, 25; builds mansion
on East Hill, 12, 80

Van Hook, James M. excrement
witness, 77
Van Loon, Hendrik, Dutch
student, 63
Van Order, Sylvester, xi, xiv
Van Wert Gas Light Company, 15
Van Wyck, Robert, defeated for
re-election as mayor of New
York, 44
Van Zoil, Alice, 112
Van Zoil, Lillian, 112
Vassar College, 106
Vaughan, Major Victor C., 39
Vermeule, Cornelius, 188–90, 197
Vinton, James C., Cornell typhoid
victim, 113
Vinton, Thomas M., 71, 75; pursues
libel suit against *Ithaca Daily
News,* xvi, *see also* Tucker &
Vinton
von Drigalski, Wilhelm, assistant to
Koch, Dr. Robert, 86
Vonnegut, Anton, 62
Vonnegut, Arthur, 62
Vonnegut, Kurt, Jr., 62
Vonnegut, Walter, 62
Vonnegut Hardware Company, 62

W

Wanke, Paul, Cornell typhoid
victim, 143
Warner, Bill, 79
Warner, Glenn S. "Pop," 79
Warren, Frederick, 177

water filtration, 121, 127, 156; sand vs. mechanical filtration, 52; Senate hearings, 52; typhoid deaths reduced, 51; William T. Morris rejects filtration, 56–57

water issues in Ithaca; high water rates, 24, 130; illnesses among Cornell freshmen, 46; low water pressure, 9, 23, 32; private wells, 9, 46, 92; sewage discharges into Cayuga Lake, 47

Waterman, Jeannie Treman, 9, 11, 22, 125

Waterman, Louisa M. 125

water referendum of 1902, 54–55, 183

water referendum of 1903, 182–84

Water Supply Engineering (Folwell), 50

water testing results, 54, 110, 119

Weather Bureau, U.S. 81

Wesleyan University, 84

Wessman, George A., Cornell typhoid victim, 113

Western Union, 145

Whetzel, Herbert H., excrement witness, 77

White, Andrew Dickson, co-founder and first president of Cornell University, ix, 3, 37, 58 62, 106, 124, 147, 170, 176; early life and education, 4; McGraw–Fiske affair, 6, 7; U.S. ambassador to Germany, x

White, E. B., 59

White, Frederick, son of Andrew, 62

Widal, George Fernand Isidor, 85, 95

Widal Reaction, 85, 95–96, 123; technique, 95–96

Wilder, Burt G., 65, 106; townie baseball incident, 65

Williams, Charles A., 112

Williams, Emmons L., 31, 65, 98, 128, 203

Williams, Gardner S., designer of dam, 49, 53–54, 56–57, 70–75, 88–89, 121, 128, 156, 163, 187; admits workers fouled stream, 77; denies Ithaca Water Works responsible for typhoid outbreak, 101; designs Magnitogorsk Dam for Stalin, 49; designs Six Mile Creek dam for Morris, 49–50; fields questions about dam design, 74; recomends first building filtration plant, 50–51; tells public Six Mile Creek okay to drink, 53

Williams, George R., 42, 136, 188, 207

Williams, Roger B., 98, 129, 136

Williams, Dr. Walter L., 121

Williamson, Samuel T., 103

Williard State Hospital Board of Managers, 210

Willkie, Wendell, GOP presidential candidate, 104

Winslow, Charles-Edward Amory, writer, xv
Women's Christian Temperance Union, 78
Wood, Butler & Morris law firm, 13–14; linoleum incident, 14, 16
Wood, Graham B., Cornell typhoid victim, 61, 79, 142, 144
Wood, Jarvis A., father of Graham, 61, 143, 179
Wood, Ralph T., 14
Woodford, Ambassador Stewart L., 153
Woodford, John R., Board of Health inspector 122
Woodward, Theodore E., 214
Work Book in Surgery (Coville), 95
Wright, Lynn George, student newspaper stringer, 133
Wright, Wilbur, 83
Wyckhoff, Edward G., 32
Wyvell, Manton M., 67, 136, 138

Y
Yale University typhoid outbreak, 160, 170, 179
Yeo, Dr. J. Burney, 89

Z
Zeek, Charles A., xi–xii
Zinck, Edmond, nephew of Theodor, xviii, 120
Zinck, Emelie, wife of Theodor, 119–20
Zinck, Louise, typhoid victim, xii, xiii, 119–20, 132
Zinck, Theodor, father of Louise, 65, 92, 119–20, 195; body recovered by Leonard brothers, xvii; death of Louise, xii; disappears from boat, xi; early life, xii; efforts to recover body, xvii; funeral, xviii; proprietor of Hotel Brunswick, xii–xiii, 65; walk to lake, xiii–xiv